T0344434

Eating Disorders and Obesity in Children and Adolescents

Eating Disorders and Obesity in Children and Adolescents

JOHANNES HEBEBRAND, MD
Professor
Department of Child and Adolescent Psychiatry, Psychosomatics and Psychotherapy
University Hospital Essen
University of Duisburg-Essen
Essen, Germany

BEATE HERPERTZ-DAHLMANN, MD
Professor
Department of Child And Adolescent Psychiatry, Psychosomatics and Psychotherapy
Technical University Aachen (RWTH)
Aachen, Germany

ELSEVIER

ELSEVIER

3251 Riverport Lane
St. Louis, Missouri 63043

Publisher: Patrick Manley
Acquisition Editor: Lauren Boyle
Editorial Project Manager: Jennifer Horigan
Project Manager: Kiruthika Govindaraju
Cover Designer: Alan Studholme

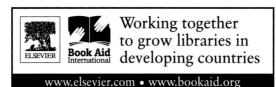

Working together
to grow libraries in
developing countries

www.elsevier.com • www.bookaid.org

List of Contributors

Evelyn Attia, MD
Director
Eating Disorders Research Program
New York State Psychiatric Institute
New York, NY, United States

Director
Columbia Center for Eating Disorders
Columbia University Medical Center
New York, NY, United States

John Baines, PhD
Professor
Institute for Experimental Medicine
Christian-Albrechts-University Kiel & Max Planck
    Institute for Evolutionary Biology
Kiel, Germany

Jennifer L. Baker, PhD
Associate Professor
Department of Clinical Epidemiology
Bispebjerg and Frederiksberg Hospital
Frederiksberg, Denmark

Associate Professor
Novo Nordisk Foundation Center for Basic Metabolic
    Research, Section on Metabolic Genetics
University of Copenhagen
Copenhagen, Denmark

Jessica H. Baker, PhD
Assistant Professor
Psychiatry
UNC
Chapel Hill, NC, United States

Manuela Barona, MSc
GOSH Institute of Child Health
University College London
London, United Kingdom

Tatyana Bidopia, BA
Department of Psychology and Neuroscience
Duke University
Durham, NC, United States

Lise G. Bjerregaard, MSc, PhD
Center for Clinical Research and Disease Prevention
Bispebjerg and Frederiksberg Hospital
Copenhagen, Denmark

John E. Blundell, PhD
Professor
Psychology
University of Leeds
Leeds, United Kingdom

Abigail R. Cooper, BA
School of Psychology
Fairleigh Dickinson University
Teaneck, NJ, United States

Riccardo Dalle Grave, MD
Director
Department od Eating and Weight Disorders
Villa Garda Hospital
Garda (VR), Italy

Nandini Datta, MA
Department of Psychology and Neuroscience
Duke University
Durham, NC, United States

Savannah Erwin, BS
Department of Psychology and Neuroscience
Duke University
Durham, NC, United States

Manfred M. Fichter, MD, Dipl-Psych
Professor
Schoen Klinik Roseneck
Prien, Germany

Department of Psychiatry and Psychotherapy
Ludwig-Maximilians-University (LMU)
Munich, Germany

Katrin Fischer, PhD
Institute for Diabetes and Obesity
Helmholtz Diabetes Center (HDC)
Helmholtz Zentrum München and German National
    Diabetes Center (DZD)
Neuherberg, Germany, Division of Metabolic Diseases
Department of Medicine
Technische Universität München
Munich, Germany

Michaela Flynn, BPsy (Hons)
Department of Psychological Medicine
Institute of Psychiatry, Psychology & Neuroscience
King's College London
London, United Kingdom

Johanna Giuranna, MSc
Department of Child and Adolescent Psychiatry,
    Psychosomatics and Psychotherapy
University Hospital Essen
University of Duisburg-Essen
Essen, Germany

Johannes Hebebrand, MD
Professor
Department of Child and Adolescent Psychiatry,
    Psychosomatics and Psychotherapy
University Hospital Essen
University of Duisburg-Essen
Essen, Germany

Beate Herpertz-Dahlmann, MD
Professor
Department of Child And Adolescent Psychiatry,
    Psychosomatics and Psychotherapy
Technical University Aachen (RWTH)
Aachen, Germany

Anja Hilbert, PhD
Professor
Integrated Research and Treatment Centre Adiposity
    Diseases
Department of Medical Psychology and Medical
    Sociology
Department of Psychosomatic Medicine and
    Psychotherapy
University of Leipzig Medical Center
Leipzig, Germany

Anke Hinney, PhD
Associate Professor
Department of Child and Adolescent Psychiatry,
    Psychosomatics and Psychotherapy
University Hospital Essen
University of Duisburg-Essen
Essen, Germany

Ashley F. Jennings, BS
School of Psychology
Fairleigh Dickinson University
Teaneck, NJ, United States

Aviva Johns, MA
Research Associate II
Eating Recovery Center
The University of Texas
Austin, TX, USA

**Carol Kan, BA (Cantab), MA, MBBS,
MRCPsych, PhD**
Institute of Psychiatry
King's College London
London, United Kingdom

Anna Keski-Rahkonen, MD, PhD, MPH
Associate Professor
Department of Public Health
University of Helsinki
Helsinki, Finland

Stephanie Laviani, MSc
Division of Paediatric Endocrinology and Diabetes
Department of Paediatrics and Adolescent Medicine
Ulm University Hospital
Ulm, Germany

Daniel Le Grange, PhD
Professor
Department of Psychiatry and Behavioral
    Neuroscience
The University of Chicago
Chicago, IL, United States

Department of Psychiatry
University of California, San Francisco
San Francisco, CA, United States

Katharine L. Loeb, PhD
School of Psychology
Fairleigh Dickinson University
Teaneck, NJ, United States

Maria G. Martini, MD, MSc
GOSH Institute of Child Health
University College London
London, United Kingdom

Adrian Meule, PhD
Department of Psychology
University of Salzburg
Salzburg, Austria

Nadia Micali, MD, PhD, MRCPsych
Department of Psychiatry
University of Geneva
Geneva, Switzerland

Child and Adolescent Psychiatry Division
Department of Child and Adolescent Health
University Hospital Geneva
Geneva, Switzerland

GOSH Institute of Child Health
University College London
London, United Kingdom

Alexandra J. Miller, BS
Department of Psychology and Neuroscience
University of North Carolina
Chapel Hill, NC, United States

Yvonne Mühlig, PhD
Department of Child and Adolescent Psychiatry,
    Psychosomatics and Psychotherapy
University Hospital Essen
University of Duisburg-Essen
Essen, Germany

Timo D. Müller, PhD
Institute for Diabetes and Obesity
Helmholtz Zentrum München
German Research Center for Environmental Health
    (GmbH)
Neuherberg, Germany

Nina Nelson, MD, PhD
Director
Kvalitet och Patientsäkerhet
Karolinska Universitetssjukhuset
Solna, Sweden

Dasha Nicholls, MBBS, MD(Res)
Reader in Child Psychiatry
Centre for Psychiatry
Imperial College
London, United Kingdom

Dorthe C. Pedersen, MSc
Center for Clinical Research and Disease Prevention
Bispebjerg and Frederiksberg Hospital
Frederiksberg, Denmark

Hans-Christian Puls, MSc
Integrated Research and Treatment Centre Adiposity
    Diseases
Department of Medical Psychology and Medical
    Sociology
Department of Psychosomatic Medicine and
    Psychotherapy
University of Leipzig Medical Center
Leipzig, Germany

Norbert Quadflieg, PhD
Department of Psychiatry
Ludwig-Maximilians-University
Munich, Germany

Miriam Remy, MSc Psych
Department of Psychiatry, Psychosomatics and
    Psychotherapy of Childhood and Adolescence
University Hospital Essen
Essen, Germany

Alannah Rivera-Cancel, BA
Department of Psychology and Neuroscience
Duke University
Durham, NC, United States

Katie Rowlands, BSc
Institute of Psychiatry, Psychological Medicine,
    Section of Eating Disorders
King's College London
London, United Kingdom

Justin R. Ryder, PhD
Assistant Professor
Pediatrics
University of Minnesota
Minneapolis, MN, United States

Erik Savereide, BS
Department of Psychology and Neuroscience
Duke University
Durham, NC, United States

Ulrike Schmidt, MD, PhD, FRCPsych
Department of Psychological Medicine
Institute of Psychiatry, Psychology & Neuroscience
King's College London
London, United Kingdom

Eating Disorders Unit
South London and Maudsley NHS Foundation Trust
London, United Kingdom

Jochen Seitz, MD
Department of Child and Adolescent Psychiatry,
    Psychosomatics and Psychotherapy
Technical University Aachen (RWTH)
Aachen, Germany

Yasmina Silén, MD
Department of Public Health
Clinicum Helsinki
University of Helsinki, Helsinki, Finland

Eric Stice, BS, MS, PhD
Senior Research Scientist
Psychology
Oregon Research Institute
Eugene, OR, United States

Thorkild I.A. Sørensen, MD
Professor of Genetic and Metabolic Epidemiology
Department of Public Health
University of Copenhagen
Copenhagen, Denmark

Professor of Genetic and Metabolic Epidemiology
Novo Nordisk Foundation Center for Basic Metabolic
    Research
University of Copenhagen
Copenhagen, Denmark

Paula Tabares, MD
Department of Psychiatry
Columbia University
New York, NY, United States

Katherine A. Thompson, MA
Department of Psychology and Neuroscience
University of North Carolina
Chapel Hill, NC, United States

Eline Tombeur, MSc
Child and Adolescent Psychiatry Division
Department of Child and Adolescent Health
University Hospital Geneva
Geneva, Switzerland

Janet Treasure, PhD, FRCP, FRCPsych
Professor
Institute of Psychiatry, Psychological Medicine,
    Section of Eating Disorders
King's College London
London, United Kingdom

Jolanda S. Van Vliet, PhD
Department of Clinical and Experimental Medicine
Pediatrics
Linköping, Sweden

Martin Wabitsch, MD, PhD
Division Chief
Division of Pediatric Endocrinology
Ulm University Medical Center
Ulm, Germany

Professor in Pediatrics
Department of Pediatrics and Adolescent Medicine
Ulm University Medical Center
Ulm, Germany

Samantha Wilkinson, BA
Research Assistant II
University of Texas at Austin
San Antonio, TX, United States

Nancy Zucker, PhD
Associate Professor
Psychiatry and Behavioral Science
Duke University
Durham, NC, United States

Associate Professor
Psychology and Neuroscience
Duke University
Durham, NC, United States

Director
Duke Center for Eating Disorders
Duke University
Durham, NC, United States

Eating and Weight Disorders at the Beginning of the Third Millennium

Many societies worldwide have been confronted with increasing rates of obesity over the past 50 years, thus rendering prevention and treatment of this weight disorder a top societal and healthcare priority. Within this same time range, eating disorders, too, have become highly relevant because of their debilitating effects on mostly young females. Recent research has provided further evidence that weight and eating disorders are related; particularly, genetic and imaging research has, for instance, revealed that anorexia nervosa and obesity in part represent opposite sides of underlying causal mechanisms. Accordingly, it is timely to provide healthcare professionals with an overview of these disorders at the beginning of the third millennium, while at the same time keeping in mind that both weight and eating disorders have only recently gained recognition as major health problems in today's societies.

Eating disorders (anorexia nervosa, bulimia nervosa, binge eating disorder) represent serious mental disorders, which have a high impact on the individual, the families, and wider society. When anorexia and bulimia nervosa were included in the Global Burden of disease study in 2013, many clinicians and researchers experienced this as a watershed moment in the recognition of eating disorders in global healthcare. About 20 million persons in the European Union currently suffer from an eating disorder. Moreover, anorexia nervosa is one of the most common chronic diseases in adolescence. Its mortality risk is higher than for other serious diseases in adolescence, such as asthma, type 1 diabetes, or any other psychiatric disorder. In contrast, obesity per se is not necessarily a serious disease. However, because of the evolvement of comorbid disorders, many and, in particular, older individuals experience a deteriorating health and premature death as a result of the excess fat accumulation and its systemic effects.

As early diagnosis and intervention are key issues for the outcome of these debilitating disorders, it was the aim of our book to provide clinicians and therapists from a broader range of disciplines with a sufficient knowledge on detection and treatment with a focus on those with onset in childhood and adolescence. We tried to include most eating disorders depicted in *DSM-5* with a special emphasis on developmental aspects, as the majority of these diseases begin in the age period from puberty till early adulthood. Moreover, there are rising frequencies in childhood. Besides a detailed overview on new epidemiological data, we made some effort to highlight the most recent scientific findings on etiology and pathophysiology to provide the reader with a deeper knowledge of the interplay between mind and body. As many of us are working with children, adolescents, and their families, it was our particular objective to give appropriate space to describe different treatment and prevention strategies. Although much progress has been made in developing new treatment modalities, there are still a high proportion of patients who do not respond to any intervention.

Looking at this comprehensive book, we would like to thank all contributors who gave their time, expertise, and passion to improve our knowledge on childhood and adolescent eating disorders and obesity. It was a great pleasure for us to work with all of you and exchange and discuss new promising ideas. We would also like to thank the publisher to give us the chance to edit this book as well as Laureen Boyle and Jennifer Horigan for their support.

We both hope that this book will be helpful for all clinicians and researchers who want to help children and adolescents to overcome their disorder and to improve their quality of life.

Aachen and Essen, Germany, September 2018
Beate Herpertz-Dahlmann and Johannes Hebebrand

References

Schmidt U, Adan R, Böhm I, et al. Eating disorders: the big issue. *Lancet Psychiatry*. 2016;3:313–315

Erskine HE, Whiteford HA, Pike KM. The global burden of eating disorders. *Curr Opin Psychiatr*. 2016;29:346–353. doi: 0.1097/YCO.0000000000000276

Beate Herpertz-Dahlmann, MD
Professor
Department of Child And Adolescent Psychiatry,
Psychosomatics and Psychotherapy
Technical University Aachen (RWTH)
Aachen, Germany

Johannes Hebebrand, MD
Professor
Department of Child and Adolescent Psychiatry,
Psychosomatics and Psychotherapy
University Hospital Essen
University of Duisburg-Essen
Essen, Germany

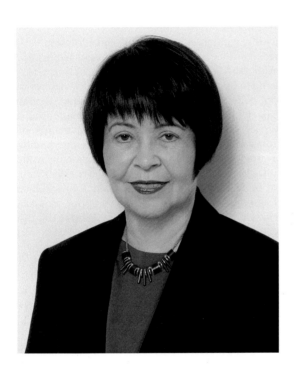

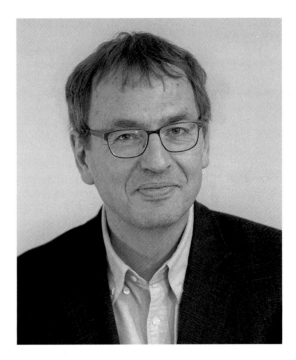

Contents

SECTION I
INTRODUCTION

1 **Overarching Key Issues for Feeding, Eating, and Weight Disorders,** *1*
Johannes Hebebrand, MD

SECTION II
DEVELOPMENTAL ASPECTS

2 **Developmentally Appropriate Assessment of Body Weight and Body Composition From Childhood to Adulthood With a Focus on Eating and Weight Disorders,** *9*
Johannes Hebebrand, MD

3 **Appetite Control—Biological and Psychological Factors,** *17*
John E. Blundell, PhD

4 **Emerging Change in Body Perception During Growth and Development Among Children and Adolescents,** *23*
Jolanda S. Van Vliet, PhD and Nina Nelson, MD, PhD

SECTION III
SYMPTOMATOLOGY: EATING DISORDERS OF INFANCY AND EARLY CHILDHOOD

5 **ARFID and Other Eating Disorders of Childhood,** *29*
Dasha Nicholls, MBBS, MD(Res)

6 **Loss of Control Eating in Children,** *35*
Nancy Zucker, PhD, Erik Savereide, BS, Savannah Erwin, BS, Tatyana Bidopia, BA, Nandini Datta, MA, and Alannah Rivera-Cancel, BA

SECTION IV
ADOLESCENT EATING DISORDERS

7 **Adolescent Eating Disorders— Definition, Symptomatology, and Comorbidity,** *39*
Beate Herpertz-Dahlmann, MD

8 **Adolescent Obesity and Comorbidity,** *47*
Martin Wabitsch, MD, PhD, Stephanie Laviani, MSc, Johannes Hebebrand, MD, and Yvonne Mühlig, PhD

SECTION V
EPIDEMIOLOGY

9 **Incidence and Prevalence of Eating Disorders Among Children and Adolescents,** *53*
Anna Keski-Rahkonen, MD, PhD, MPH and Yasmina Silén, MD

10 **Development, Tracking, Distribution, and Time Trends in Body Weight During Childhood,** *63*
Lise G. Bjerregaard, MSc, PhD, Jennifer L. Baker, PhD, and Thorkild I.A. Sørensen, MD

SECTION VI
ETIOLOGY AND PATHOPHYSIOLOGY

11 **Genetics of Eating and Weight Disorders,** *67*
Anke Hinney, PhD and Johanna Giuranna, MSc

12 **Influence of Hormones on the Development of Eating Disorders,** *73*
Katherine A. Thompson, MA, Alexandra J. Miller, BS, and Jessica H. Baker, PhD

13 **Endocrine Mechanisms in Obesity,** *79*
Katrin Fischer, PhD and Timo D. Müller, PhD

14 **Microbiome and Inflammation in Eating Disorders,** *87*
Jochen Seitz, MD, John Baines, PhD, and Beate Herpertz-Dahlmann, MD

15 **Eating Disordered Mothers and Their Children: Intergenerational Effects,** *93*
Nadia Micali, MD, PhD, MRCPsych, Maria G. Martini, MD, MSc, Manuela Barona, MSc, and Eline Tombeur, MSc

16 **An Addiction Perspective on Eating Disorders and Obesity,** *99*
Adrian Meule, PhD

17 **Stigmatization Associated With Obesity in Children and Adolescents,** *105*
Anja Hilbert, PhD and Hans-Christian Puls, MSc

SECTION VII
TREATMENT

18 **Cognitive-Behavioral Therapy in Adolescent Eating Disorders,** *111*
Riccardo Dalle Grave, MD

19 **Family-Based Treatment for Adolescent Eating Disorders,** *117*
Abigail R. Cooper, BA, Ashley F. Jennings, BS, Katharine L. Loeb, PhD, and Daniel Le Grange, PhD

20 **Inpatient and Day Patient Treatment of Adolescents With Eating Disorders,** *123*
Beate Herpertz-Dahlmann, MD

21 **Early Intervention for Eating Disorders in Young People,** *129*
Michaela Flynn, BPsy (Hons) and Ulrike Schmidt, MD, PhD, FRCPsych

22 **Pharmacotherapy of Eating Disorders in Children and Adolescents,** *135*
Evelyn Attia, MD and Paula Tabares, MD

23 **Conventional Weight Loss Programs,** *143*
Yvonne Mühlig, PhD, Miriam Remy, MSc Psych, Martin Wabitsch, MD, PhD and Johannes Hebebrand, MD

24 **Metabolic and Bariatric Surgery as a Treatment for Adolescent Severe Obesity,** *149*
Justin R. Ryder, PhD

SECTION VIII
COURSE AND OUTCOME

25 **Staging Model of Eating Disorders,** *153*
Janet Treasure, PhD, FRCP, FRCPsych, Carol Kan, BA (Cantab), MA, MBBS, MRCPsych, PhD, and Katie Rowlands, BSc

26 **Outcomes of Anorexic and Bulimic Eating Disorders,** *159*
Manfred M. Fichter, MD, Dipl-Psych and Norbert Quadflieg, PhD

27 **Outcome of Childhood Obesity,** *165*
Dorthe C. Pedersen, MSc, Thorkild I.A. Sørensen, MD, and Jennifer L. Baker, PhD

SECTION IX
PREVENTION

28 **Eating Disorder Prevention Programs,** *171*
Eric Stice, BS, MS, PhD, Aviva Johns, MA, and Samantha Wilkinson, BA

INDEX, *179*

CHAPTER 1

Overarching Key Issues for Feeding, Eating, and Weight Disorders

JOHANNES HEBEBRAND, MD

PHENOMENOLOGY AND CLASSIFICATION SYSTEMS

Feeding and Eating Disorders

Phenomenology in the context of contemporary psychiatry provides the basis for nosology, or the development of disease definitions, diagnostic categories, or dimensional classifications.[1] Most of the symptoms of anorexia nervosa (AN), interestingly excluding body weight and shape concerns, were first described in 1873[2] and thus predated modern psychiatry; bulimia nervosa (BN) was delineated in 1979.[3] The third major eating disorder, binge eating disorder (BED), has only recently gained acceptance as a formal eating disorder.[4]

In contrast to most other psychiatric disorders the symptomatology of eating disorders transcends psychopathology in that body weight and somatic symptoms including amenorrhea and other starvation or obesity-related symptoms are also important for the respective clinical phenotypes. Accordingly, the intertwining of the primary behaviors with the psychological and somatic consequences of starvation can be viewed as constituting the core symptomatology of AN.[5,6] Because body weight also warrants consideration in BN and BED, clinicians need to have a solid grasp of both the core psychopathology and the associated somatic, anthropometric, and pathophysiological features. Furthermore, knowledge of the neuroendocrine dysregulations, heritability, and genetic correlations between eating disorders and other associated psychiatric and nonpsychiatric phenotypes complement our insight into this group of disorders.

DSM-5[4] for the first time created the overarching category Feeding and Eating Disorders, which are characterized by "a persistent disturbance of eating or eating related behavior that results in the altered consumption or absorption of food and that significantly impairs physical health or psychosocial functioning."

ICD-11[7] also makes use of the same term to define the respective category and lists the same disorders albeit in a different order (Table 1.1). According to ICD-11, abnormal eating or feeding behaviors are "not explained by another health condition and are not developmentally appropriate or culturally sanctioned. Feeding disorders involve behavioral disturbances that are not related to body weight and shape concerns, such as eating of non-edible substances or voluntary regurgitation of foods. Eating disorders include abnormal eating behavior and preoccupation with food as well as prominent body weight and shape concerns."

In comparison with feeding disorders, eating disorders have been the subject of much more research due to their higher prevalence rates, their longer durations, and the overall greater medical relevance. A brief discussion of the current definitions of AN reveals that despite the recent/ongoing revisions of the criteria for this disorder, problems persist with respect to the conceptualization of the core phenotype and the clinical usefulness of the criteria (compare DSM-5 with ICD-11 definitions in Table 1.2): (1) Although the words refusal and denial (see DSM-IV A and C criteria) have been removed in DSM-5 as originally suggested by Hebebrand and coworkers,[5,6] the ICD-11 definition[7] still refers to behaviors *aimed* at reducing energy intake and increasing energy expenditure, thus suggesting a strong *intentional* component. However, the evidence for such intentions is weak at best and not in line with the purely descriptive symptomatology of other mental disorders.[5,6] (2) Although obesity experts have become more and more reluctant to reduce obesity to an excess energy intake in relationship to energy expenditure in light of the multitude and complexity of factors involved in body weight regulation,[8] the DSM-5 definition (see A criterion) of AN focuses on this somewhat

TABLE 1.1
Comparison of the Classification of Feeding and Eating Disorders in DSM-5[4] and ICD-11[7]

CLASSIFICATION SYSTEM	
DSM-5	**ICD-11**

Pica	Pica
	    Trichophagia
	    Trichobezoar

Rumination disorder	Rumination-regurgitation disorder
Avoidant restrictive food intake disorder	Avoidant restrictive food intake disorder

Anorexia nervosa
    Restricting type
    Binge-eating/purging type
	Anorexia nervosa (AN)
	    AN with significantly low body weight
	        AN with significantly low body weight, restricting pattern
	        AN with significantly low body weight, binge-purge pattern
	    AN with dangerously low body weight
	    AN in recovery with normal body weight

Bulimia nervosa	Bulimia nervosa
Binge eating disorder	Binge eating disorder
Other specified feeding or eating disorder	Other specified feeding or eating disorder
Unspecified feeding or eating disorder	Feeding or eating disorders, unspecified

To enhance comparisons the ICD-11 ranking was adjusted according to DSM-5.

TABLE 1.2
DSM-5[4] and ICD-11[7] Criteria for Anorexia Nervosa

DSM-5	ICD-11
A. Restriction of energy intake relative to requirement, leading to a significantly low body weight in the context of age, sex, developmental trajectory, and physical health. B. Intense fear of gaining weight or of becoming fat, or persistent behavior that interferes with weight gain, even though at a significantly low weight. C. Disturbance in the way in which one's body weight or shape is experienced, undue influence of body weight or shape on self-evaluation, or persistent lack of recognition of the seriousness of the current low body weight.	Anorexia nervosa is characterized by significantly low body weight for the individual's height, age, and developmental stage (body mass index [BMI] less than 18.5 kg/m² in adults and BMI-for-age under fifth percentile in children and adolescents) that is not due to another health condition or to the unavailability of food. Low body weight is accompanied by a persistent pattern of behaviors to prevent restoration of normal weight, which may include behaviors aimed at reducing energy intake (restricted eating), purging behaviors (e.g., self-induced vomiting, misuse of laxatives), and behaviors aimed at increasing energy expenditure (e.g., excessive exercise), typically associated with a fear of weight gain. Low body weight or shape is central to the person's self-evaluation or is inaccurately perceived to be normal or even excessive.

outdated concept of an impaired energy balance. Clinicians cannot and do not validly measure energy intake and expenditure of their patients. They observe underweight, associated cognitions and behaviors, and mental and somatic symptoms related to starvation. (3) A discussion is required as to whether underweight should continue to be a core feature of the phenotype. Apparently, in contrast to only a few decades ago, a higher number of severely eating disordered and premorbidly overweight patients with a restricting eating behavior present for clinical treatment with a body weight in the normal range. These patients have lost substantial amounts of weight and show symptoms of starvation including amenorrhea; their clinical picture strongly resembles that of patients with AN. As such, an inclusion of starvation-related symptoms - instead of underweight - in the diagnostic criteria would appear appropriate. (4) If underweight is to remain the cardinal symptom of AN, it should be conceptualized in a way to enable all health professionals to readily and consistently diagnose this weight category, thus also enabling comparisons of epidemiologically based prevalence data. The cutoffs should be operationalized in such a way as to allow all healthcare professionals to easily understand and assess the respective criterion. Because other symptoms need to be present for a diagnosis of AN, a rather high weight cutoff criterion should be employed. In this context, the use of the fifth BMI centile in ICD-11[7] is so low, that many patients who would have previously been diagnosed as having AN would no longer qualify for this diagnosis.

Slight differences exist with respect to the subclassification of AN. DSM-5[4] differentiates between the *restricting* and *binge eating/purging* types and includes the specifiers "in partial remission" and "in full remission" for those individuals, who no longer have a low body weight. For those with a low body weight, the current severity is subdivided into mild (BMI$\geq$17 kg/m^2), moderate (16.0–16.9), severe (15.0–15.9), and extreme (BMI <15 kg/m^2); the level of severity may be complemented to allow staging of clinical symptoms, the degree of functional disability, and the need for supervision. The ICD-11[7] subdivision is based on *AN of significantly low body weight* (18.5–14.0 kg/m^2) and *AN of dangerously low body weight* (<14 kg/m^2) in addition to *AN in recovery with normal body weight*. Both classification systems point to the use of BMI-age centiles for the assessment of body weight of children and adolescents. However, BMI centiles cannot further differentiate height-adjusted weight of patients with a BMI centile <1; absolute BMI values or BMI z-scores would offer the possibility to more precisely assess the degree of underweight.[9] Furthermore, it is unclear what percentages of childhood, adolescent, and adult patients with AN fulfill the ICD-11 or DSM-5 subgroups defined via the different BMI cutoffs.

Overall, discussion is warranted as to the appropriateness of the sole use of cognitions and behaviors for eating disorders that include somatic and metabolic symptoms, which in the case of AN can be life-threatening and strongly impact the prognosis—the mere recognition of mental symptoms does not sufficiently capture the essence of this disorder. Furthermore, in the light of frequent intraindividual transitions from one eating disorder to another, diagnostic categories could attempt to come up with overarching criteria and allow for subtypes based on symptom patterns.[6] Consensus should be reached as to how to optimally categorize types and severity of AN.

Weight Disorders

ICD-11[7] refers to "Overweight, obesity or specific nutrient excesses" within the overarching category "Endocrine, nutritional or metabolic diseases" as conditions, in which body size is excessive. Overweight (BMI between 25 and 30 kg/m^2) and obesity (BMI $\geq$ 30 kg/m^2) represent the two major weight disorders according to ICD-11. For children and adolescents the BMI categories used to define overweight or obesity vary by age and gender in infants, children and adolescents. The WHO[10] had previously defined obesity as a condition of abnormal or excessive fat accumulation in adipose tissue to the extent that health may be impaired." However, BMI does not allow direct assessment of adiposity (see chapter 2). An alternative categorization and different definitions for ICD-11 have been proposed to circumvent some of the problems inherent to the previous conceptualization and definition of both overweight and obesity[8]; this alternative proposal is based on etiology, degree of adiposity, and health risk.

The World Health Organization does not consistently use the term overweight; according to a previous definition, overweight defined via a BMI $\geq$25 kg/m^2 encompasses preobesity (25–29.9 kg/m^2) and obesity grades 1 (35–34.9), 2 (35–39.9), and 3 ($\geq$40 kg/m^2).[10] The prevalence rates for BMI $\geq$25 and$\geq$ 30 kg/m^2 are in the range of 50%–60% and 20%–30% in Western countries.[8] It is thus clearly debatable if more than 50% of peoples of different countries should be labeled as having an excessive body size or a disorder as such, in particular because many overweight and obese individuals do not experience symptoms or a functional impairment related to a BMI $\geq$25 kg/m^2. Furthermore, health risks have been found to only start to increase with a BMI >30 or 35 kg/m^2.[8] Although obesity is not a mental disorder, DSM-5[4] points to the "robust associations between obesity and a number of mental disorders." Furthermore, "obesity may be a risk factor for the development of some mental disorders." The European Association for the Study of Obesity[8] included *Obesity arising from or aggravated by major depressive disorder* (MDD) within the overarching category *Obesity attributable to a certain defined etiological factor*, thus acknowledging the weight gain in a subgroup of patients with MDD as one of the certain defined etiological factors for obesity.

GETTING A GRIP ON THE IMPLICATIONS OF THE POLYGENIC DISSECTION OF EATING AND WEIGHT DISORDERS

Genetic research has resulted in substantial progress with respect to the elucidation of pathways involved in body weight regulation and obesity in particular. On the one hand, the detection of rare monogenic forms of obesity has allowed an insight into major pathways operative in weight regulation such as the leptin-melanocortinergic-brain-derived neurotrophic factor pathway.[11,12] It has become evident that a voracious appetite and excessive overeating can be the result of monogenic disorders such as in leptin deficiency syndromes; this knowledge has entailed novel drug therapies for single rare inborn disorders.[11] On the other hand, the elucidation of the polygenic basis of body weight has taken off over the past few years. More than 700 BMI loci have been identified in the most recent meta-analysis of genome-wide association studies (GWAS) based on over 700,000 probands.[13] Progress in eating disorders lags behind due to the difficulties inherent to ascertaining tens of thousands of patients. The most recent GWAS based on 3495 AN cases and 10,982 controls picked up a single genome-wide significant locus.[14]

Currently, four major overarching themes appear relevant for our understanding of weight and eating disorders and AN in particular. (1) The genetic architectures of both BMI including underweight and obesity and AN are complex. A large number of loci with small effect sizes, which according to current knowledge act in an additive manner (nonadditive mechanisms have not yet been detected, but appear probable), account for the respective genetic predispositions at the level of the DNA. The elucidation of BMI loci lags substantially behind that for body height, for which roughly 25% of the genetic predisposition can be explained upon analysis of the same data set as used for the most recent GWAS meta-analysis for BMI.[13] The apparent lack of major gene effects in AN[15,16] potentially suggests that multiple pathways exist into this eating disorder. It appears safe to conclude that apart from monozygotic twins the underlying polygenic contribution will hardly ever completely overlap in two obese or eating disordered individuals. The high number of polygenic loci involved and the intersubject variation of the molecular genetic predisposition along with the high number of subjects required to detect loci raise questions as to the chances of detecting environmental factors other than those with major effects. If the environmental factors are as multiple and of similarly small effect sizes, the elucidation of these disorders appears a formidable task indeed. (2) The female preponderance in AN is partially explained by polygenic loci, which affect body weight in females only.[12,14,17] The total extent to which the female predominance to develop both AN and BN can be explained by genetic factors remains to be elucidated. It is, however, noteworthy that sex-specific polygenic loci have not only been detected for BMI but also for body composition and shape. For example, 20 of the 49 waist-to-hip ratios adjusted for BMI loci demonstrated significant sexual dimorphism, 19 of which displayed a stronger effect in females.[18] (3) Genetic correlations based on GWAS data have not only confirmed known clinical associations but have also detected novel overlapping genetic predispositions. For example, negative genetic correlations have been observed between BMI and educational attainment, schizophrenia and AN, as well as between AN and insulin, glucose and certain lipid phenotypes.[14,19] Positive genetic correlations have been detected between AN and schizophrenia, neuroticism, educational attainment, and serum concentrations of high-density lipoprotein cholesterol.[14] According to these novel results,[14,17] the genetic predisposition to underweight overlaps with that for AN. The genetic correlations between AN and metabolic traits have led to the hypothesis that AN in part is a metabolic disease.[14] However, a word of caution is warranted. The loci responsible for underweight, which overlap with AN, may very well also underlie the genetic correlations with metabolic traits. Causality needs to be established by adjusting genetic correlations for BMI. (4) For a number of complex phenotypes, substantial genetic correlations between childhood and adult onset have been detected; for instance, this holds true for childhood and adult obesity.[19] The mechanisms underlying the age at the onset of a particular disorder require further elucidation; it remains to be seen if a higher polygenic loading leads to an earlier age at onset.

THE URGENT NEED TO IMPROVE THE TREATMENT OF FEEDING, EATING, AND WEIGHT DISORDERS

Despite the recent exciting novel insights into the complex regulation of body weight and the molecular genetic etiologies of weight and eating disorders, the treatment of these disorders has not substantially progressed. However, the novel insights do offer the possibility to develop hypotheses for the treatment of eating disorders.[20-23] A brief delineation of but one example related to the potential of a novel treatment of AN with recombinant leptin serves to illustrate the need to implement research aiming from bench to bedside.

The major physiological function of leptin is to signal states of negative energy balance and decreased energy stores, thus coregulating the adaptation of the organism to starvation.[24-26] This hormone is synthesized in adipocytes; after weight loss, both its synthesis and secretion into circulating blood are reduced; serum levels in patients with AN are mostly below those of age and/or BMI matched controls ($\leq 2\,\mu g/L$; 28–30). As a result, the leptin signal weakens due to a reduced binding of leptin to leptin receptors in the nucleus accumbens of the hypothalamus, thus inducing a cascade of central alterations including those involving the leptin-melanocortinergic-BDNF pathway,[11,20,24-26] which serves to induce energy intake and reduce energy expenditure. Some of the major effects of subthreshold levels of leptin subsequently referred to as hypoleptinemia are conveyed via the hypothalamic-pituitary-adrenal, hypothalamic-pituitary-gonadal, hypothalamic-pituitary-thyroid, and hypothalamic-pituitary-growth hormone axes.[24-26] As a result of the hypoleptinemia-induced alterations of these axes, levels of corticotropin-releasing factor, ACTH, and cortisol increase, thus amounting to a stress response to starvation; levels of gonadotropin-releasing hormone and further downstream of luteinizing (LH) and follicle-stimulating hormone (FSH) decrease, entailing amenorrhea, T3, and to a lesser extent T4 decrease in response to a lowered level of thyroid-stimulating hormone (frequently levels of T3, T4, and TSH are in the low normal range in patients with AN). Finally, growth hormone is upregulated to enhance carbohydrate metabolism as a result of an increased secretion of growth hormone–releasing hormone.

In animal models, obesity in *ob/ob* mice whose phenotype arises from leptin deficiency can successfully be "cured."[30] Both antidepressant[31] and anxiolytic[32] effects of leptin treatment have been observed in these mice. In rats with anorexia-based activity, which results from food restriction over 23 h and ad libitum access for the remaining hour of the day over a period of several days, the development of hyperactivity is suppressed by recombinant leptin; furthermore, leptin can also be used to "treat" hyperactivity in this rat model.[33-35]

In humans, recombinant leptin has been used to very successfully treat patients with inborn leptin deficiency.[36,37] The voracious hunger of such treated patients is normalized within days; during the following months and years, patients lose substantial amount of body weight. Volumes of specific brain regions increase, indicating a neurotrophic function of leptin.[38] Attempts to treat patients with multifactorial obesity largely failed[39]; the induced weight loss was nonsignificant in comparison with placebo treatment. Recombinant leptin applied over a period of 3 months has been used to treat eight females with hypothalamic amenorrhea of at least 6 months duration in a pilot study[40]; the mean BMI was $20\,kg/m^2$. Although the investigators excluded patients with an eating disorder, it is conceivable that a subgroup had recovered a normal body weight after AN. In some females, ovulations set in, in others follicles grew in size. A slight degree of weight loss was observed as a side effect in the third treatment month. In patients with AN, leptin levels have been associated with activity levels,[33,41] although not consistently.[42]

Recombinant leptin has been approved by the Food and Drug Administration to treat lipodystrophy,[43] the approval of the European Medical Agency is upcoming shortly.[44] Lipodystrophy is associated with a reduced fat mass and hypoleptinemia; treatment with leptin entails a substantial metabolic improvement.[45] The annual treatment costs are over half a million US dollars.[46]

Can recombinant leptin benefit patients with AN who have hypoleptinemia?[27-29,47] Recombinant leptin could reduce hyperactivity and entail earlier resumption of menstruation. It could also be helpful for those patients whose hematopoiesis has been reduced to a clinically relevant degree.[48] Depending on the mechanisms involved in this eating disorder or in subgroups of patients with AN, recombinant leptin could increase the leptin level and thus alleviate the metabolic state of starvation. It may very well be that subgroups of patients have become "addicted" to this metabolic state. And finally, if the patients perceive a reward by their control of hunger, what would happen if the amount of control exerted to overcome hunger is substantially decreased with recombinant leptin? Could females, in whom the disorder has just begun, profit from a rapid increment of serum leptin levels, thus reducing the rewarding effect of weight loss?

We need clinical trials to address these questions and to assess side effects.[22,23] The use of recombinant leptin in the treatment of patients with AN could prove to be ineffective or unsafe but might also represent a major step forward toward making use of our increased knowledge related to the advances in understanding appetite and weight regulation and the neuroendocrine mechanisms underlying the adaptation to starvation.

REFERENCES

1. Andreasen NC. DSM and the death of phenomenology in America: an example of unintended consequences. *Schizophr Bull.* 2007;33:108–112.
2. Vandereycken W, van Deth R. Who was the first to describe anorexia nervosa: Gull or Lasègue? *Psychol Med.* 1989;19(4):837–845.
3. Russell G. Bulimia nervosa: an ominous variant of anorexia nervosa. *Psychol Med.* 1979;9(3):429–448.
4. American Psychiatric Association. *Diagnostic and Statistical Manual of Mental Disorders.* 5th ed. 2013. Washington, D.C.
5. Hebebrand J, Casper R, Treasure J, Schweiger U. The need to revise the diagnostic criteria for anorexia nervosa. *J Neural Transm.* 2004;111(7):827–840.
6. Hebebrand J, Bulik CM. Critical appraisal of the provisional DSM-5 criteria for anorexia nervosa and an alternative proposal. *Int J Eat Disord.* 2011;44(8):665–678.
7. World Health Organization. https://icd.who.int/browse11/l-m/en.
8. Hebebrand J, Holm JC, Woodward E, et al. A proposal of the European association for the study of obesity to improve the ICD-11 diagnostic criteria for obesity based on the three dimensions etiology, degree of adiposity and health risk. *Obes Facts.* 2017;10(4):284–307.
9. Hebebrand J. Body weight and body composition in childhood and adolescence: diagnostic issues and current controversies. In: Herpertz-Dahlmann B, Hebebrand J, ed. *Eating Disorders and Obesity in Children and Adolescents.* Elsevier, [this book].
10. World Health Organization. *Obesity. Preventing and Managing the Global Epidemic. Report of a WHO Consultation (WHO Technical Report Series 894);* 2000. www.who.int/nutrition/publications/obesity/WHO_TRS_894/en/.
11. Farooqi IS, O'Rahilly S. The genetics of obesity in humans[Updated 2017 Dec 23] In: De Groot LJ, Chrousos G, Dungan K, et al., eds. *Endotext [Internet].* South Dartmouth (MA): Inc.; 2000. Available from: https://www.ncbi.nlm.nih.gov/books/NBK279064/MDText.com.
12. Hinney A, Giuranna J. The genetics of eating and weight disorders. In: Herpertz-Dahlmann B, Hebebrand J, eds. *Eating Disorders and Obesity in Children and Adolescents.* Elsevier, [this book].
13. Yengo L, Sidorenko J, Kemper KE, et al. *Meta-analysis of Genome-wide Association Studies for Height and Body Mass Index in ~700,000 Individuals of European Ancestry;* 2018. https://doi.org/10.1101/274654.
14. Duncan L, Yilmaz Z, Gaspar H, et al. Significant locus and metabolic genetic correlations revealed in genome-wide association study of anorexia nervosa. *Am J Psychiat.* 2017;174(9):850–858.
15. Cui H, Moore J, Ashimi SS, et al. Eating disorder predisposition is associated with ESRRA and HDAC4 mutations. *J Clin Invest.* 2013;123(11):4706–4713.
16. Huckins LM, Hatzikotoulas K, Southam L, et al. Investigation of common, low-frequency and rare genome-wide variation in anorexia nervosa. *Mol Psychiatry.* 2018;23(5):1169–1180.
17. Hinney A, Kesselmeier M, Jall S, et al. Evidence for three genetic loci involved in both anorexia nervosa risk and variation of body mass index. *Mol Psychiat.* 2017;22(2):192–201.
18. Shungin D, Winkler TW, Croteau-Chonka DC. New genetic loci link adipose and insulin biology to body fat distribution. *Nature.* 2015;518(7538):187–196.
19. Bulik-Sullivan B, Finucane HK, Anttila V, et al. An atlas of genetic correlations across human diseases and traits. *Nat Genet.* 2015;47(11):1236–1241.
20. Hebebrand J, Muller TD, Holtkamp K, Herpertz-Dahlmann B. The role of leptin in anorexia nervosa: clinical implications. *Mol Psychiat.* 2007;12:23–35.
21. Müller TD, Föcker M, Holtkamp K, Herpertz-Dahlmann B, Hebebrand J. Leptin-mediated neuroendocrine alterations in anorexia nervosa: somatic and behavioral implications. *Child Adolesc Psychiat Clin N Am.* 2009;18(1):117–129.
22. Hebebrand J, Albayrak Ö. Leptin treatment of patients with anorexia nervosa? The urgent need for initiation of clinical studies. *Eur Child Adolesc Psychiat.* 2012;21(2):63–66.
23. Hebebrand J, Antel J, Herpertz-Dahlmann B. Basic mechanisms and potential for treatment of weight and eating disorders. In: Geddes JR, Andreasen NC, Goodwin GM, eds. *The New Oxford Textbook of Psychiatry.* 3rd ed. Oxford, UK: Oxford University Press; 2019. [in press].
24. Ahima RS, Prabakaran D, Mantzoros C, et al. Role of leptin in the neuroendocrine response to fasting. *Nature.* 1996;382(6588):250–252.
25. Ahima RS, Flier JS. Leptin. *Annu Rev Physiol.* 2000;62:413–437.
26. Rosenbaum M, Leibel RL. 20 years of leptin: role of leptin in energy homeostasis in humans. *J Endocrinol.* 2014;223(1):T83–T96.
27. Hebebrand J, Blum WF, Barth N, et al. Leptin levels in patients with anorexia nervosa are reduced in the acute stage and elevated upon short-term weight restoration. *Mol Psychiat.* 1997;2(4):330–334.
28. Köpp W, Blum WF, von Prittwitz S, et al. Low leptin levels predict amenorrhea in underweight and eating disordered females. *Mol Psychiat.* 1997;2(4):335–340.
29. Föcker M, Timmesfeld N, Scherag S, et al. Screening for anorexia nervosa via measurement of serum leptin levels. *J Neural Transm.* 2011;118(4):571–578.
30. Halaas JL, Gajiwala KS, Maffei M, et al. Weight-reducing effects of the plasma protein encoded by the obese gene. *Science.* 1995;269(5223):543–546.
31. Lu XY, Kim CS, Frazer A, Zhang W. Leptin: a potential novel antidepressant. *Proc Natl Acad Sci USA.* 2006;103:1593–1598.
32. Asakawa A, Inui A, Inui T, Katsuura G, Fujino MA, Kasuga M. Leptin treatment ameliorates anxiety in ob/ob obese mice. *J Diabetes Complicat.* 2003;17:105–107.

33. Exner C, Hebebrand J, Remschmidt H, et al. Leptin suppresses semi-starvation induced hyperactivity in rats: implications for anorexia nervosa. *Mol Psychiat.* 2000;5(5):476–481.
34. Verhagen LA, Luijendijk MC, Adan RA. Leptin reduces hyperactivity in an animal model for anorexia nervosa via the ventral tegmental area. *Eur Neuropsycho Pharmacol.* 2011;21(3):274–281.
35. Hebebrand J, Exner C, Hebebrand K, et al. Hyperactivity in patients with anorexia nervosa and in semistarved rats: evidence for a pivotal role of hypoleptinemia. *Physiol Behav.* 2003;79(1):25–37.
36. Farooqi IS, Jebb SA, Langmack G, et al. Effects of recombinant leptin therapy in a child with congenital leptin deficiency. *N Engl J Med.* 1999;341(12):879–884.
37. Wabitsch M, Funcke JB, Lennerz B, et al. Biologically inactive leptin and early-onset extreme obesity. *N Engl J Med.* 2015;372(1):48–54.
38. Matochik JA, London ED, Yildiz BO, et al. Effect of leptin replacement on brain structure in genetically leptin-deficient adults. *J Clin Endocrinol Metab.* 2005;90:2851–2854.
39. Hukshorn CJ, Saris WH, Westerterp-Plantenga M, Farid AR, Smith FJ, Campfield LA. Weekly subcutaneous pegylated recombinant native human leptin (PEG-OB) administration in obese men. *J Clin Endocrinol Metab.* 2000;85:4003–4009.
40. Welt CK, Chan JL, Bullen J, et al. Recombinant human leptin in women with hypothalamic amenorrhea. *N Engl J Med.* 2004;351(10):987–997.
41. Holtkamp K, Herpertz-Dahlmann B, Hebebrand K, Mika C, Kratzsch J, Hebebrand J. Physical activity and restlessness correlate with leptin levels in patients with adolescent anorexia nervosa. *Biol Psychiat.* 2006;60:311–313.
42. Stengel A, Haas V, Elbelt U, Correll CU, Rose M, Hofmann T. Leptin and physical activity in adult patients with anorexia nervosa: failure to demonstrate a simple linear association. *Nutrients.* 2017;9(11). https://doi.org/10.3390/nu9111210.
43. *Food and Drug Administration.* 2014. https://www.fda.gov/downloads/drugs/drugsafety/postmarketdrugsafetyinformationforpatientsandproviders/ucm388903.pdf.
44. Murphy A. *MYALEPTA® (Metreleptin) Receives Positive CHMP Opinion in Patients with Generalized and Partial Lipodystrophy;* 2018. https://globenewswire.com/news-release/2018/06/01/1515454/0/en/MYALEPTA-metreleptin-Receives-Positive-CHMP-Opinion-in-Patients-with-Generalized-and-Partial-Lipodystrophy.html.
45. Tsoukas MA, Farr OM, Mantzoros CS. Leptin in congenital and HIV-associated lipodystrophy. *Metabolism.* 2015;64(1):47–59.
46. Radke, 2015. http://www.raredr.com/news/Myalept-Price-500K-600K.
47. Monteleone AM, Castellini G, Volpe U, et al. Neuroendocrinology and brain imaging of reward in eating disorders: a possible key to the treatment of anorexia nervosa and bulimia nervosa. *Prog Neuro-Psychopharmacol Biol Psychiat.* 2018;80(Pt B):132–142.
48. Cioffi JA, Shafer AW, Zupancic TJ, et al. Novel B219/OB receptor isoforms: possible role of leptin in hematopoiesis and reproduction. *Nat Med.* 1996;2(5):585–589.

CHAPTER 2

Developmentally Appropriate Assessment of Body Weight and Body Composition From Childhood to Adulthood With a Focus on Eating and Weight Disorders

JOHANNES HEBEBRAND, MD

USE AND LIMITATIONS OF THE BODY MASS INDEX

The body mass index (BMI; kg/m^2) is widely used to assess body weight adjusted for height. Among adults the correlations between BMI and height and weight are in the range of −0.15 and 0.6–0.8, respectively.[1] However, in children the correlation between BMI and height is positive (r = 0.3); in older adolescents the correlation is close to zero.[1,2] In children, adolescents, and adults, the BMI distribution is shifted to the right, indicating that body mass in the upper range is less tightly regulated. Indeed, body mass and BMI have exceeded 500 kg and 150 kg/m^2, respectively, in single extremely obese individuals.[3]

In medical terms, the major drawback of the index is that it does not distinguish between fat-free mass and fat mass. BMI is nevertheless widely used as a simple surrogate marker of fat mass; at the adult population level correlations between fat mass and BMI are sufficiently high (r≈0.6–0.9; 1). In children and adolescents, BMI has in general proven to be a superior index to other weight-height or other anthropometric indices for prediction of both current[2] and future adiposity.[4] BMI, however, does not sufficiently predict fat mass or percent fat mass in subjects, whose BMI clusters in a narrow range as in patients with anorexia nervosa (AN) or obesity. Hence, an individual assessment is crucial. In patients with AN or in individuals with class III obesity (BMI ≥ 40 kg/m^2), usually both fat-free and fat mass are beyond the normal range. Regional fat deposits can be assessed with magnetic resonance imaging. Dual-energy X-ray absorptiometry, underwater weighing, and air displacement plethysmography measure whole body fat and fat-free mass reliably but are expensive and available in specialized centers only. Skinfold measurements and bioelectrical impedance analysis provide less reliable estimates but are easy to implement.[1]

BODY MASS INDEX AND HEALTH RISKS

A medically relevant low BMI in most cases is associated with a subnormal level of adiposity as during a famine or acute AN. The physiological adaptation to starvation is largely based on the altered endocrine function of the adipose tissue. Serum hypoleptinemia represents the most physiologically important circulating marker of starvation-related weight loss and upregulates or downregulates the hypothalamus-pituitary-end organ axes, thus entailing many of the endocrine symptoms of starvation.[5] As such, the serum leptin level can serve as a proxy for fat mass in patients with AN.[6] In starvation regions, an exponential increase in mortality rates among adult males and females sets in after BMI drops to below 13 and 12 kg/m^2, respectively.[7] In both famines and acute AN, BMIs of below 10 kg/m^2 have been observed [7–9]; for any given degree of starvation, females have a lower mortality risk.[7]

In contrast, a high BMI is usually indicative of a high level of adiposity, which entails the major associated health risks, including type 2 diabetes mellitus (T2DM), cardiovascular disorders, and different types of cancer.[10,11] The World Health Organization (WHO) defines obesity as "a condition of abnormal or excessive fat accumulation in adipose tissue, to the extent that health may be impaired."[12] This impairment not only depends on the amount but also on the distribution, tissue-specific deposition (e.g., ectopic fat in muscle or liver), and type of fat mass (white vs. brown adipose tissue); health risks are higher for visceral (apple-shaped) as compared with gluteofemoral (pear-shaped) fat distribution. As a consequence, waist circumference should be measured in addition to BMI in overweight patients (see Refs. 13 and 14 for US and German centiles). Estimates for the population-attributable risks of obesity range from 5% to 15% for all-cause mortality, −0.2%–8% for all-cancer incidence, 7%–44% for cardiovascular disease incidence, and 3%–83% for T2DM incidence.[11] Cardiovascular disease accounts for more than two-thirds of deaths related to a high BMI.[10]

Nevertheless, it is important to point out that over a wide range of the BMI distribution the BMI does not allow any conclusion as to its implications for health of the respective individual. Major mediators of the link between high BMI/adiposity and the respective disorders include raised blood pressure, hyperinsulinemia, elevated cholesterol, and inflammation markers. The longer term medical risks are most pronounced in young and middle-aged individuals. It is a matter of ongoing debate if metabolically healthy obesity indeed exists or if it represents a transitory state prior to the initial onset of metabolic alterations.[10]

BMI AND WEIGHT CATEGORIES AND THEIR PREVALENCES

BMI is used to define the adult weight categories into underweight (BMI < 18.5 kg/m^2), normal weight (18.5–24.9), and overweight (≥25), which is subdivided into preobesity (25–29.9) and obesity classes I (30–34.9), II (35–39.9), and III (≥40 kg/m^2; 10). In global terms, 462 million adults worldwide are underweight, while 1.9 billion have a BMI ≥25 kg/m^2.[15] Overweight occurs in >50% of most European and the US adult populations; obesity (all classes) prevalence rates are in the range of 20%–40% in most (post)industrialized countries and also affect a substantial proportion of the populations of developing countries; rates for obesity are similar in males and females. However, class III obesity (BMI ≥ 40 kg/m^2) is more common in US adult females (9.5%) in comparison with males (5.5%; 16).

For children and adolescents, different definitions of childhood overweight and obesity are used, which are based upon national or international reference samples. Sex-specific BMI age centiles are most frequently used to define the respective weight categories. In the United States, overweight and obesity in children and adolescents are defined via BMI between the 85th and 95th centiles and ≥95th centile, respectively (reference data based on the five national health examination surveys and supplemental data)[17] (see Fig. 2.1a,b). US prevalence rates for obesity and extreme obesity (BMI ≥ 120% of the 95th centile on the CDC growth chart for BMI) were 17% and 5.8%, respectively; rates were comparable between males and females.[18] Globally, obesity rates in children and adolescents increased from less than 1% in 1975 to nearly 6% in girls and almost 8% in boys in 2016. Combined, the number of obese 5- to 19-year-olds rose more than 10-fold, from 11 million in 1975 to 124 million in 2016.[19]

In Germany and other European countries, overweight and obesity are defined via a BMI between the 90th and 97th centile and ≥97th centile, respectively[20]; extreme obesity has been defined via a BMI ≥99.5 centile. Cross-country comparisons are hampered by the differences in absolute values that constitute BMI age- and sex-specific centiles, especially in the upper range.[10] International age- and sex-specific definitions by the WHO and the International Obesity Task Force are available for use in clinical practice and research[21]; they also enable the study of cross-country comparisons and allow determination of secular increases in rates of childhood and adolescent overweight and obesity.

To compare relative weight among individuals with a very high or low body weight, the use of BMI-standard deviation scores (SDSs) or z-scores has been recommended.[22] Thus, many patients with AN have a BMI below the first BMI age centile, thus rendering the use of BMI-SDS or z-scores for further differentiation of this extreme weight group helpful. However, depending on the clinical situation, nutritional status will be assessed more accurately using methods that accurately measure body fat percentage (see above[23]).

DEVELOPMENTAL ASPECTS

Childhood BMI tracks into adulthood: correlations between adult BMI at an age of 35 years and BMI at infancy, aged 10 and 18 years, are in the range of r = 0.15, 0.35, and 0.7, respectively.[24] An obese child is more likely to remain obese as an adult (1) the older the child, (2) the more extreme the overweight, and (3) if one or both parents are obese.[25] On average, in young adults body weight increases by approximately 200–800 g annually with higher weight increments

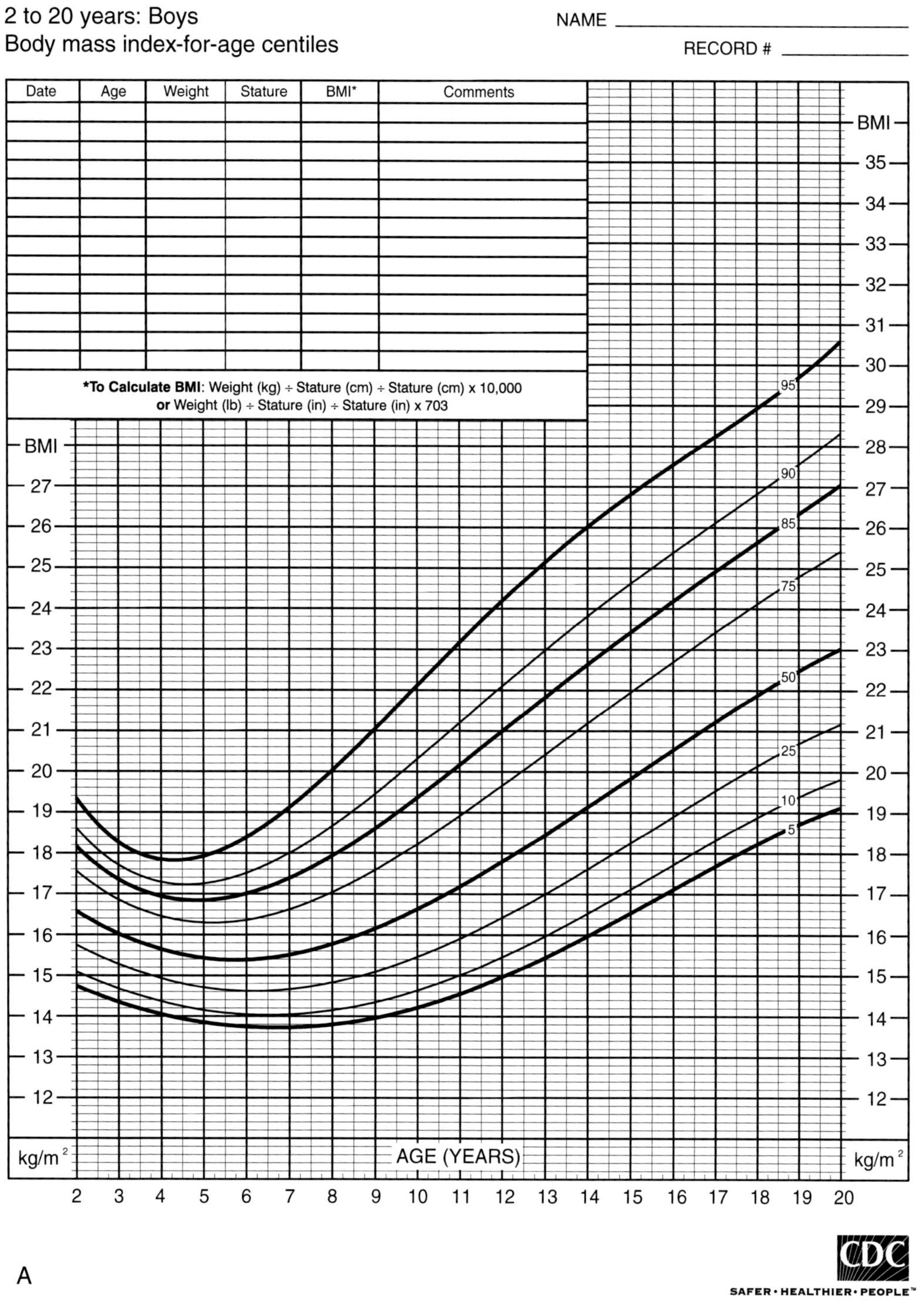
2 to 20 years: Boys
Body mass index-for-age centiles
NAME
RECORD #
Date
Age
Weight
Stature
BMI*
Comments
*To Calculate BMI: Weight (kg) ÷ Stature (cm) ÷ Stature (cm) x 10,000
or Weight (lb) ÷ Stature (in) ÷ Stature (in) x 703
BMI
95
90
85
75
50
25
10
5
kg/m2
AGE (YEARS)
2 3 4 5 6 7 8 9 10 11 12 13 14 15 16 17 18 19 20
A
CDC
SAFER • HEALTHIER • PEOPLE

FIG. 2.1 **(A)** and **(B)**: Centiles for body mass index (BMI; kg/m^2) of the Centers for Disease Control for boys and girls aged 2 to 20 years.[17]

2 to 20 years: Girls
Body mass index-for-age centiles

NAME _____

RECORD # _____

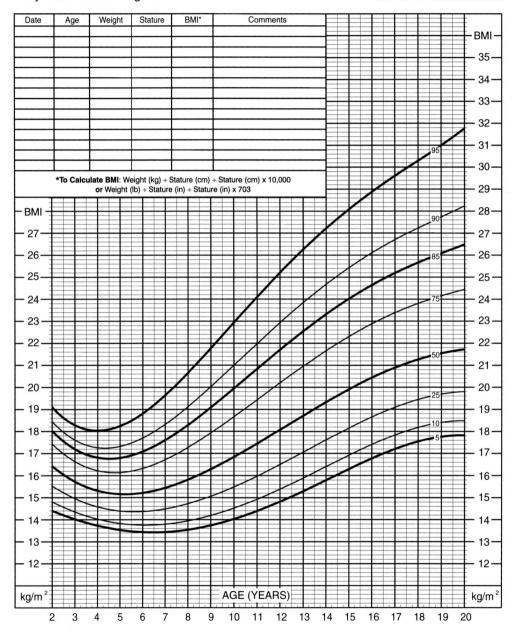

B

FIG. 2.1, cont'd

among the initially overweight subjects,[26,27] thus resulting in substantially divergent prevalence rates of underweight and obesity as defined via the rigid WHO cutoffs of BMI $<18.5\,kg/m^2$ and $\geq30\,kg/m^2$ in young adulthood and old age.[10,28] Apart from initial BMI and age, smoking, physical activity, and early socioeconomic status have been determined to account for most of the explained variance in weight change in Swedish females.[29] Puberty, pregnancy, and menopause represent time periods for steeper weight gains in predisposed females. National anthropometric reference data (2007–10) for children and adults of the US population allow the assessment of several anthropometric indices across the age span[13]; for other countries, national references are recommended.

The fetus has minimal fat mass until 24 weeks of gestation; at birth %BF has been found to range from 7% to 23%.[30] The steep BMI increment observed in the first 6 months of life is largely due to the increase in fat mass, afterward lean body mass intermittently increases disproportionately. A transient drop in mean BMI values sets in at an age of 6 months until around 6 years due to substantial growth in height. The adiposity rebound marks the time period at which BMI starts to increase after this transient BMI drop; an earlier adiposity rebound strongly predicts adolescent overweight and obesity.[31]

Slight gender differences in body composition exist prior to puberty with a higher percent body fat in females already evident at birth. By later childhood, girls begin to gain fat more readily; at the age of 10 years, girls average 2 kg more fat mass than boys, who in turn have approximately 1 kg more of fat-free mass. During puberty, girls gain more fat mass than males, and by the end of puberty, they have about 5–6 kg more absolute fat mass. In contrast, boys maintain their absolute fat-free mass throughout puberty. Their weight gain in this developmental phase is due to an increment in fat-free mass. Sex differences with respect to the development of %BF and fat distribution are relevant for the sex-dependent induction of the prepubertal neuroendocrine mechanisms that result in fertility and in female menarche in particular.[1,32]

BODY WEIGHT IN FEEDING AND EATING DISORDERS

The higher percent body fat in prepubertal and adolescent females may partially account for the female predominance of AN; fat mass can be reduced with less medical sequelae than a comparative loss of fat-free mass. In AN, but also in other feeding and eating disorders, the inadequate increment in fat mass or (intermittent) loss of fat mass can result in a complex derangement of the neuroendocrine circuits particularly affecting the regulation of the female hypothalamus-pituitary-gonadal axis. This derangement not only affects somatic growth and health but also impinges on mental health. Interestingly, because extreme obesity is almost twice as common in adult females,[16] females are more prone to develop both a low and high extreme weight.

In avoidant/restrictive food intake disorder (ARFID), the underweight associated with insufficient intake commonly starts in early childhood.[33] Children seemingly initially show picky eating to then develop full-blown ARFID. The underweight typically persists over prolonged periods of time and may continue into adulthood.

The data related to premorbid body weight in AN are somewhat conflicting. A preponderance of both underweight [34] and overweight [35] has been reported in addition to studies that report a normal premorbid weight distribution.[36] A clear reason for this divergence is not evident; however, the time point for premorbid weight assessment may play a role. BMI at referral for inpatient treatment has repeatedly been shown to correlate ($r\approx0.5$–0.6) with the BMI prior to the onset of the disorder; in contrast, the amount of weight loss is negatively correlated with the BMI at referral.[36]

In AN, BMI remains below average after recovery,[9,37] potentially reflecting a "scarring effect" on the mechanisms underlying body weight regulation including the persistence of a restrictive/rigid type of eating behavior. An alternative explanation is that specific genetic mechanisms predisposing to AN (and a subsequent low body weight) become operative during adolescence and persist thereafter. Indeed, a genetic correlation between AN and underweight has recently been uncovered.[38,39]

Parental and childhood obesity has been shown to be more common among patients with bulimia nervosa and binge eating disorder (BED) than in controls.[40] BED occurs in individuals of all weight categories albeit with a clear preponderance among overweight individuals.[1,33,41] BED is very strongly associated with overweight (including obesity) in treatment-seeking individuals; most overweight patients with BED were already overweight prior to the onset of the eating disorder with overweight/obesity potentially tracking from childhood.

OUTLOOK

Despite obvious limitations, BMI, BMI age centiles, and BMI z-scores should be used for assessment of relative weight in children, adolescents, and adults. Personalized risk prediction needs to be improved for the medical evaluation of the effects of both high and low body weight and adiposity, respectively, on somatic and mental health. General practitioners and experts in the fields of eating and weight disorders require guidance as to how to assess BMI, BMI centile, fat mass, and endocrine parameters to best evaluate the risks for an individual patient. The weight development of patients with eating disorders prior to the onset, during the disorder, and after recovery warrants further research. The female preponderance at both ends of the adult body weight distribution requires explanation.

REFERENCES

1. Hebebrand J. Diagnostic issues in eating disorders and obesity. *Child Adolesc Psychiatr Clin N Am.* 2009;18(1):1–16.
2. Mei Z, Grummer-Strawn LM, Pietrobelli A, et al. Validity of body mass index compared with other body-composition screening indexes for the assessment of body fatness in children and adolescents. *Am J Clin Nutr.* 2002;75:978–985.
3. Wikipedia. https://en.wikipedia.org/wiki/List_of_the_heaviest_people.
4. Freedman DS, Khan LK, Serdula MK, Dietz WH, Srinivasan SR, Berenson GS. Inter-relationships among childhood BMI, childhood height, and adult obesity: the Bogalusa Heart Study. *Int J Obes Relat Metab Disord.* 2004;28(1):10–16.
5. Hebebrand J, Muller TD, Holtkamp K, Herpertz-Dahlmann B. The role of leptin in anorexia nervosa: clinical implications. *Mol Psychiat.* 2007;12(1):23–35.
6. Mathiak K, Gowin W, Hebebrand J, et al. Serum leptin levels, body fat deposition, and weight in females with anorexia or bulimia nervosa. *Horm Metab Res.* 1999;31(4):274–277.
7. Collins S. The limit of human adaptation to starvation. *Nat Med.* 1995;1(8):810–814.
8. Born C, de la Fontaine L, Winter B, et al. First results of a refeeding program in a psychiatric intensive care unit for patients with extreme anorexia nervosa. *BMC Psychiatr.* 2015;24(15):57.
9. Hebebrand J, Himmelmann GW, Herzog W, et al. Prediction of low body weight at long-term follow-up in acute anorexia nervosa by low body weight at referral. *Am J Psychiat.* 1997;154(4):566–569.
10. Hebebrand J, Holm JC, Woodward E, et al. A proposal of the European association for the study of obesity to improve the ICD-11 diagnostic criteria for obesity based on the three dimensions etiology, degree of adiposity and health risk. *Obes Facts.* 2017;10(4):284–307.
11. Flegal KM, Panagiotou OA, Graubard BI. Estimating population attributable fractions to quantify the health burden of obesity. *Ann Epidemiol.* 2015;25:201–207.
12. World Health Organization. *Obesity: Preventing and Managing the Global Epidemic. Report of a WHO Consultation (WHO Technical Report Series 894);* 2000. www.who.int/nutrition/publications/obesity/WHO_TRS_894/en/.
13. Fryar CD, Gu Q, Ogden CL. Anthropometric reference data for children and adults: United States, 2007–2010. National Center for Health Statistics. *Vital Health Stat.* 2012;11(252). https://www.cdc.gov/nchs/data/series/sr_11/sr11_252.pdf.
14. Kromeyer-Hauschild K, Dortschy R, Stolzenberg H, et al. Nationally representative waist circumference percentiles in German adolescents aged 11.0-18.0 years. *Int J Pediatr Obes.* 2011;6(2–2):e129–e137.
15. World Health Organization: Malnutrition. http://www.who.int/news-room/fact-sheets/detail/malnutrition.
16. Flegal KM, Kruszon-Moran D, Carroll MD, Fryar CD, Ogden CL. Trends in obesity among adults in the United States, 2005 to 2014. *J Am Med Assoc.* 2016;315(21):2284–2291.
17. Centers for Disease Control and Prevention. https://www.cdc.gov/growthcharts/index.htm.
18. Ogden CL, Carroll MD, Lawman HG, et al. Trends in obesity prevalence among children and adolescents in the United States, 1988–1994 through 2013–2014. *J Am Med Assoc.* 2016;315(21):2292–2299.
19. Abarca-Gómez L, et al. Worldwide trends in body-mass index, underweight, overweight, and obesity from 1975 to 2016: a pooled analysis of 2416 population-based measurement studies in 128.9 million children, adolescents, and adults. *Lancet.* 2017;390(10113):2627–2642.
20. Kromeyer-Hauschild K, Wabitsch M, Kunze D, et al. Percentiles of body mass index in children and adolescents evaluated from different regional German studies (in German). *Monatsschr Kinderheilkd.* 2001;149:80.
21. Cole TJ, Lobstein T. Extended international (IOTF) body mass index cut-offs for thinness, overweight and obesity. *Pediatr Obes.* 2012;7:284–294.
22. Brannsether B, Eide GE, Roelants M, Bjerknes R, Júlíusson PB. Interrelationships between anthropometric variables and overweight in childhood and adolescence. *Am J Hum Biol.* 2014;26(4):502–510.
23. Fusch G, Raja P, Dung NQ, Karaolis-Danckert N, Barr R, Fusch C. Nutritional status in sick children and adolescents is not accurately reflected by BMI-SDS. *J Am Coll Nutr.* 2013;32(6):407–416.
24. Guo SS, Roche AF, Chumlea WC, Gardner JD, Siervogel RM. The predictive value of childhood body mass index values for overweight at age 35 y. *Am J Clin Nutr.* 1994;59(4):810–819.
25. Whitaker RC, Wright JA, Pepe MS, Seidel KD, Dietz WH. Predicting obesity in young adulthood from childhood and parental obesity. *N Engl J Med.* 1997;337(13):869–873.
26. Yanovski JA, Yanovski SZ, Sovik KN, Nguyen TT, O'Neil PM, Sebring NG. A prospective study of holiday weight gain. *N Engl J Med.* 2000;342(12):861–867.

27. Malhotra R, Ostbye T, Riley CM, Finkelstein EA. Young adult weight trajectories through midlife by body mass category. *Obesity*. 2013;21(9):1923–1934.

28. Hemmelmann C, Brose S, Vens M, Hebebrand J, Ziegler A. Percentiles of body mass index of 18–80-year-old German adults based on data from the Second National Nutrition Survey. *Dtsch Med Wochenschr*. 2010;135(17):848–852.

29. Lahmann PH, Lissner L, Gullberg B, Berglund G. Sociodemographic factors associated with long-term weight gain, current body fatness and central adiposity in Swedish women. *Int J Obes Relat Metab Disord*. 2000;24(6):685–694.

30. Toro-Ramos T, Paley C, Pi-Sunyer F, Gallagher D. Body composition during fetal development and infancy through the age of 5 years. *Eur J Clin Nutr*. 2015;69(12):1279–1289. https://doi.org/10.1038/ejcn.2015.117.

31. Hughes AR, Sherriff A, Ness AR, Reilly JJ. Timing of adiposity rebound and adiposity in adolescence. *Pediatrics*. 2014;134(5):e1354–e1361.

32. Loomba-Albrecht LA, Styne DM. Effect of puberty on body composition. *Curr Opin Endocrinol Diabetes Obes*. 2009;16(1):10–15.

33. American Psychiatric Association. *Diagnostic and Statistical Manual of Mental Disorders (DSM-5)*. American Psychiatric Press; 2013.

34. Stice E, Gau JM, Rohde P, Shaw H. Risk factors that predict future onset of each DSM-5 eating disorder: predictive specificity in high-risk adolescent females. *J Abnorm Psychol*. 2017;126(1):38–51.

35. Berkowitz SA, Witt AA, Gillberg C, Rastam M, Wentz E, Lowe MR. Childhood body mass index in adolescent-onset anorexia nervosa. *Int J Eat Disord*. 2016;49(11):1002–1009.

36. Föcker M, Bühren K, Timmesfeld N, et al. The relationship between premorbid body weight and weight at referral, at discharge and at 1-year follow-up in anorexia nervosa. *Eur Child Adolesc Psychiat*. 2015;24(5):537–544.

37. Fichter MM, Quadflieg N, Hedlund S. Twelve-year course and outcome predictors of anorexia nervosa. *Int J Eat Disord*. 2006;39(2):87–100.

38. Hinney A, Kesselmeier M, Jall S, et al. Evidence for three genetic loci involved in both anorexia nervosa risk and variation of body mass index. *Mol Psychiat*. 2017;22:321–322.

39. Duncan L, Yilmaz Z, Gaspar H, et al. Significant locus and metabolic genetic correlations revealed in genome-wide association study of anorexia nervosa. *Am J Psychiat*. 2017;174(9):850–858.

40. Fairburn CG, Doll HA, Welch SL, Hay PJ, Davies BA, O'Connor ME. Risk factors for binge eating disorder: a community-based, case-control study. *Arch Gen Psychiat*. 1998;55(5):425–432.

41. Herpertz-Dahlmann B. Adolescent eating disorders: update on definitions, symptomatology, epidemiology, and comorbidity. *Child Adolescent Psychiat Clin N Am*. 2015;24(1):177–196.

Appetite Control—Biological and Psychological Factors

JOHN E. BLUNDELL, PHD

Appetite is a field of study concerned with eating, hunger, food behavior, and energy intake. This set of operations is influenced by both biological and environmental factors, and can be regarded as a system. This system of appetite control is complex. Both biological and environmental aspects are of significance for understanding the problems that we face.

At the outset we can envisage two scenarios. For obesity, it can be inferred that no one is actually trying to become fat; obesity happens to people against their wishes. People are not intending to eat more; the overconsumption is passive and the weight gain (fat gain) follows without any personal effort or intention. In contrast, a weight (fat) loss is invariably deliberate and requires a mental effort. Undereating does not simply happen; it is intentional and purposeful. These two situations reflect the operations of the appetite system. Overeating is readily permitted and leads to fat gain. In contrast, the system defends itself strongly against a reduction of energy intake which is difficult to maintain and requires personal effort. The appetite system operates asymmetrically: readily allowing an energy surfeit but preventing an energy deficit. What is known about the processes of appetite control that can help to understand these situations?

HUMANS ARE OMNIVORES

The fact that humans are omnivores is of huge significance for understanding the appetite system. Humans are not restricted in their food habits to the same extent as herbivores or carnivores, and consequently they are capable of consuming a huge range of nutritional materials. Humans are generalists rather than specialists. Of course, this ability has been of enormous evolutionary significance and has enabled humans to colonize a wide variety of environments and habitats. Just as different groups of humans can exist on widely divergent types of foods (profiles of nutrition) in different parts of the world, the patterns of behavior that bring these nutrients into the mouth can differ widely. It can be appreciated that developing a science that encompasses such complexity is a daunting proposition. A science has therefore developed around a more restricted range of environments and behavioral types. Not surprisingly, this science has focused on the nutrition and behavioral types relevant to technologically industrialized societies in which we live and to the preoccupations of people living in these societies.

This position means that appetite control cannot be dissociated from the nutritional environment and the availability of foods.[2] This is relevant when considering that behavior can be seen as the agency that mediates in meeting two nutritional demands, namely, what to eat and how much to eat. Both are important for obesity. The problem of what to eat arises because of a combination of our omnivorous nature and the abundance of foods in the environment. This is the issue of food choice and involves the conscious or automatic selection among potential edible materials. Interestingly, this food choice is not strongly programmed biologically but is dependent upon factors such as geography, climate, religion, ethnicity, economics (price, affordability), social class, and culture. In contrast, the issue of how much to eat has always been conceptualized with reference to homeostatic principles of energy requirements of the body, with a stronger link to biology. This means that appetite control, for theoretical and methodological reasons, can be divided into issues of food choice and homeostasis.

FOOD CHOICE AND HEDONIC PROCESSES

The complexity of the issue of human food choice has been elegantly described by the Rozin's behavioral science approach. This has defined human food selection as the interaction of biology, culture, and individual experience.[22] Indeed, the importance of food selection for the overall control of appetite cannot be underestimated. As an addition to the complexity of human food preferences provided by the work of Rozin, a common perception about food choice is that it is dominated by the attribute of palatability. In simple terms, this means that people eat for pleasure. Indeed there are strong logical and biological reasons why the pleasurable taste of food should influence preference and consumption, and it is clearly a major issue in the manufacture and appeal of food products in the commercial market. This introduces the field of food hedonics which illustrates the intimate relationship between the behavioral aspect of appetite control (namely eating) and the nutritional characteristics of the available foods. Some extreme ideas have raised the idea that foods could be blessed with the quality of hyperpalatability designed with a combination of manufactured tastes, textures, and mouthfeel and exerting effects on brain neurotransmitters similar to (but much weaker than) the effects generated by drugs.[18] These ideas gave public support to claims for the existence of food addiction. However, the application of critical reviews and analyses is now showing that this concept of food addiction lacks strong evidential support and is much different from drug addiction.[21,19] Other writers have proposed the concept of "eating addiction" as an alternative to food addiction.[16]

A significant advance in the area of hedonics came about with the objective demonstration that in animals the notion of pleasure was not a unitary process.[1] Of course, in this area, the terms pleasure, reward, and reinforcement have particular meanings and it is important to be semantically clear. However, a key distinction made concerns separate identities for "liking" and "wanting." Liking is defined as a source of pleasure or reinforcement, while wanting is regarded as having a motivational component (technically referred to as incentive salience). It follows that a food that generates a combination of liking plus wanting would exert a strong influence over food choice. It is immediately apparent that a person can have a liking for a food, but not want (to eat) that food at that particular time or place. Therefore, the distinction between liking and wanting is meaningful.

Importantly, a procedure has been developed to simultaneously measure both liking and wanting for foods in humans.[13] The procedure avoids semantic confusion by using a nonverbal technique to measure wanting and also incorporates a covert (nonconscious) element known as implicit wanting.[12] With this procedure, food choice can be tracked to changes in liking or wanting independently or in combinations of both.

As Mela[20] has pointed out, this type of procedure allows a behavioral discrimination for foods that may underlay obesity and is a powerful device for investigating the level of risk associated with the consumption, and overconsumption, of certain foods and nutrients.

WHAT IS HOMEOSTATIC APPETITE CONTROL?

Homeostatic appetite control embodies both excitatory and inhibitory signals that stimulate and suppress appetite and food intake, and incorporates both tonic (long-term) and episodic (short-term) control mechanisms. Tonic effects are those with an enduring and stable influence over appetite and food intake that do not fluctuate significantly between or within day. These tonic control mechanisms have traditionally centred around the inhibitory action of insulin and leptin, but it now appears that the energy expenditure of metabolically active tissue also provides an enduring signal to eat. Episodic influences covary with the consumption of food across the day and respond acutely to the presence (or absence) of nutrients in the gastrointestinal (GI) tract. The classic satiety peptides cholecystokinin (CCK), glucagon-like peptide-1 (GLP-1), and peptide tyrosine tyrosine (PYY), along with the orexigenic peptide ghrelin, are thought to acutely influence the timing, type, and amount of food consumed across the day. However, the physiology of the postprandial state is complex and there is certainly not one single satiety peptide.[15] It is more likely that a group of peptides, fluctuating with separate patterns, can act conjointly to contribute to the encoding of a state of satiety.

EPISODIC PROCESSES AND THE SATIETY CASCADE

It is possible that the issue of satiety is the most heavily researched phenomenon in appetite control relevant to nutrition. It is conceived as being fundamental to the control over how much people eat, and is therefore crucial in the attempt to understand food consumption (and overconsumption) underlying obesity and the gain of adipose tissue. In its simplest form, the issue of satiety is about the feeling of fullness and the suppression of hunger and eating. A formulation devised 30 years[5] ago—called the "satiety cascade"—created a framework for thinking about the problem. In fact, this formulation identifies two distinct elements, namely satiation and satiety. Satiation refers to the operation of those processes ongoing during an episode of eating (such as a meal) and brings that episode to an end. Satiety refers to the inhibition of eating (and the suppression of hunger and augmentation of fullness) when an episode of consumption has ended. This is what people normally have in mind when they speak of satiety. In principle, the sequential operation of satiation and satiety influence the size and frequency of eating episodes—including the susceptibility to snacking between meals. Both of these processes are crucial for the control over the amount of food energy ingested.

A significant feature of the satiety cascade is the identification of different—but overlapping—psychological and physiological processes in the control of eating. These include physiological sensory factors arising from the smell and taste of food; psychological factors such as cognitions, beliefs, and expectations; and physiological factors in the stomach and other parts of the GI tract. See Fig. 3.1.

All features of foods (taste, texture, smell, palatability, amount, color, variety) have the potential to influence food choice, the perception of hunger, and eating itself. It appears obvious that the properties of foods exert a major influence over how much food energy will be consumed. In recent years the dietary variables of portion size and energy density have received attention because of their potential to lead people to

overconsume more (food) energy than is either wished for or required, and therefore to cause weight gain or obesity. Because of the nature of these dietary variables, their actions will be exerted during the actual process of eating (rather than after consumption) and the effects are therefore on satiation rather than satiety.

There is broad agreement on the effects of energy density on appetite control and its effects are profound. The action is mediated at the subconscious level. Because energy density is heavily dependent on the macronutrient composition of foods, most people are unaware of the nutritional composition of much of what is eaten and have a tendency to consume food based on weight or volume rather than on the nutrient composition (which is not easily perceived). Energy density, expressed as energy per unit of weight, is a property of every single food. It has been demonstrated by Stubbs et al.[24,25] that fat has the strongest positive relationship with energy density and the water content of foods has the strongest inverse association. The contribution of fat to the overconsumption of energy was experimentally demonstrated by Stubbs and others.[24] This phenomenon was termed high-fat hyperphagia[25] or passive overconsumption.[7] Normally, people are not actively endeavoring to consume more energy; this is unwanted energy intake

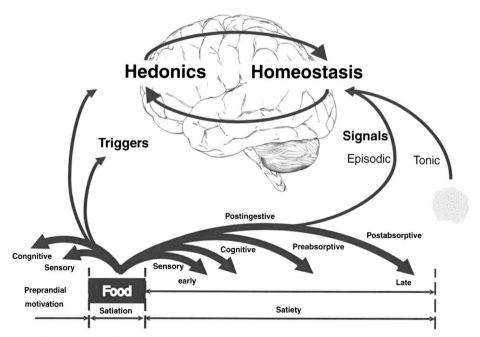

FIG. 3.1 The concept of the satiety cascade showing the separation of the processes of satiation (controlling meal size) and satiety (controlling the postmeal state of hunger). The model also shows the way in which the hedonic and homeostatic processes interact in the overall control of eating.

that happens as a consequence of the property of the foods chosen. "This passive overconsumption of energy leading to obesity is a predictable outcome of market economies predicated on consumption-based growth" and has been identified as a major contributor of the obesogenic environment on weight gain.[26]

It is noteworthy that the effects of fat and energy density are also observed in children. When energy density was raised by doubling the amount of fat in meals (but keeping protein and carbohydrate constant) a highly significant effect on energy intake was observed.[14] A further extension of this diet-induced effect on behavior can be seen in combinations of nutrients and tastes. Here, a potent combination is the subcategory of high-energy dense foods comprising high-fat and high-sugar products. This category of food items exerts a particularly strong effect on consumption through actions on both explicit liking and implicit wanting. In this particular case, there is an active "want" to eat these foods (induced by the potent combination of taste and texture), which is strongly apparent in binge eaters.[9]

TONIC PROCESSES OF APPETITE AND THE DRIVE TO EAT

An important feature, often overlooked, is that the motivation to eat is one of our strongest psychological experiences and is based on biological processes. This drive is clearly of evolutionary significance and it is extremely difficult to control. This drive is common to all living organisms but the strength, timing, and direction of the drive vary from species to species, and there is considerable variability within species. In humans the strength of the drive to eat cannot be denied except under special cultural or pathological conditions. The strength of the drive obliges an engagement with the environment which is the source of food. The power of the drive and its unrelenting presence suggest the operation of important biological processes.

In recent years the issue of the drive to eat has been investigated within an energy balance framework. Energy expenditure and energy intake are not independent of each other, they interact. This concept can be traced back to the work of pioneers of nutritional physiology in the United Kingdom such as Edholm and Widdowson who postulated that "the differences between the intakes of food (of individuals) must originate in the differences in the expenditure of energy."[10] Evidence now indicates that we can think of energy expenditure as a drive for energy intake.[4] In turn, we can envisage two forms of energy expenditure: the metabolic and the

behavioral. Energy expenditure arising from metabolism is normally referred to as resting metabolic rate (RMR), and it accounts for approximately 70% of total energy expenditure (metabolic plus behavioral). It is also known that the major contributor to RMR is lean mass or fat-free mass (FFM), which accounts for about 60% of the variance in RMR. In contrast, fat mass (FM) accounts for only about 7%. FFM comprises tissues such as skeletal muscle, heart, brain, liver, kidneys, and the GI tract organs. Consequently, this new approach to appetite control stipulates that the energy required to maintain the functioning of the body's vital organs constitutes a drive for energy, in other words, the motivation to seek and eat food.[6,17] See Fig. 3.2.

IMPLICATIONS

This conceptual scheme, described above, makes sense in the light of evolutionary theory and has strong biological plausibility. In contrast to the action of FFM which can drive eating via RMR, adipose tissue (FM) can be regarded as having an inhibitory purpose—in keeping with one of its main functions as a store of energy. An important corollary is that, as FM accumulates due to a positive energy balance, the inhibitory action becomes weaker—due to leptin and insulin resistance. This means that as a person becomes fatter he or she get no help from the increasing adipose tissue mass for controlling his or her appetite; in fact appetite becomes more difficult to control. This inference resonates with the experience of many people as they become fatter. Obese people not only have more FM but also more FFM to support the fat tissue; consequently, we can expect them to have a stronger drive to eat. Many personal testimonies support this. In addition, because of a weakened inhibitory effect of accumulated fat tissue, they are less able to resist the increased drive for food. This is one reason why obesity is regarded as a "wicked" problem since as people gain fat, it becomes more difficult, not less, to resist eating. It seems that only certain drugs—such as glucagon-like-peptide (GLP1) agonists—have the power to substantially overcome the drive to eat.[3]

Most, but not all, studies in this area have been carried out on adults. What is known about the source of the drive to eat in younger age groups? Interestingly, there is strong evidence for the operation of the same tonic mechanisms underlying the drive to eat. First, it has been shown that skeletal muscle mass (one of the largest components of FFM) is a strong predictor of energy intake in obese adolescents.[8] Second, in a brain imaging study in 7- to 10-year-old children, it was

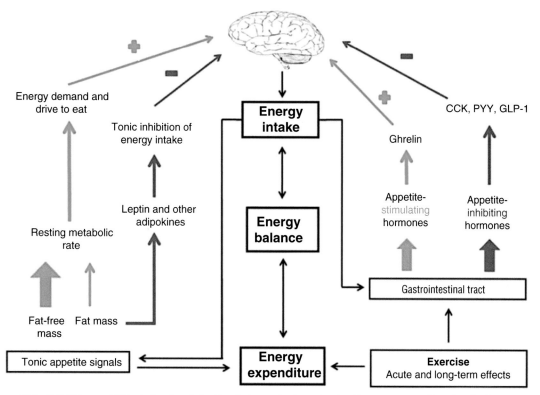

FIG. 3.2 This model illustrates the distinction between tonic and episodic processes, with episodic signals arising as a consequence of food consumption whereas tonic signals arise from body tissues and metabolism. The metabolic demand for energy arises from energy requirements generated by the major energy using organs of the body (heart, liver, brain, gastrointestinal tract, skeletal muscle) and is reflected in resting metabolic rate. The overall strength of the drive for food is the balance between the tonic excitatory and inhibitory processes. The effect of fat mass on energy intake reflects a lipostatic view of appetite control; leptin is a key mediator of the inhibitory influence of fat on brain mechanisms. See text for discussion.

found that FFM was a driver of appetite and was associated with a greater intake of high-energy dense foods—especially in an area of the brain with dense dopamine signalling.[11] More recently, a prospective study on children aged 6 to 8 years and from 8 to 10 years indicated that muscle mass predicted lower levels of the trait of satiety responsiveness while FM predicted higher levels of the trait of food responsiveness.[23] These findings are in keeping with the elements of the appetite control model in Fig. 3.2 and indicate how a combination of FFM and FM in obese children acts conjointly to promote a tendency to overconsume.

SUMMARY

Appetite control represents the outcome of a complex set of interactions between biology and the environment; both play a role in determining how appetite is expressed. Neither single statement nor set of statements can definitively define how appetite will be expressed in different individuals and in differing circumstances. Individual variability in the expression of appetite (quantitative and qualitative) is huge, and average values are often misleading. The descriptions set out in this chapter indicate how it is meaningful to conceptualize some of the key processes that influence the way in which people eat and how much is eaten. Appetite reflects energy intake, but it is now recognized that energy expenditure has a major influence on the drive for energy (food). This indicates the importance of energy balance and shows how appetite control can best be understood within a framework of energy balance. This framework is also highly relevant for obesity, and since the metabolic drive to eat is so powerful, it is an important consideration in various types of eating disorders. The strength of the drive to eat is a powerful biological and psychological force underlying the etiology and the management of both obesity and the eating disorders.

REFERENCES

1. Berridge K, Kringelbach M. Affective neuroscience of pleasure: reward in humans and animals. *Psychopharmacology.* 2008;199(3):457–480.
2. Blundell J. The contribution of behavioural science to nutrition: appetite control. *Nutr Bull.* 2017;42(3): 236–245.
3. Blundell J, Finlayson G, Axelsen MB, et al. Effects of once-weekly semaglutide on appetite, energy intake, control of eating, food preference and body weight in subjects with obesity. *Diabetes Obes Metabol.* 2017.
4. Blundell J, Gibbons C, Caudwell P, Finlayson G, Hopkins M. Appetite control and energy balance: impact of exercise. *Obes Rev.* 2015;16(S1):67–76.
5. Blundell J, Rogers P, Hill A. Evaluating the satiating power of foods: implications for acceptance and consumption. In: *Food Acceptance and Nutrition.* London: Academic Press; 1987:205–219.
6. Blundell JE, Caudwell P, Gibbons C, et al. Role of resting metabolic rate and energy expenditure in hunger and appetite control: a new formulation. *Dis Models Mech.* 2012;5(5):608–613.
7. Blundell JE, MacDiarmid JI. Passive overconsumption fat intake and short-term energy balancea. *Ann N Y Acad Sci.* 1997;827(1):392–407.
8. Cameron JD, Sigal RJ, Kenny GP, et al. Body composition and energy intake—skeletal muscle mass is the strongest predictor of food intake in obese adolescents: the HEARTY trial. *Appl Physiol Nutr Metabol.* 2016.
9. Dalton M, Finlayson G. Psychobiological examination of liking and wanting for fat and sweet taste in trait binge eating females. *Physiol Behav.* 2014;136:128–134.
10. Edholm OG, Fletcher JG, Widdowson EM, McCance RA. The energy expenditure and food intake of individual men. *Br J Nutr.* 1955;9(03):286–300.
11. Fearnbach SN, English LK, Lasschuijt M, et al. Brain response to images of food varying in energy density is associated with body composition in 7-to 10-year-old children: results of an exploratory study. *Physiol Behav.* 2016;162:3–9.
12. Finlayson G, King N, Blundell J. The role of implicit wanting in relation to explicit liking and wanting for food: implications for appetite control. *Appetite.* 2008;50(1): 120–127.
13. Finlayson G, King NA, Blundell JE. Liking vs. wanting food: importance for human appetite control and weight regulation. *Neurosci Biobehav Rev.* 2007;31(7):987–1002.
14. Fisher JO, Liu Y, Birch LL, Rolls BJ. Effects of portion size and energy density on young children's intake at a meal. *Am J Clin Nutr.* 2007;86(1):174–179.
15. Gibbons C, Caudwell P, Finlayson G, et al. Comparison of postprandial profiles of ghrelin, active GLP-1 and total PYY to meals varying in fat and carbohydrate, and their association with hunger and the phases of satiety. *J Clin Endocrinol Metabol.* 2013;98(5):E847–E855.
16. Hebebrand J, Albayrak Ö, Adan R, et al. "Eating addiction", rather than "food addiction", better captures addictive-like eating behavior. *Neurosci Biobehav Rev.* 2014;47:295–306.
17. Hopkins M, Blundell JE. Energy balance, body composition, sedentariness and appetite regulation: pathways to obesity. *Clin Sci.* 2016;130(18):1615–1628.
18. Kessler DA. *The End of Overeating: Taking Control of the Insatiable American Appetite, Rodale;* 2010.
19. Long CG, Blundell JE, Finlayson G. A systematic review of the application and correlates of YFAS-diagnosed 'food addiction' in humans: are eating-related 'addictions'a cause for concern or empty concepts? *Obes Facts.* 2015;8(6):386–401.
20. Mela DJ. Eating for pleasure or just wanting to eat? Reconsidering sensory hedonic responses as a driver of obesity. *Appetite.* 2006;47(1):10–17.
21. Rogers PJ. Food and drug addictions: similarities and differences. *Pharmacol Biochem Behav.* 2017;153:182–190.
22. Rozin P. *Towards a Psychology of Food Choice.* Institut Danone; 1998.
23. Steinsbekk S, Llewellyn CH, Fildes A, Wichstrøm L. Body composition impacts appetite regulation in middle childhood. A prospective study of Norwegian community children. *Int J Behav Nutr Phys Activ.* 2017;14(1):70.
24. Stubbs R. Macronutrient effects on appetite. *Int J Obes Relat Metab Disord.* 1995;19:S11.
25. Stubbs R, Whybrow S. Energy density, diet composition and palatability: influences on overall food energy intake in humans. *Physiol Behav.* 2004;81(5):755–764.
26. Swinburn BA, Sacks G, Hall KD, et al. The global obesity pandemic: shaped by global drivers and local environments. *Lancet.* 2011;378(9793):804–814.

Emerging Change in Body Perception During Growth and Development Among Children and Adolescents

JOLANDA S. VAN VLIET, PHD • NINA NELSON, MD, PHD

INTRODUCTION

The transition from childhood to adolescence is characterized by rapid physical, psychological, social, and behavioral changes.[1] During this period, it is important that young people maintain a healthy balance between body perception and objective body measurements to help avoid inappropriate weight control behaviors.[2]

A negative interpretation of the body and pronounced body dissatisfaction can result in dietary restraint and compensatory behaviors. A biased interpretation of body-related information has been found to be associated with the specific psychopathology of eating disorders (EDs) such as anorexia nervosa (AN) and bulimia nervosa (BN).[3–5] The core symptoms of AN and BN are shape and weight preoccupation as well as shape overvaluation associated with energy restriction and weight loss.[4] An unbalanced body perception can be considered as one of the key factors of maladaptive cognitions and behaviors in both EDs.[3–5]

The literature uses various terms to describe perception of physical appearance,[6] the most common of which is body image. *Body image* is a construct that combines estimation of body size with subjective evaluation of the mental image. Body image as a psychological construct is part of self-image and self-esteem.[7] Body image, as used in the literature, can refer to either body satisfaction or body perception.[6] *Body satisfaction* is the extent to which an individual is content with his/her body size and shape. Incorporated into the concept of body satisfaction are terms such as body confidence, body esteem, and body dissatisfaction.[6] *Body perception* is defined as the assessment by an individual of the physical aspects of the body and the extent to which this assessment is accurate.[6] Our studies use the term *overweight perception* to describe the assessment by the individual that the physical appearance of the body is "too fat" or "far too fat."[8–11] To establish the accuracy of individual assessments, we compared overweight perception with anthropometric measurements, using the internationally accepted parameters of waist circumference (WC) and Body Mass Index (BMI) as references for overweight/obesity. The international reference values in children and adolescents for BMI and WC are adjusted for age and gender since both measures increase with chronological age and vary according to gender and stage of pubertal maturation.[12,13] This chapter uses the term body perception, since our findings compare individual assessment of physical appearance with actual physical aspects of the body during growth and development. However, we also use the other terms mentioned when appropriate in relation to the research described and discussed.

We focus on emergence of body perception in relation to actual body and weight measurements. A better understanding of this relationship may help children and adolescents to avoid additional weight gain in cases of underestimation and to prevent unhealthy weight control behaviors in cases of overestimation of body size.

MAJOR FINDINGS
Body Perception Related to Gender- and Age-Specific Body Measurements

The prevalence of overweight perception has increased over time, especially among girls, but also among boys[11,14] and so, too, has the prevalence of actual overweight, especially among boys.[11,15,16] Indeed, overweight is a strong predictor of overweight perception. As shown in Table 4.1, there were no age- or gender-related differences regarding the absence of overweight perception when overweight had been established by

TABLE 4.1
Prevalence of Misconception 1 and Misconception 2 for Boys and Girls, Respectively

				BOYS			GIRLS		
	All boys [n=98]	All girls [n=141]	P-value	<13y [n=62]	≥13y [n=34]	P-value	<13y [n=74]	≥13y [n=67]	P-value
MISCONCEPTION 1[a]:									
IsoBMI	4.1%	16.3%	0.003	3.2%	5.9%	0.533	1.4%	32.8%	0.000
WC	4.1%	11.5%	0.043	3.2%	5.9%	0.533	0.0%	24.2%	0.000
MISCONCEPTION 2[b]:									
IsoBMI	6.1%	6.4%	0.935	4.8%	8.8%	0.440	9.5%	3.0%	0.116
WC	16.3%	20.9%	0.381	17.7%	14.7%	0.703	26.0%	15.2%	0.115

[a]Misconception 1: Perception of overweight unsupported by measured overweight/obesity according to IsoBMI and WC, respectively.
[b]Misconception 2: Perception of nonoverweight despite presence of overweight/obesity as measured by IsoBMI and WC.
IsoBMI, age- and gender-specific Body Mass Index; *WC*, waist circumference.

objective measurements,[10] which suggests that perception of actual overweight may be both age- and gender-independent.

However, several studies on overweight perception claim a gender difference in which girls are more inclined to feel fat and dissatisfied with their bodies than boys, suggesting that cultural influences pertaining to slimness may play a role.[17–20] Girls were found to be at nearly three times the risk for perception of overweight compared with boys.[10] Misperception of overweight was particularly common among girls aged 13 years and above, who have a significantly higher prevalence of feeling too fat despite measured normal weight, compared with boys and younger girls (see also Table 4.1).[10,20] In girls, particularly those aged 13 years and above, overweight perception seems to be strongly influenced by determinants for body perception other than actual overweight.[10,16,20]

One interesting finding in our study was that girls, particularly those age 13 years and above, were less likely to form a misconception of overweight based on their WC than on IsoBMI (i.e., age- and gender-specific BMI for children up to 18 years), suggesting that girls are more likely to assess their weight according to WC than according to IsoBMI when forming opinions on body perception (see Table 4.1),[8,10] possibly because WC is more clearly related to abdominal fat and changes in body shape at different ages.[16,21] The focus on various aspects of the body other than more objective parameters, such as height, weight, and body shape, may reflect current physical ideals, as suggested by other investigators.[22] It is likely that adolescent girls use WC, a characteristic of body

shape rather than body size, as a basis for assessment of body size. The weak agreement between subjective body perception and objective determinants in girls may be attributable to the more ambiguous cut-off points for BMI in adolescence than in the adult population since normal BMI parameters increase with age and vary with gender, stage of pubertal maturation, and body composition.[8] Correct interpretation of BMI requires consideration of both lean body mass and fat body mass since lean body mass contributes relatively more to total body weight.[23] When evaluating the accuracy of body perception among children and adolescents, WC must also be taken into account since it appears to be more relevant than BMI,[8,10] and like BMI, is also related to health outcomes such as overweight and other health-related issues.[21]

Body Perception and Characteristics of Female Pubertal Development

Female pubertal characteristics such as acne and breast growth were found to increase the likelihood of overweight perception significantly among girls, even after adjusting for actual overweight based on WC, as shown in Table 4.2.[9] Furthermore, the perception of being too fat was more likely to occur among nonoverweight girls who perceive breast growth than among overweight girls.[9] This finding supports earlier studies that visible physiological changes affect body perception in girls.[24–26] Physical changes in body fat distribution and breast growth are generally more obvious in nonoverweight girls. Girls may initially experience breast growth in particular as a positive change but may find it distressing later in the developmental process because it is associated

TABLE 4.2

Logistic Univariate Regression Model Predicting Odds Ratios (OR), 95% Confidence Intervals (CI), and Significance of Perceived Emergence of Each of the Secondary Pubertal Characteristics for Overweight Perception.

Perceived emergence of secondary pubertal characteristics	OR FOR OVERWEIGHT PERCEPTION			OR ADJUSTED FOR OVERWEIGHT BASED ON WC	
	OR when emergence of the pubertal characteristic is not perceived	OR when emergence of the pubertal characteristic is perceived	CI when emergence of the pubertal characteristic is perceived	OR when emergence of the pubertal characteristic is perceived	CI when emergence of the pubertal characteristic is perceived
Breast growth (n = 220)	1.00	2.83[a]	1.51–5.31	2.73[a]	1.36–5.47
Acne (n = 203)	1.00	2.56[a]	1.42–4.60	2.02[a]	1.07–3.82
Pubic hair growth (n = 214)	1.00	1.33	0.73–2.42	1.37	0.70–2.66
Growth spurt (n = 173)	1.00	1.30	0.72–2.35	1.04	0.55–1.99
Menstruation (n = 220)	1.00	1.55	0.88–2.74	1.45	0.77–2.73

In a multiple regression model, the OR for each of the characteristics of overweight perception is predicted and adjusted for overweight based on waist circumference (WC).

[a]$P < 0.05$.

with characteristic female accumulation of body fat—not just around the breasts, but throughout the body.[27]

The natural increase in body fat that accompanies puberty in girls often conflicts with stereotypes of the ideal female body.[7] Therefore, girls in puberty tend to develop a negative body perception, which is confirmed by the high prevalence of misconceptions of feeling fat despite normal weight measurements. These misconceptions relate to both WC and IsoBMI, as shown in Table 4.1.[10] In contrast, boys undergoing puberty naturally become more muscular and develop broader shoulders following their growth spurt, both of which contribute to the positive ideal of the male body.[28,29] Boys aged 13 years and above may therefore develop a more positive self-image with age and pubertal development, which might help to explain the relative lack of misconceptions about feeling fat among nonoverweight boys.[10] Gender differences in body perception have also been shown to reflect how male and female adolescents evaluate their bodies: girls tend to view their bodies primarily as a means of attracting others, while boys perceive their bodies as a means of effectively operating in the external environment.[19,29]

Adolescence is a period of rapid physiological change, so it is not surprising that the majority of disturbances in body perception can be found during this period.[7,30,31] Individuals often find it difficult to make appropriate judgments and to draw correct conclusions about their weight and body size, especially during puberty, when the rapid pace of developmental changes are not always synchronized among peers. Several studies show that individuals who mature early or more rapidly tend to have more subcutaneous truncal fat, as well as overweight and obesity, compared with their same-aged peers.[31,32] Consequently, the timing of pubertal maturation in girls has been shown to influence body perception, where girls who mature early more often report feeling too fat.[33]

When considering age at onset of pubertal development, it is therefore important to note the secular trend toward earlier development over the past century. Age at menarche dropped dramatically during the first half of the 20th century in Western nations. However, since 1960 the trend toward earlier onset of menarche has slowed and even reversed in some societies.[34] Nevertheless, modern studies found that breast development occurs significantly earlier among girls who were born more recently.[35] Meanwhile, higher BMI at younger ages was found to be related to earlier breast development.[36,37] However, the possible role of factors other than BMI, such as nutrition, physical activity, or endocrine disrupting chemicals, have also been suggested as potential causes.[37,38] In any case, the secular trend toward earlier breast development should raise some concerns, considering the association between breast development and inappropriate overweight perception as discussed in this chapter.[9]

CONCLUSION

Actual overweight surpasses overweight perception, at least among boys and girls younger than 13 years. Among girls, age and the visible physical changes that accompany female pubertal development, such as acne and breast growth, are related to overweight perception. In addition, WC, more so than IsoBMI, influences body and overweight perception, possibly due to its correlation with abdominal fat measurements at different ages.

OUTLOOK

The emergence of body perception serves as a pathway for children and adolescents to better understand the changes that normally accompany growth and development. Educational interventions aimed at boys and girls, their parents, schools, and healthcare services are needed to improve understanding of these natural physical changes and how to appropriately interpret them.

To narrow the gap between measured and perceived body size, WC is a relevant measurement for children and adolescents in addition to BMI. Both health professionals and individuals may wish to obtain WC in adolescents to serve as an additional objective measurement of body size and as a common target for intervention.

Among girls, the use of self-reported breast growth (indicator of accumulation of body fat) and age at menarche as measurements for female pubertal development may help girls to increase their understanding of the natural body changes occurring during pubertal development and thereby could lower the risk for overweight perception. At the same time, for health professionals, self-reported breast growth and age at menarche could serve as indicators and targets for intervention.

REFERENCES

1. Berenbaum SA, Beltz AM, Corley R. The importance of puberty for adolescent development. *Adv Child Dev Behav.* 2015;48:53–92.
2. Bucchianeri MM, Fernandes N, Loth K, et al. Body dissatisfaction: do associations with disordered eating and psychological well-being differ across race/ethnicity in adolescent girls and boys? *Cult Divers Ethn Minor Psychol.* 2016;22(1): 137–146.
3. Brockmeyer T, Anderle A, Schmidt H, et al. Body image related negative interpretation bias in anorexia nervosa. *Behav Res Ther.* 2018;104:69–73.
4. Forrest LN, Jones PJ, Ortiz SN, et al. Core psychopathology in anorexia nervosa and bulimia nervosa: a network analysis. *Int J Eat Disord.* Epub April 2018.
5. Duarte C, Ferreira C, Trindade IA, et al. Normative body dissatisfaction and eating psychopathology in teenage girls: the impact of inflexible eating rules. *Eat Weight Disord Stud Anorexia Bulim Obes.* 2016;21(1): 41–48.
6. Burrowes N. *Body Image – a Rapid Evidence Assessment of the Literature a Project on Behalf of the Government Equalities Office;* 2013;48p.
7. Eisenberg ME, Neumark-Sztainer D, Paxton SJ. Five-year change in body satisfaction among adolescents. *J Psychosom Res.* 2006;61(4):521–527.
8. Van Vliet JS, Kjölhede EA, Duchén K, et al. Waist circumference in relation to body perception reported by Finnish adolescent girls and their mothers. *Acta Paediatr.* 2009;98(3):501–506.
9. Van Vliet JS, Räsänen L, Gustafsson PA, et al. Overweight perception among adolescent girls in relation to appearance of female characteristics. *Paediatr Health.* 2014;2:1. http://dx.doi.org/10.7243/2052-935X-2-1.
10. van Vliet J, Gustafsson P, Duchen K, et al. Social inequality and age-specific gender differences in overweight and perception of overweight among Swedish children and adolescents: a cross-sectional study. *BMC Public Health.* 2015;15(1):628. http://dx.doi.org/10.1186/s12889-015-1985-x.
11. Van Vliet JS, Gustafsson PA, Nelson N. Feeling "too fat" rather than being "too fat" increases unhealthy eating habits among adolescents - even in boys. *Food Nutr Res.* 2016;60. https://doi.org/10.3402/fnr.v60.29530.
12. Cole TJ, Bellizzi MC, Flegal KM, et al. Establishing a standard definition for child overweight and obesity worldwide: international survey. *BMJ.* 2000;320(7244): 1240–1243.
13. McCarthy HD, Jarrett KV, Crawley HF. The development of waist circumference percentiles in British children aged 5.0-16.9 y. *Eur J Clin Nutr.* 2001;55(10):902–907.
14. Whitehead R, Berg C, Cosma A, et al. Trends in adolescent overweight perception and its association with psychosomatic health 2002-2014: evidence from 33 countries. *J Adolesc Health.* 2017;60(2):204–211.
15. Matthiessen J, Stockmarr A, Biltoft-Jensen A, et al. Trends in overweight and obesity in Danish children and adolescents: 2000-2008 – exploring changes according to parental education. *Scand J Public Health.* 2014;42(4):385–392.
16. Buscemi S, Marventano S, Castellano S, et al. Role of anthropometric factors, self-perception, and diet on weight misperception among young adolescents: a cross-sectional study. *Eat Weight Disord Stud Anorexia Bulim Obes.* 2018;23(1): 107–115.
17. Calzo JP, Sonneville KR, Haines J, et al. The development of associations among body mass Index, body dissatisfaction, and weight and shape concern in adolescent boys and girls. *J Adolesc Heal.* 2012;51(5):517–523.

18. Mäkinen M, Puukko-Viertomies L-R, Lindberg N, et al. Body dissatisfaction and body mass in girls and boys transitioning from early to mid-adolescence: additional role of self-esteem and eating habits. *BMC Psychiatry.* 2012;12(1):35. http://dx.doi.org/10.1186/1471-244X-12-35.

19. Tatangelo GL, Ricciardelli LA. A qualitative study of preadolescent boys' and girls' body image: gendered ideals and sociocultural influences. *Body Image.* 2013;10(4):591–598.

20. Martini MCS, Assumpção D de, Barros MB de A, et al. Are normal-weight adolescents satisfied with their weight? *Sao Paulo Med J.* 2016;134(3):219–227.

21. McCarthy HD. Body fat measurements in children as predictors for the metabolic syndrome: focus on waist circumference. *Proc Nutr Soc.* 2006;65(4):385–392.

22. Thoma ME, Hediger ML, Sundaram R, et al. Comparing apples and pears: women's perceptions of their body size and shape. *J Womens Heal.* 2012;21(10):1074–1081.

23. Eissa MA, Dai S, Mihalopoulos NL, et al. Trajectories of fat mass Index, fat free–mass Index, and waist circumference in children. *Am J Prev Med.* 2009;37(1):S34–S39.

24. Szamreta EA, Qin B, Ohman-Strickland PA, et al. Associations of anthropometric, behavioral, and social factors on level of body esteem in peripubertal girls. *J Dev Behav Pediatr.* 2017;38(1):58–64.

25. Knowles A-M, Niven AG, Fawkner SG, et al. A longitudinal examination of the influence of maturation on physical self-perceptions and the relationship with physical activity in early adolescent girls. *J Adolesc.* 2009;32(3):555–566.

26. Brooks-Gunn J. Antecedents and consequences of variations in girls' maturational timing. *J Adolesc Health Care.* 1988;9(5):365–373.

27. Hillman JB, Biro FM. Dynamic changes of adiposity during puberty: life may not be linear. *J Adolesc Health.* 2010;47(4):322–323.

28. Lubans DR, Cliff DP. Muscular fitness, body composition and physical self-perception in adolescents. *J Sci Med Sport.* 2011;14(3):216–221.

29. Smolak L, Stein JA. The relationship of drive for muscularity to sociocultural factors, self-esteem, physical attributes gender role, and social comparison in middle school boys. *Body Image.* 2006;3(2):121–129.

30. Pinyerd B, Zipf WB. Puberty-timing is everything! *J Pediatr Nurs.* 2005;20(2):75–82.

31. de Guzman NS, Nishina A. A longitudinal study of body dissatisfaction and pubertal timing in an ethnically diverse adolescent sample. *Body Image.* 2014;11(1):68–71.

32. Li W, Liu Q, Deng X, et al. Association between obesity and puberty timing: a systematic review and meta-analysis. *Int J Environ Res Public Health.* 2017;14(12):1266. https://doi:10.3390/ijerph14101266.

33. Voelker DK, Reel JJ, Greenleaf C. Weight status and body image perceptions in adolescents: current perspectives. *Adolesc Health Med Ther.* 2015;6:149–158.

34. Biro FM, Khoury P, Morrison JA. Influence of obesity on timing of puberty. *Int J Androl.* 2006;29(1):272–277–290.

35. Aksglaede L, Sorensen K, Petersen JH, et al. Recent decline in age at breast development: the copenhagen puberty study. *Pediatrics.* 2009;123(5):e932–e939.

36. Biro FM, Greenspan LC, Galvez MP, et al. Onset of breast development in a longitudinal cohort. *Pediatrics.* 2013;132(6):1019–1027.

37. Juul A, Teilmann G, Scheike T, et al. Pubertal development in Danish children: comparison of recent European and US data. *Int J Androl.* 2006;29(1):247–255.

38. Villamor E, Jansen EC. Nutritional determinants of the timing of puberty. *Annu Rev Public Health.* 2016;37(1):33–46.

CHAPTER 5

ARFID and Other Eating Disorders of Childhood

DASHA NICHOLLS, MBBS, MD(RES)

Avoidant restrictive food intake disorder, or ARFID, is conceptualized as an umbrella term, which aimed to bring together various terminologies that preceded it in order to stimulate high-quality research in a neglected area.[1] Since first being named in the DSM-5, there has been a rush to publish research in this "new" area. Nonetheless, at the time of writing there are still less than 100 articles on PubMed using the search term ARFID, so knowledge remains limited. Most publications are based on populations presenting to eating disorder (ED) clinics. Yet ARFID is a reconceptualization of the DSM-IV diagnosis of feeding disorder of infancy or early childhood (FDIEC), expanded beyond childhood to include a range of eating disturbances that lead to deficits in nutritional intake and/or psychosocial function as a result of food restriction. A recent review article by Kennedy et al. asked, "Is ARFID a feeding disorder or an eating disorder, and what are the implications for practice?"[2] The fact that ICD-11 is not yet published contributes further confusion, since FDIEC remains a common diagnosis in countries and within disciplines where ICD-10 rather DSM-5 dominate the diagnostic discourse.

Research to date has focused on characterizing and subtyping ARFID in middle childhood and adolescence, and on measuring prevalence, with a small amount of attention to treatment in the same age group.

EPIDEMIOLOGY

ARFID is still quite a new diagnosis with a lack of reliable measurement tools. Questions about the validity of parent report, self-report, and objective measures of eating problems are also applicable. Many standard epidemiology screening tools for mental health do not pick up feeding and eating disorders (FEDs). A multiformat tool, the Pica, ARFID, Rumination Disorder Interview (PARDI), is in development and a self-report screening instrument, the Eating Disturbances in Youth-Questionnaire (EDY-Q), validated in 8- to 13-year-olds.[3]

Data available to date suggest that rates of ARFID differ according to context as well as measurement method. In a community sample of German children aged 8–13 years, rates of 3.2% have been reported based on using the EDY-Q.[3] Hay et al.[4] reported ARFID in 0.3% of older adolescents and adults in Australia on the basis of two screening questions: "Are you currently avoiding or restricting eating any foods to the degree that you have lost a lot of weight and/or become lacking in nutrition (e.g., have low iron) and/or had problems with family, friends or at work?" and "Yes – for any other reason e.g., food dislike or fear of swallowing." Numbers with ARFID were too low to draw conclusions regarding gender distribution.

Among a large sample of pediatric gastroenterology patients, only 1.5% were classified as having ARFID, with a further 2.4% having some features.[5] This important study, based on clinical case material, raises questions about potential thresholds for clinical significance. For example, picky or selective eating (sensory subtype) is common in the population, and factors associated with help seeking or clinical compromise may be independent of the eating phenomenology itself.

Higher rates of ARFID are reported in other clinic populations, particularly ED clinics. Among adolescents hospitalized in US ED programs, 12.4%–22% have ARFID,[6,7] and in adolescent medicine outpatient clinics between 5% and 14% have ARFID.[8–10] Using surveillance methodology in three separate national samples, 25% and 34% of children aged <13 years had a form of restrictive ED without weight/shape concerns and would now be classified ARFID.[11] Meanwhile in adults, rates of 11% in patients aged 15–40 years in a Japanese ED clinic[12] and 9.2% of adults in a US ED service[13] have been reported. Interestingly, almost all the Japanese clinic samples were female, by contrast with other studies, and no cases presented with the sensory subtype, suggesting developmental differences in presentation and potential overlap with non-fat phobic anorexia nervosa.

SUBTYPING ARFID

DSM-5 proposes three subtypes of ARFID. The first, ARFID associated with lack of appetite and limited intake, was previously encompassed by terms such as restricted eating, food avoidance emotional disorder, infantile anorexia, and failure to thrive. Key characteristics include low overall appetite, lack of interest in eating, difficulties with the physical act of feeding (e.g., small bite sizes, prolonged mealtimes). Weight loss tends to be insidious, often resulting in compromised growth rather than acute medial compromise. In the 8- to 17-year age group, Norris et al.[14] found that 39% of young people presenting to an ARFID clinic fell into this group.

The second subtype, ARFID associated with limited variety secondary to the sensory characteristics of food, was previously encompassed by terms such as selective eating, perseverative feeding disorder and sensory feeding disorder. Restricted eating is typically longstanding, i.e., a normal range of foods has never been eaten and food neophobia and/or picky eating present since the age of weaning. Manifestations include problems with food color, smell, texture and temperature, and profoundly rigid eating behavior, e.g., food items on a plate cannot touch or must be a specific brand. Eighteen percent of 8- to 17-year-olds fell into this group,[14] but prevalence is highly age dependent.

The third proposed subtype, ARFID associated with fear of aversive consequences of eating, was previously encompassed by terms such as functional dysphagia (fear of choking), or emetophobia (fear of vomiting). Unlike sensory food avoidance, food phobias are usually secondary events, sometimes with a clear trigger and follow a period of normal eating for developmental stage. Of 8- to 17-year-olds with ARFID, 43% fell into this category.[14]

While the three subtype model is dominant in the literature and has been validated in community as well as clinical populations,[15] ARFID phenotypes have not been empirically derived and remain the subject of discussion and debate. Fisher et al.,[9] using an etiological framework, examined the prevalence of five proposed subtypes of ARFID: generalized anxiety; gastrointestinal symptoms; fears of eating secondary to fears of choking or vomiting; food allergies; and restrictive eating for "other" reasons.

Not only is the "correct" subgroup classification unclear, the extent to which these subgroups are distinct is too, with almost a quarter of patients of "mixed type."[14] Comorbid anxiety is common across the subtypes. For example, non-help-seeking children with sensory food aversions develop an avoidance-reinforced anxiety associated with new foods. They may then develop anticipatory nausea (with sight or smell triggers), fear of vomiting (due to textures), or a fear of choking, such that a minor eating specific event or a nonspecific rise in anxiety precipitates restriction to the point of medical compromise.

One option is a dimensional approach, looking at underlying factors across specified domains of interest. Thomas et al.[16] have hypothesized a three-dimensional model wherein neurobiological abnormalities in sensory perception, homeostatic appetite, and negative valence systems underlie the three primary ARFID presentations of sensory sensitivity, lack of interest in eating, and fear of aversive consequences respectively, but each element can occur to a greater or lesser degree in any presentation. This model, which awaits empirical validation, has been used to inform a cognitive behavioral approach to assessment and treatment (CBT-AR). A question arises as to whether the model might be applicable across the restrictive EDs.

THE BOUNDARY BETWEEN ARFID AND EATING DISORDERS

Central to the diagnosis of ARFID is the absence of weight and shape concern as the driver for food restriction. While distinction has face validity, it is not hard to find areas where the interface can be difficult to discern. Examples include younger patients and patients with non–fat phobic (NFP) anorexia nervosa (AN).

The challenge of diagnosing AN in children is well described.[17] Not uncommonly the reasons for restriction only become apparent when food intake is challenged, i.e., during weight restoration. Even so, it can be difficult to distinguish AN from ARFID, and careful assessment is needed to ascertain whether specific cognitions are maintaining the eating problem. Patients with ARFID tend to have a longer duration of illness prior to diagnosis and a younger age of onset. Underlying medical conditions and dependence on nutritional supplements are more common. Both ARFID and AN are associated with significant anxiety and distress around mealtimes. In a chart review of 205 patients presenting to an ED service 12% of patients with ARFID transitioned to a diagnosis of AN during treatment,[8] reminding us that some ARFID features are a risk factor for the development of AN.[18,19] It is therefore important to keep reassessing the diagnosis, particularly if treatment is not progressing as expected.

Given that DSM-5 AN can be diagnosed on the basis of behaviors preventing weight gain and lack of recognition of the seriousness of low weight but without body image disturbance, some cases of ARFID can be difficult to distinguish from NFP-AN. Becker et al.[20] described cases where restriction of food intake was due to religious beliefs or because of somatic discomfort. "Orthorexia," or "clean eating" is another example on the boundary between NFP-AN and ARFID. A distinction that has been made is the aversion to weight gain in NFP-AN, the so called "ego-syntonic" nature. Experience suggests, however, that resistance to change can be just as extreme in some patients with ARFID.

Commonalities between ARFID and AN in terms of neurodevelopmental underpinnings are also noted,[2] e.g., autism spectrum traits, heightened sensory sensitivity, reduced interoceptive awareness, and alexithymia. Long-term data on outcome for ARFID are needed to know whether expressed weight and shape concern is significant for prognosis or whether a transdiagnostic approach to restrictive EDs may be more helpful in understanding etiology and mechanisms. Such an approach would further shift the emphasis away from cultural and gender-based understandings toward neurobiological etiological models.

TREATMENT

Given its heterogeneous nature, treatment must be tailored to the specifics of the presentation, based on a psychological and systemic formulation that takes into consideration relevant medical comorbidity, such as food allergies. Approaches include those focused on the patient, on caregivers, on relationships between the child and caregivers and other family members, and on the patient's wider context, e.g., school.

Nutritional compromise can be at the macro- and micronutrient level, and if associated with underweight, this should be addressed as a priority, bearing in mind the person's premorbid weight and height and his or her genetic potential. In a retrospective review of 700 adolescents attending ED programs, Forman et al.[6] found that treatment of ARFID did not differ from that of AN or atypical AN with respect to refeeding protocol or family involvement, although children with ARFID require nasogastric feeding more often than those with AN and demonstrate less distress regarding this process.

For patients where range rather than quantity of food is the problem, careful consideration of treatment goals and expectations is important. The application of family-based treatment approaches advocated for ED has begun to be explored, especially in underweight patients. Others favor a cognitive behavioral approach, with the patient in the driving seat, as would befit diagnoses primarily understood in terms of anxiety. As for other ED, engagement, identifying specific drivers for motivation, as well as realistic pacing are key to successful systematic desensitization to feared or new foods.

OTHER EATING DISORDERS OF EARLY CHILDHOOD

Pica and rumination disorder (RD) were previously classified as "disorders primarily occurring in infancy, early childhood, and adolescence" but, like ARFID, are now applicable across the age range. Pica, or the eating of nonnutritive substances that are outside the range of socially or developmentally sanctioned norms, occurs in around 12% of children aged 7–14 years (by self and parent report), for around 40% of whom the behavior is recurrent.[21] In adolescent and adult patients seeking treatment for ED or obesity rates were lower, at 0%–1.3%[22] The literature and clinical experience suggests that severe complications can arise but these are infrequent events. No clinical trials have been undertaken.

Where RD was once considered a relatively rare self-soothing behavior seen in cases of severe neglect and some people with intellectual disability, RD is now recognized as a relatively common functional gastrointestinal disorder characterized by effortless and repetitive regurgitation of recently ingested food from the stomach to the oral cavity followed by either reswallowing or spitting.[23] Patients often report this as vomiting or reflux, so direct observation and manometry may be needed to confirm the diagnosis. Increase in intragastric pressure followed by regurgitation is the most important characteristic to distinguish rumination from other disorders such as gastroesophageal reflux. The mainstay of the treatment is behavioral therapy incorporating diaphragmatic breathing techniques alongside psychoeducation. Occasionally, symptoms are so severe that medical intervention, including enteral feeding, is necessary to medically stabilize before psychological interventions can begin. Hartmann et al.[21] found RD in 11.5% (1.5% recurrent) of 7- to 14-year-olds.

Pica and RD show a small but significant correlation with one another and also with ARFID.[21] Both are also associated with other emotional and behavioral problems.

CHILDHOOD ONSET ANOREXIA NERVOSA

Although the diagnostic criteria and clinical features of AN are, by definition, comparable in children,[24] there are preliminary suggestions that the genetic and environmental risk (and therefore etiology),[25] and the course and outcome may differ in children from adolescent or older onset.[26] Given that rates of childhood AN appear to be increasing, this is an area where further investigation is needed.

CONCLUSION

ARFID is a diagnosis applicable to a number of presentations where food restriction compromises nutrition and function. Data from patients and from community samples are limited and the integration of knowledge from the ED and feeding disorders literature in its early days. Priority areas for future research include an improved developmental understanding of acquisition of eating skills, including prospective longitudinal clinical studies to clarify the course and outcomes of feeding and eating problems. Big datasets on ARFID patients would enable ARFID subtypes to be empirically derived. A transdiagnostic approach to restrictive eating behavior may reveal new insights relevant to AN.

REFERENCES

1. Bryant-Waugh R, Markham L, Kreipe RE, et al. Feeding and eating disorders in childhood. *Int J Eat Disord.* 2010;43:98–111.
2. Kennedy GA, Wick MR, Keel PK. Eating disorders in children: is avoidant-restrictive food intake disorder a feeding disorder or an eating disorder and what are the implications for treatment? *F1000Res.* 2018;7:88. https://doi.org/10.12688/f1000research.13110.1. 2018/02/06.
3. Kurz S, van Dyck Z, Dremmel D, et al. Early-onset restrictive eating disturbances in primary school boys and girls. *Eur Child Adolesc Psychiatry.* 2015;24:779–785. https://doi.org/10.1007/s00787-014-0622-z.
4. Hay P, Mitchison D, Collado AEL, et al. Burden and health-related quality of life of eating disorders, including avoidant/restrictive food intake disorder (ARFID), in the Australian population. *J Eat Disord.* 2017;5:21. https://doi.org/10.1186/s40337-017-0149-z. 2017/07/07.
5. Eddy KT, Thomas JJ, Hastings E, et al. Prevalence of DSM-5 avoidant/restrictive food intake disorder in a pediatric gastroenterology healthcare network. *Int J Eat Disord.* 2015;48:464–470. https://doi.org/10.1002/eat.22350.
6. Forman SF, McKenzie N, Hehn R, et al. Predictors of outcome at 1 year in adolescents with DSM-5 restrictive eating disorders: report of the national eating disorders quality improvement collaborative. *J Adolesc Health.* 2014;55:750–756. https://doi.org/10.1016/j.jadohealth.2014.06.014.
7. Nicely TA, Lane-Loney S, Masciulli E, et al. Prevalence and characteristics of avoidant/restrictive food intake disorder in a cohort of young patients in day treatment for eating disorders. *J Eat Disord.* 2014;2:21. https://doi.org/10.1186/s40337-014-0021-3.
8. Norris ML, Robinson A, Obeid N, et al. Exploring avoidant/restrictive food intake disorder in eating disordered patients: a descriptive study. *Int J Eat Disord.* 2014;47:495–499. https://doi.org/10.1002/eat.22217.
9. Fisher MM, Rosen DS, Ornstein RM, et al. Characteristics of avoidant/restrictive food intake disorder in children and adolescents: a "new disorder" in DSM-5. *J Adolesc Health.* 2014;55:49–52. https://doi.org/10.1016/j.jadohealth.2013.11.013.
10. Ornstein RM, Rosen DS, Mammel KA, et al. Distribution of eating disorders in children and adolescents using the proposed DSM-5 criteria for feeding and eating disorders. *J Adolesc Health.* 2013;53:303–305. https://doi.org/10.1016/j.jadohealth.2013.03.025.
11. Pinhas L, Nicholls D, Crosby RD, et al. Classification of childhood onset eating disorders: a latent class analysis. *Int J Eat Disord.* 2017. https://doi.org/10.1002/eat.22666.
12. Nakai Y, Nin K, Noma S, et al. Clinical presentation and outcome of avoidant/restrictive food intake disorder in a Japanese sample. *Eat Behav.* 2017;24:49–53. https://doi.org/10.1016/j.eatbeh.2016.12.004. 2016/12/26.
13. Nakai Y, Nin K, Noma S, et al. Characteristics of avoidant/restrictive food intake disorder in a cohort of adult patients. *Eur Eat Disord Rev.* 2016;24:528–530. https://doi.org/10.1002/erv.2476. 2016/10/28.
14. Norris ML, Spettigue W, Hammond NG, et al. Building evidence for the use of descriptive subtypes in youth with avoidant restrictive food intake disorder. *Int J Eat Disord.* 2018;51:170–173. https://doi.org/10.1002/eat.22814. 2017/12/08.
15. Kurz S, van Dyck Z, Dremmel D, et al. Variants of early-onset restrictive eating disturbances in middle childhood. *Int J Eat Disord.* 2016;49:102–106. https://doi.org/10.1002/eat.22461.
16. Thomas JJ, Lawson EA, Micali N, et al. Avoidant/restrictive food intake disorder: a three-dimensional model of neurobiology with implications for etiology and treatment. *Curr Psychiatry Rep.* 2017;19:54. https://doi.org/10.1007/s11920-017-0795-5. 2017/07/18.
17. Bravender T, Bryant-Waugh R, Herzog D, et al. Classification of eating disturbance in children and adolescents: proposed changes for the DSM-V. *Eur Eat Disord Rev.* 2010;18:79–89.
18. Nicholls DE, Viner RM. Childhood risk factors for lifetime anorexia nervosa by age 30 years in a national birth cohort. *J Am Acad Child Adolesc Psychiatry.* 2009;48:791–799.
19. Marchi M, Cohen P. Early childhood eating behaviors and adolescent eating disorders. *J Am Acad Child Adolesc Psychiatry.* 1990;29:112–117.
20. Becker AE, Thomas JJ, Pike KM. Should non-fat-phobic anorexia nervosa be included in DSM-V? *Int J Eat Disord.* 2009;42:620–635.

21. Hartmann AS, Poulain T, Vogel M, et al. Prevalence of pica and rumination behaviors in German children aged 7-14 and their associations with feeding, eating, and general psychopathology: a population-based study. *Eur Child Adolesc Psychiatry.* 2018. https://doi.org/10.1007/s00787-018-1153-9. 2018/04/21.

22. Delaney CB, Eddy KT, Hartmann AS, et al. Pica and rumination behavior among individuals seeking treatment for eating disorders or obesity. *Int J Eat Disord.* 2015;48:238–248. https://doi.org/10.1002/eat.22279. 2014/04/15.

23. Absah I, Rishi A, Talley NJ, et al. Rumination syndrome: pathophysiology, diagnosis, and treatment. *Neuro Gastroenterol Motil.* 2017;29. https://doi.org/10.1111/nmo.12954. 2016/10/22.

24. Nicholls DE, Lynn R, Viner RM. Childhood eating disorders: British national surveillance study. *Br J Psychiatry.* 2011;198:295–301. https://doi.org/10.1192/bjp.bp.110.081356. 198/4/295.

25. Klump KL, Culbert KM, Slane JD, et al. The effects of puberty on genetic risk for disordered eating: evidence for a sex difference. *Psychol Med.* 2012;42:627–637. https://doi.org/10.1017/S0033291711001541.

26. Herpertz-Dahlmann B, Dempfle A, Egberts KM, et al. Outcome of childhood anorexia nervosa-the results of a five- to ten-year follow-up study. *Int J Eat Disord.* 2018;51:295–304. https://doi.org/10.1002/eat.22840. 2018/02/17.

CHAPTER 6

Loss of Control Eating in Children

NANCY ZUCKER, PHD • ERIK SAVEREIDE, BS • SAVANNAH ERWIN, BS • TATYANA BIDOPIA, BA • NANDINI DATTA, MA • ALANNAH RIVERA-CANCEL, BA

DEFINITION AND PHENOMENOLOGY OF LOSS OF CONTROL

The construct "loss of control" (LOC) in the domain of eating is defined as feeling as though one cannot stop eating or control what or how much one is eating. For children, LOC is often elaborated with examples to clarify the term. For example, in semistructured interviews, such as the Eating Disorders Examination 12oD/C.2 adapted for children,[1] LOC is initially explained as a sense of lack of control overeating and food seeking in the absence of hunger or after satiation. Then, a concrete example may be offered, such as "a ball rolling down a hill, going faster and faster."[2] Given that the construct LOC is difficult to conceptualize even for an adult sample, care is taken to make sure children understand what LOC around eating may feel like before assessing for frequency of LOC eating episodes.

Children who engage in LOC eating episodes have been shown to endorse aspects of disordered eating aligned with the adult criteria for binge eating disorder.[3] As in adult research, the experience of LOC appears to be a noxious clinical feature, irrespective of the amount of food consumed. Children (aged 6.1–13.8 years) who reported LOC eating, with or without the consumption of objectively large amounts of food, tended to endorse greater levels of anxiety, depression, and poorer self-esteem compared with their same-aged peers.[2] Similarly, in community-based samples, youths reporting LOC eating were heavier and more likely to endorse disordered eating cognitions, depressive symptoms, poorer social functioning, and emotional stress than those without binge eating.[2] Taken together, this body of literature suggests that children experiencing LOC during eating likely concurrently feel other negative emotions both in the moment and after an LOC eating episode.

DEVELOPMENTAL CONSIDERATIONS FOR THE EXPERIENCE OF LOC

In adults, classic theories of the maintenance of binge eating episodes have focused on three primary functions of LOC eating episodes: compensation for dietary restraint; attention diversion; and affect regulation. In children, it is conceivable that these functions are similar, but (1) may have developmentally sensitive expressions, (2) have unique functions for LOC eating, or (3) the form and function of binge eating looks the same across ages. Evidence to date supports all three hypotheses.

Developmental Contributions to Dietary Restraint in Children and Adolescents

The role of dietary restraint in precipitating an LOC eating episode is complicated by parental control of the eating environment. In adults, rigid and/or extreme dietary rules are proposed to promote LOC eating. Hypotheses about this association include that "forbidden foods" may be perceived as increasingly rewarding and/or that extreme caloric depletion may make it challenging to regulate intake when food is available.[4] For children, parents primarily control the types and amounts of food brought into the household. As such, foods that typically constitute a binge (e.g., high-fat/high-sugar foods) may not be readily available. The feeding style of a parent, i.e., how a parent attempts to regulate their child's eating behavior, may also contribute to LOC eating in children. A body of work has supported an association between maternal restrictive feeding and their daughters' increased consumption of food after reported satiation following a meal.[5] However, the direction of causality is unclear. Some studies show that parents may impose different feeding strategies in children who seem more responsive to food in the environment. Given these constraints, it is not surprising that youth reporting secretive eating are more likely to also report LOC.[6] Taken together, these findings raise the possibility that dietary restriction does not have to be self-imposed to contribute to LOC eating episodes.

Developmental Considerations of Emotion Dysregulation and Distraction in Children

Family mealtimes may be a unique trigger for LOC eating in children. As mealtimes are also a setting for family interactions, conflictual communications may add to the experience of increased emotional intensity at mealtimes. In fact, maladaptive family functioning during mealtime predicts LOC and faster chewing in children.[7] This association may suggest that children use food and/or eating behavior as a way to manage intense situational affect: for example, using food to improve mood or eating faster to escape the meal more quickly. Thus, family meals may be a unique setting for children's LOC eating to function as a means of emotion regulation.

There is some evidence that LOC eating serves as a strategy to deal with negative emotions by either providing distraction or replacing one negative emotion with a less aversive one.[8,9] Greater emotion dysregulation has been observed to correlate with more self-reported LOC eating, suggesting that more frequent negative emotions and turning to food as a coping strategy could be factors contributing to the development of LOC.[10]

Parents may inadvertently teach their children to associate emotions with eating. A recent longitudinal study observed that emotional eating was uncommon in a sample of 3- to 5-year-olds regardless of whether they received food as a reward. However, when observed 2 years later, the children whose parents had reported using food as a reward at the first assessment consumed significantly more calories when exposed experimentally to emotional stressors than children whose parents had not used food as a reward.[11] These results suggest parents may facilitate learned associations between affect and eating. Further, children have reported the experience of feeling numb during an LOC episode, suggesting that it may function similarly to adults in helping to escape from aversive self-awareness.[3] Thus, there may be critical windows for intervention in young childhood, a period in which children have not yet learned to associate eating and emotions.

The Course of Loss of Control Episodes

The stability of LOC episodes throughout development is not currently well understood. Once a child experiences an LOC episode, it is difficult to predict whether they will subsequently experience more. One study found that most children experience only one LOC episode.[8] If future studies of children find LOC episodes to be primarily one-time occurrences, this may suggest temporary vulnerability to LOC during development and improvement over time.

Measurement of loss of control eating

The child version of the Eating Disorder Examination (ChEDE),[1] a semistructured interview validated for use in children aged 8–14 years, is the most widely utilized

assessment of LOC in children and adolescents.[12] The ChEDE contains simpler terminology than the adult version and has developmentally sensitive methods to assess diagnostic criteria that are abstract or cognitively complex. Episodes of eating are assessed along dimensions of quantity of food consumed (whether it was excessive given the situational context) and whether the individual experienced LOC while eating. Crossing these two dimensions (excessive Y/N and LOC Y/N) results in four potential categories of eating episodes. These are assessed in the prior 28 days and include (1) objective binge eating (OBE), an episode involving both LOC and the consumption of an unambiguously large quantity of food; (2) subjective binge eating (SBE) episode involving LOC and the consumption of a subjectively large quantity of food (as determined by the interviewer), i.e., children feel they have overeaten, but the actual quantity of food is not deemed to be excessive; (3) objective overeating (OO), episodes involving the consumption of an objectively large amount of food but no experience of LOC; and (4) no experience of overeating or LOC. Youth experiencing at least one episode of OBE or SBE are classified as experiencing LOC eating. The interview consists of four subscales: restraint, eating concern, shape concern, and weight concern and a global score that independently measures disordered eating attitudes held by the child or adolescent. The ChEDE is associated with high reliability ($\alpha = 0.53$–0.84)[13] and validity and involves clear instruction on interview items, ameliorating the pitfalls of self-report questionnaires in measuring LOC eating in children and adolescents.[1,14]

Several self-reported measures have acceptable psychometric properties and can be employed when the use of interview is not feasible. For example, the child version of the Eating Disorder Examination Questionnaire (ChEDE-Q) was developed for children/adolescents aged 8–14 years but also evaluated in adolescents up to 17 years[14,15]; the child version of the Eating Attitudes Test (ChEAT) was designed for 8- to 13-year-olds[16]; the adolescent version of the Questionnaire on Eating and Weight Patterns (QEWP-A) was designed for 10- to 8-year-olds[17]; the Youth Eating Disorder Examination-Questionnaire (YEDE-Q) has been evaluated in adolescents aged 7–17 years.[6,12]

Despite the strengths of these measures, consideration of specific limitations may aid in the selection of the best measure for a given research question. The ChEDE-Q has demonstrated adequate reliability ($\alpha = 0.62$–0.88); however, it was shown to overestimate eating disorder psychopathology in youth, consistent with evidence that children/adolescents have difficulties identifying binge eating/LOC eating episodes without verbal instruction on assessment items.[14,18] Additionally, the ChEAT is a reliable measure ($\alpha = 0.68-0.80$) but did not adequately capture the guilt and preoccupation associated with LOC eating in adolescents.[13,17] Compared with the ChEDE, the QEWP-A showed limited convergent validity in the detection of objective or subjective bulimic episodes in this same sample of adolescents.[17] The YEDE-Q was also found to be limited in detecting SBE and OO episodes in overweight adolescents, identifying fewer true cases of LOC eating than the ChEDE but showing high internal consistency across studies ($\alpha = 0.63-0.89$).[6,12,13] Although these questionnaires were associated with high internal consistency and reliability measures overall, the cited limitations in their validity with regard to assessing all features of LOC eating may necessitate the use of a semistructured interviews, particularly in studies that intend to better understand the phenomenology of LOC in children and adolescents.

TREATMENT OF LOSS OF CONTROL EATING IN CHILDREN

LOC eating is a key feature of binge eating disorder (BED), a disorder that can emerge in childhood. Treatments that are efficacious in the treatment of BED, by corollary, improve LOC eating. There is an emerging literature on incorporating families in treatment of childhood BED. Shomaker et al.[19] evaluated family-based interpersonal psychotherapy (FB-IPT) for children (aged 8–13 years) with LOC eating who were also overweight or obese. FB-IPT involved 12 weekly sessions with parent-child dyads focused on psychoeducation and skill training; specific skills targeted included communication and conflict resolution between the parent and child. In this study, the children who received FB-IPT showed greater improvement in symptoms of depression, anxiety, and LOC eating at posttreatment compared with children who received a family-based health education program.[19]

Treatments with a primary goal of weight loss can have secondary benefits of reducing LOC eating, provided that the dietary rigidity mentioned earlier is avoided. Behavior therapy for pediatric obesity targets behaviors that may contribute to unhealthy weight regulation (e.g., altering contingencies to make exercise more rewarding). Under this model, inappropriate weight gain is minimized by identifying behavioral cues that trigger LOC eating and learning different responses to those cues, thereby extinguishing the behavior of LOC eating. Behavior therapy has been shown to prevent further weight gain as well as reduce the frequency of binge eating episodes in children aged 8–12 years.[20]

Other treatments specifically target LOC eating in an effort to prevent weight gain. In a randomized controlled trial, Boutelle et al.[21] introduced two treatments designed to reduce overeating and prevent weight gain in overweight and obese children. One treatment, "Volcravo," is an exposure therapy that incorporates mindfulness skills. Volcravo teaches parent-child dyads to recognize craving (wanting in the absence of hunger) and identify antecedents of craving, and offers opportunities to practice enduring the experience of craving ("riding the wave") in response to a food cue until the urge to eat is lessened. After eight weekly sessions, children reported significantly fewer episodes of overeating and eating in the absence of hunger, and reduced LOC overeating; these results held at a 6-month follow-up. The second treatment by Boutelle and colleagues was adapted from an adult-oriented appetite awareness training program by Craighead and Allen,[22] which promotes recognition and response to internal food-related cues. The adapted program, called children's appetite awareness training (CAAT), focused on increasing awareness of internal states of hunger and satiety and using this awareness to inform food consumption choices. In CAAT sessions, parent-child dyads learned to monitor hunger and satiety cues and identify potential situations in which eating in the absence of hunger might occur, and practiced coping skills to manage these situations. Treatment sessions incorporated experiential exercises to solidify these skills during a mealtime. CAAT was shown to reduce binge eating (both subjective and objective binge episodes) after 8 weeks of treatment and 12 months after treatment termination.[21,22]

FUTURE DIRECTIONS IN UNDERSTANDING LOC EATING

Improving the quality and frequency of family meals may be a strategic way to address multiple vulnerabilities associated with LOC eating. Improved parent-child communication during mealtimes can enhance emotion awareness and reduce family conflict, a trigger for LOC episodes. Educating parents about surges in appetite that accompany growth spurts may lessen parental anxiety about child weight gain. Given evidence that parents may impose feeding styles based on their perception of their child's capacity to regulate their intake, parents' misperception of normative developmental changes in appetite may contribute to inappropriate environmental regulation. If a child fears that food is not readily available to satiate hunger, strategies of secretive eating may be an adaptive form of compensation. Interventions that focus on helping children and families to savor food by eating more slowly and to saver interactions during mealtimes may lessen both maladaptive food consumption and loneliness, thereby precluding the need for LOC eating as a means of emotion regulation.

REFERENCES

1. Bryant-Waugh RJ, Cooper PJ, Taylor CL, Lask BD. The use of the eating disorder examination with children: a pilot study. *Int J Eat Disord*. 1996;19(4):391–397.
2. Tanofsky-Kraff M, Yanovski SZ, Wilfley DE, Marmarosh C, Morgan CM, Yanovski JA. Eating-disordered behaviors, body fat, and psychopathology in overweight and normal-weight children. *J Consult Clin Psychol*. 2004;72(1):53–61.
3. Tanofsky-Kraff M, Goossens L, Eddy KT, et al. A multisite investigation of binge eating behaviors in children and adolescents. *J Consult Clin Psychol*. 2007;75(6):901–913.
4. Wilson GT, Fairburn CC, Agras WS, Walsh BT, Kraemer H. Cognitive-behavioral therapy for bulimia nervosa: time course and mechanisms of change. *J Consult Clin Psychol*. 2002;70(2):267–274.
5. Birch LL, Fisher JO, Davison KK. Learning to overeat: maternal use of restrictive feeding practices promotes girls' eating in the absence of hunger. *Am J Clin Nutr*. 2003;78(2):215–220.
6. Kass AE, Wilfley DE, Eddy KT, et al. Secretive eating among youth with overweight or obesity. *Appetite*. 2017;114:275–281.
7. Czaja J, Hartmann AS, Rief W, Hilbert A. Mealtime family interactions in home environments of children with loss of control eating. *Appetite*. 2011;56(3):587–593.
8. Hilbert A, Hartmann AS, Czaja J, Schoebi D. Natural course of preadolescent loss of control eating. *J Abnorm Psychol*. 2013;122(3):684–693.
9. Stojek MMK, Tanofsky-Kraff M, Shomaker LB, et al. Associations of adolescent emotional and loss of control eating with 1-year changes in disordered eating, weight, and adiposity. *Int J Eat Disord*. 2017;50(5):551–560.
10. Kelly NR, Tanofsky-Kraff M, Vannucci A, et al. Emotion dysregulation and loss-of-control eating in children and adolescents. *Health Psychol*. 2016;35(10):1110–1119.
11. Farrow CV, Haycraft E, Blissett JM. Teaching our children when to eat: how parental feeding practices inform the development of emotional eating-a longitudinal experimental design. *Am J Clin Nutr*. 2015;101(5):908–913.
12. Goldschmidt A, Wilfley DE, Eddy KT, et al. Overvaluation of shape and weight among overweight children and adolescents with loss of control eating. *Behav Res Ther*. 2011;49(10):682–688.
13. Bryant M, Ashton L, Brown J, et al. Systematic review to identify and appraise outcome measures used to evaluate childhood obesity treatment interventions (CoOR): evidence of purpose, application, validity, reliability and sensitivity. *Health Technol Asses*. 2014;18(51).
14. Decaluwé V, Braet C. Assessment of eating disorder psychopathology in obese children and adolescents: interview versus self-report questionnaire. *Behav Res Ther*. 2004;42(7):799–811.
15. Sören K, Ricarda S, Mandy V, Andreas H, Wieland K, Anja H. An 8-item short form of the eating disorder examination-questionnaire adapted for children (ChEDE-Q8). *Int J Eat Disord*. 2017;50(6):679–686.
16. Maloney MJ, McGuire JB, Daniels SR. Reliability testing of a children's version of the eating attitude test. *J Am Acad Child Adolesc Psychiatry*. 1988;27(5):541–543.
17. Marian TK, Morgan MC, Yanovski ZS, Cheri M, Wilfley DE, Yanovski JA. Comparison of assessments of children's eating-disordered behaviors by interview and questionnaire. *Int J Eat Disord*. 2003;33(2):213–224.
18. Le Grange D, Lock J, eds. *Eating Disorders in Children and Adolescents: A Clinical Handbook*. Guilford Press; 2011.
19. Shomaker LB, Tanofsky-Kraff M, Matherne CE, et al. A randomized, comparative pilot trial of family-based interpersonal psychotherapy for reducing psychosocial symptoms, disordered-eating, and excess weight gain in at-risk preadolescents with loss-of-control-eating. *Int J Eat Disord*. 2017;50(9):1084–1094.
20. Epstein LH, Paluch RA, Saelens BE, Ernst MM, Wilfley DE. Changes in eating disorder symptoms with pediatric obesity treatment. *J Pediatr*. 2001;139(1):58–65.
21. Boutelle KN, Zucker NL, Peterson CB, Rydell SA, Cafri G, Harnack L. Two novel treatments to reduce overeating in overweight children: a randomized controlled trial. *J Consult Clin Psychol*. 2011;79(6):759–771.
22. Craighead LW, Allen HN. Appetite awareness training: a cognitive behavioral intervention for binge eating. *Cogn Behav Pract*. 1995;2(2):249–270.

CHAPTER 7

Adolescent Eating Disorders— Definition, Symptomatology, and Comorbidity

BEATE HERPERTZ-DAHLMANN, MD

INTRODUCTION

Anorexia nervosa (AN) and bulimia nervosa (BN) combined ranked as the 12th leading cause of disability-adjusted life years (DALYS) of more than 300 physical and mental disorders in adolescent females in high-income countries[1,2] (Global Burden of Disease Study 2013). Prevalence of eating disorders (EDs) was highest in Western countries, especially in the United States and Europe. According to DSM-5, eight categories are described: pica, rumination disorder, avoidant/restrictive food intake disorder (ARFID), AN, BN, binge eating disorder (BED), other specified feeding or eating disorder (OSFED), and unspecified feeding or eating disorder. In this chapter, most of the emphasis will be on AN and BN, while ARFID and BED (including loss of control (LOC) of eating) will be mainly dealt within other chapters.

ANOREXIA NERVOSA

Definition

AN is listed among the most important psychiatric disorders of childhood and adolescence "with lifelong consequences" by the WHO.[3] In the transition from DSM-IV to DSM-5, classification criteria were significantly modified by omitting wording that might imply deliberate or willful action of the patient, such as, "refusal to maintain body weight at or above a minimally normal weight for age and height," or "denial of the seriousness of low body weight," and thus might have supported stigmatization of ED patients[4] (for a more detailed discussion, see Chapter 1).

DSM-5 items are listed in Table 7.1.

The former D criterion focusing on amenorrhea has been left out to not preclude applicability to males, premenarchal girls, and females on contraceptives.

For young patients, the reference weight criterion (what is the weight that can be minimally expected?) is an unresolved question. In most countries, a body mass index (BMI, calculated as weight in kilograms divided by height in meters squared) below the 10th BMI percentile is defined as the lower weight threshold for adult, adolescent, and childhood AN[6-8] (for further explanations see Chapter 1). In the draft version of ICD-11, a lower weight threshold corresponding to the fifth BMI percentile was chosen. This decision is difficult to comprehend, as many patients currently diagnosed with AN will no longer fulfill the diagnostic criteria. In addition, the protracted course of the disorder merits efforts to early diagnose the disorder. Somatic and psychological consequences might be more serious in the developing child or adolescent.

TABLE 7.1
Diagnostic Criteria for Anorexia Nervosa According to DSM-5 (Abbreviated Form[5])

A. Restriction of energy intake relative to requirements, leading to a significantly low body weight in the context of age, sex, developmental trajectory, and physical health. For children and adolescents, significantly low weight is defined as a weight that is less than minimally expected.

B. Intense fear of gaining weight or of becoming fat or persistent behavior that interferes with weight gain.

C. Body image disturbance, undue influence of weight and shape on self-confidence, or persistent lack of recognition of the seriousness of the illness.

Subtypes: Restricting and Binge Eating/Purging Type.

Eating Disorders and Obesity in Children and Adolescents. https://doi.org/10.1016/B978-0-323-54852-6.00007-0

The restricting type of AN is defined by achieving weight loss mainly by a reduced caloric intake and/or physical hyperactivity. Patients diagnosed with AN binge eating/purging type may engage in binging and purging (e.g., laxative abuse or self-induced vomiting), only binging (with intermittent periods of fasting or excessive exercising), or only purging (for a more extensive review, see Ref. 5). The presence of purging behavior was identified as a negative outcome parameter in some studies, but not all[9]; however, both subtypes (restricting and binge eating/purging) differ in somatic and psychiatric comorbidity.

Moreover, DSM-5 differentiates between "current severity states" based on absolute BMI in adults and corresponding BMI percentiles in children and adolescents. However, although there is an association between severity and number of hospitalizations and duration of illness in AN, several authors doubt the utility of these thresholds because the different categories did not distinguish between ED psychopathology, depression, or measures of impaired emotional or physical functioning.[10] Moreover, a parameter for global functioning comprising impairment and need for treatment seems to be necessary.

"DSM-5 also differentiates between two different stages of remission, partial or full remission. The latter is defined by no more fulfilling any of the diagnostic criteria of AN without defining the exact period of time. However, in the scientific literature, it is questioned whether the absence of diagnostic criteria for AN actually defines remission."

Symptomatology

At the beginning of the disorder young people with AN resist eating, often pursue a strict diet, and/or practice excessive physical training and thus become underweight; many of them view themselves as fat despite severe starvation. Certain body parts, especially the thighs and waist, are more overestimated than others. Some patients are able to realize the emaciated state of their body but find it good looking. Quite a few patients become vegetarians or even vegans. Individuals with AN are often obsessed with food, practice highly ritualized and rigid eating behavior, and develop a desperate weight phobia. Several of them count calories excessively. Not all, but the majority of subjects with AN experience their symptoms as ego-syntonic and do not wish to let their disorder go because they feel distinguished by it; however, they are often isolated and excluded from age-appropriate activities (for a review, see also Herpertz-Dahlmann[5]). Physical hyperactivity in patients with AN

is a significant obstacle in treatment and associated with more severe psychopathology, a more chronic course of illness, a lower BMI, and a higher dissatisfaction with one's own body.[11,12]

Atypical AN is characterized by a normal weight, while all other criteria of AN are met (for a more detailed description, see the chapter in this book by Hebebrand "Overarching concepts..."). Adolescents with atypical AN have similar medical and psychological complications as those of patients with "pure AN" but are at much higher risk to be overlooked in routine clinical practice.[13]

BULIMIA NERVOSA

Definition

BN is also characterized by a morbid fear of fatness and often by a body image disturbance, which leads to a deep discontent with one's own body and shape. The majority of patients weigh in the normal or upper-normal range; several have a history of being overweight. Those weighing in the lower weight range categories often report a history of AN. In contrast to AN, fasting is interrupted by binge eating episodes accompanied by a feeling of LOC. Patients with BN try to compensate for their binges with purging behavior, such as vomiting, laxative abuse, or more seldom by use of other medications that might promote weight loss (e.g., diuretics or thyroid hormones). Overweight patients with BN often not only seek help for their ED but also try to lose weight, which renders treatment difficult (Table 7.2).[14]

In comparison to DSM-IV, the symptom frequency of binge eating and subsequent purging was reduced to once a week for 3 months instead of twice a week.

TABLE 7.2

Diagnostic Criteria for Bulimia Nervosa According to DSM-5 (Abbreviated Form)

A. Recurrent episodes of binge eating.

B. Recurrent inappropriate compensatory behavior (e.g., self-induced vomiting, laxative or diuretics abuse, or fasting or excessive exercise)

C. Frequency of binge eating at least once a week for 3 months.

D. Self-confidence is contingent on weight and shape.

E. Symptoms do not only occur during in the context of AN.

Symptomatology

In comparison with AN, BN is not obviously apparent, which leads to the consequence of less access to treatment. Similar to AN, BN often starts with periods of fasting, which are interrupted by an LOC and subsequent binge attacks. In addition to the purging behavior (see above), several patients practice excessive exercising because of their dread of fatness. While in the beginning of the disorder, binging is often induced by fasting, emotional stress, feelings of loneliness, or boredom, it becomes increasingly more habitual throughout the course of the disorder and sometimes becomes even regularly scheduled in everyday life. Bulimic behavior might occur between once a week to several times a day and is mostly practiced in secret. To facilitate vomiting, patients may drink large amounts of fluids during meals. A binge might comprise more than 10,000 calories and is mostly composed of cold food that is easy to swallow, such as deserts and chocolate. When examining patients with BN, it is important to differentiate between patients with "subjective" and "objective" binges. Particularly, patients with a previous history of AN might rate a small amount of food as a binge if they experience a feeling of LOC.[5]

Binge Eating Disorder and Loss of Control Eating

BED was classified as a mental disorder for the first time in DSM-5.[15] Its main characteristics are recurrent binge attacks of large amounts of food without compensatory behavior to avoid weight gain, a feeling of LOC, and a marked distress. Most, but not all, individuals who suffer from BED are overweight or obese. Remarkably, children and adolescents might eat large amounts of food (e.g., during prepubertal or pubertal growth spurts) and will not be considered to be exhibiting clinically relevant behavior; these situations have to be differentiated from BED. The core criterion of a binge eating–associated clinical disorder is the perception of LOC in the absence of hunger. In addition, children and adolescents often do not fulfill the DSM-5 frequency criterion of BED (at least once a week for 3 months). For this reason, LOC eating in children and adolescents has been illustrated in a separate chapter in this book (by Zucker et al.).

MEDICAL CONSEQUENCES AND COMORBIDITY WITH MENTAL DISORDERS

Somatic Symptoms

Moderate to severe starvation in AN is characterized by a variety of symptoms, which are displayed in Table 7.3 (for detailed information see Ref. 16). The younger the girl, the more rapid the weight loss, the

TABLE 7.3
Physical Changes in Adolescent Eating Disorders[5,17]

	Anorexia Nervosa	Bulimia Nervosa
Physical examination findings	Dry skin Lanugo hair formation (only with severe weight loss) Jaundice (only with severe weight loss) Alopecia Brittle hair and nails Acrocyanosis Low body temperature Dehydration Retardation of growth and pubertal development	Erosion of dental enamel Periodontal disease Parotid/salivary gland enlargement Scars on the skin of the back of the hand resulting from inducing the gag reflex (Russell's sign) Dehydration
Cardiovascular system	Bradycardia ECG-abnormalities (mostly prolonged QT-interval) Pericardial effusion Heart murmur (mitral valve prolapse) Hypotension Edema (before or during refeeding)	ECG-abnormalities (cardiac arrhythmia, prolonged QT-interval) Edema
Gastrointestinal system	Impaired gastric emptying Reduced bowel sounds Constipation Pancreatitis	Esophagitis Hematemesis Pancreatitis Delayed gastric emptying
Blood	Leukopenia, thrombocytopenia, anemia	
Biochemical abnormalities	Hypokalemia Hyponatremia Hypomagnesemia Hypocalcemia Hypophosphatemia (during refeeding) Glucose ↓ Creatinine ↑, urea nitrogen ↑ AST↑, ALT↑ (with severe fasting or beginning of refeeding) Amylase↑, lipase ↑ Cholesterol ↑	Hypokalemia Hyponatremia Hypomagnesemia (caused by diarrhea) Hypocalcemia Metabolic alkalosis (in case of severe purging) Metabolic acidosis (in case of severe laxative abuse)

higher the rate of medical complications. Electrolyte changes and dehydration may be especially serious in binge eating/purging AN or BN.

Patients with AN who drink large amounts of water to increase their body weight before weighing or to appease their hunger may develop problems with their fluid balance (e.g., concentrating their urine [diabetes insipidus]). Vitamin deficits (with the exception of vitamin D) are rare in both disorders.

ENDOCRINE CHANGES

Starvation-induced endocrine alterations are the cause of medium- and long-term consequences of EDs, especially AN. The most prominent hormonal changes are described in Fig. 7.1.

ENDOCRINE CHANGES IN EATING DISORDERS[18]

Long-standing estrogen deficits, hypercortisolemia, hypoleptinemia, and reduced insulin-like growth factor (IGF-1) all contribute to the uncoupling of bone formation and bone resorption associated with osteopenia and osteoporosis, which is often not completely reversible after weight rehabilitation because of a relatively short window of opportunity of bone formation during adolescence.

Moreover, long-standing gonadal hormone deficits also impact brain development and might result in neuropsychological dysfunction and the so-called "biological scars" of the brain, possibly leading to higher vulnerability for mental disorders later in life.[19,20]

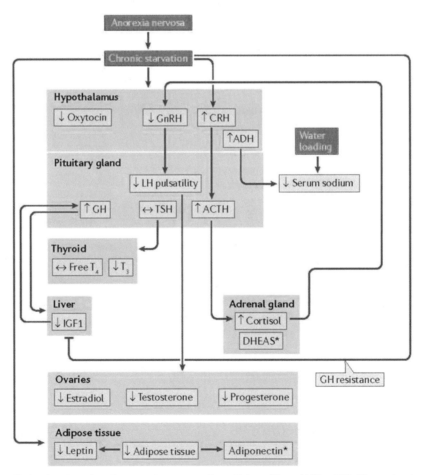

FIG. 7.1 Endocrine alterations in anorexia nervosa. From Schorr, M. and Miller, K.K. The endocrine manifestations of anorexia nervosa: mechanisms and management. Nature Reviews Endocrinology 13 (2016); with permission.

PSYCHIATRIC COMORBIDITY IN ADOLESCENT EATING DISORDERS

Children and adolescents with EDs suffer from multiple comorbid mental disorders that may begin either before or after onset of the ED. In AN and BN, prevalence rates of at least one comorbid condition vary between 40% and 90%[21] (for a review, see also Ref. 5). Rates in clinical samples are usually higher than those in epidemiological samples.

Depression/Dysthymia: A recent metaanalysis demonstrated that eating pathology is a risk factor for depression and that depression is a risk factor for eating pathology.[22]

Typical symptoms of depression in EDs, specifically in AN, are a depressive mood, low self-esteem, anhedonia, feelings of emptiness, and social withdrawal. In our own study comprising 172 adolescents with first-onset AN, approximately one-third of the patients also had a current affective disorder.[23] Patients with severe weight loss usually report more severe depressive symptoms than do those with only moderate weight loss.[24] On average, patients with EDs develop moderate levels of depression. The neurobiological changes associated with starvation and disturbed eating behavior, such as low levels of leptin and alterations in the neurotransmitters serotonin and dopamine, contribute to the development of depressive states. Thus, initiating any antidepressant medication should be delayed until the effect of weight gain can be observed. However, if depression persists despite weight rehabilitation, a medication with selective serotonin reuptake inhibitors (SSRIs) might be indicated, especially if the depression predated the ED.

In adolescent binge eating/purging AN, depressive symptoms are usually more pronounced than those in restricting AN[25]; the highest depression rates are reported for adolescents with BN. About one half of patients with BN report current mood disorder symptoms.[27] In the epidemiological study by Swanson et al.,[21] a similar proportion of the participants with BN reported some type of affective disorder in their lifetime. In both EDs, depression plays a central role for the development of suicidal behavior.[23,27]

In a minority of patients, depression precedes the ED. In our sample of 172 patients with AN about 6% reported premorbid depressive symptoms; however, long-term investigations on the relationship between EDs and depression hardly exist. Astonishingly, in the studies by Stice, negative affect did not emerge as a significant predictive factor in EDs (for more details see Chapter 28).

Anxiety Disorders

In clinical and epidemiological studies, approximately one-quarter of patients with current AN suffer from anxiety disorders (obsessive-compulsive disorders [OCDs] not included).[21] In a clinical sample of acutely ill patients with AN,[26] this rate mounted up to 60%. Apart from specific phobias, the most prevalent anxiety disorders are generalized anxiety disorders and social phobia. As with depressive states in AN, symptoms of anxiety disorders are often alleviated by weight gain.[24]

Lifetime rates of anxiety symptoms in BN are even higher than those in AN, with about two-thirds suffering from some kind of anxiety disorder.[21]

Social phobia also plays a major role in BN. In a recent metaanalysis, 12 studies, including all ED groups, were evaluated in a quantitative synthesis. There was a major difference in expression of social phobia between ED patients and controls. Individuals with both AN and BN displayed significantly more social phobia symptoms with a positive association with age; these symptoms improved with treatment solely in AN.[28] However, a significant positive association between BMI and symptoms of anxiety could not be found. The high prevalence of social phobia might underscore the importance of including social skills training in the treatment of adolescent EDs.

Corresponding to the treatment of depression in EDs a medication with SSRIs should be considered for anxiety disorders if severe symptoms persist after weight rehabilitation.

Obsessive-Compulsive Disorder

Clinical symptoms of OCD in AN are mostly either washing or ordering compulsions or the obsession that things are going wrong. Obsessions and compulsions within the context of a "true" comorbidity with OCD have to be differentiated from ED-related obsessions and rituals.

In a remarkable work,[29] females with OCD had a 16-fold increased risk of also developing AN, while males with OCD had a 37-fold risk, based on the results of a population-based study. Similarly, in the longitudinal course of AN, the risk for males to also develop OCD was nearly double compared with that for females. These results point to a common heritability model for AN and OCD with already preliminary data.[30] In another recent study, an association between OCD and subsequent development of BN was also revealed.[31] Moreover, traits such as rigidity, perfectionism, and scrupulosity related to OCD are quite common in patients with EDs, especially those with AN.

Autism Spectrum Disorder

The association between AN and autism spectrum disorder (ASD) is an emerging field of research. Comorbid ASD symptoms are overrepresented in studies of AN and often require more treatment intensity than that for pure AN. However, the prevalence of ASD symptoms in adolescents is lower than that in adult patients with AN. Social withdrawal, perseveration, and rigidity are also symptoms of severe starvation. Thus, the question is whether autistic traits are associated with a more severe and chronic course of the disorder or whether a chronic course of AN is accompanied by a more severe form of neuroprogression (for further details, see Chapter 25) followed by more distinct autistic traits.[32] In a recent study on clinical outcome in patients with AN and comorbid ASD compared with those with ASD traits social difficulties remained despite weight gain and improvement of ED symptoms.[32a] However, long-term studies in weight-recovered patients with AN are necessary to answer questions on the relationship between AN and ASD. Moreover, tools to diagnose ASD have a higher validity for the male sex than that for the female sex. Thus, autistic traits may be underdiagnosed in females with AN.

Attention-Deficit/Hyperactivity Disorder (ADHD)

Several studies have pointed to a significant positive association between EDs and attention-deficit/hyperactivity disorder (ADHD), e.g., children with ADHD are at increased risk to later develop an ED (for a review, see Ref. 33). Nazar et al.[34] found an increased risk for all EDs including restricting AN, while others reported ADHD to be most strongly associated with EDs that are characterized by binge eating.[35] However, until recently, it was not clarified whether this association was "partially or entirely due to an association with other underlying psychopathology."[36] In a large investigation comprising more than 4700 participants aged 18–44 years, lifetime ADHD was significantly associated with BN, BED, and any other ED, with the exception of AN. After adjusting for demographic variables and psychiatric comorbidities, only the association between BN and ADHD remained significant, pointing to the fact that the previously observed association between ADHD and the remaining EDs might be mainly due to some other underlying psychopathology.[36] In our own study on the association between BN and ADHD, patients with both diagnoses were more inattentive and impulsive, had more severely disturbed eating behavior, and more general psychopathology than those with BN alone.[37]

Substance Abuse Disorder

There is also a continuing debate regarding whether EDs and substance abuse disorder (SAD) share a similar disposition. In the large epidemiological sample by Swanson et al.,[21] the adjusted odds ratios for SAD were 1.3 and 2.2 for AN and BN, respectively. Accordingly, patients with the binge eating/purging type of AN are much more at risk than those with the restricting type. Some authors even consider restricting AN as a protective factor against SAD.[38] However, most of the previous studies did not control for age; as patients with BN are generally older than patients with AN, the probability to also develop SAD is higher than that for patients with AN. ED patients with comorbid ADHD appear to be especially prone to developing SAD.[39]

Suicidality and Self-Injurious Behavior

Suicide is one of the leading causes of death in adult AN. In adolescent AN, suicidal attempts are reported in 3%–7% of affected females, and suicidal ideation is reported in about one-third to one-half of the adolescent population with AN.[23,27,40] In our own study, approximately 10% of 148 adolescent patients reported previous suicidal ideation and approximately 4% reported self-injurious behavior (see below).[23]

Suicidal behavior is also elevated in BN and BED. Most, but not all, studies report a higher risk for individuals with AN in comparison with those with BN.[41] Patients with the binge eating/purging type of AN are more prone to suicidality than those with the restricting subtype.[42] Additional associations were found between concurrent depression and duration of illness.[42]

Self-injurious behavior is reported more often in patients who practice binge eating or purging or in those with a history of BN.[42] As has been well established from the study of other disorders, a history of maltreatment or abuse is more prevalent in patients with self-injurious behavior than in those without.[43] In addition, nearly all studies found an association between the severity of ED and self-injurious behavior.

CONCLUSION

EDs are severe disorders of youth that affect physical and mental health with potentially long-lasting sequelae in later life and a high tendency for chronicity. Keeping in mind that outcome may be influenced by early detection and treatment, pediatricians and general practitioners, who often serve as "gatekeepers," must be trained to identify EDs as early as possible and to facilitate referrals to ED specialists. Those who are working with children and adolescents with EDs should be well aware of the high rate of somatic and psychiatric comorbidity, which might require specifically tailored interventions.

REFERENCES

1. Hoek HW. Review of the worldwide epidemiology of eating disorders. *Curr Opin Psychiatry.* 2016;29(6):336–339.
2. GBD 2013 DALYs and HALE Collaborators, Murray CJL, Barber RM, et al. Global, regional, and national disability-adjusted life years (DALYs) for 306 diseases and injuries and healthy life expectancy (HALE) for 188 countries, 1990-2013: quantifying the epidemiological transition. *Lancet Lond Engl.* 2015;386(10009):2145–2191. https://doi.org/10.1016/S0140-6736(15)61340-X.
3. World Health Organization. In: *Mental Health: Facing the Challenges, Building Solutions: Report from the WHO European Ministerial Conference.* Copenhagen, Denmark: World Health Organization, Regional Office for Europe; 2005.
4. Hebebrand J, Bulik CM. Critical appraisal of the provisional DSM-5 criteria for anorexia nervosa and an alternative proposal. *Int J Eat Disord.* 2011;44(8):665–678. https://doi.org/10.1002/eat.20875.
5. Herpertz-Dahlmann B. Adolescent eating disorders: update on definitions, symptomatology, epidemiology, and comorbidity. *Child Adolesc Psychiatr Clin N Am.* 2015;24(1):177–196. https://doi.org/10.1016/j.chc.2014.08.003.
6. Hebebrand J, Blum WF, Barth N, et al. Leptin levels in patients with anorexia nervosa are reduced in the acute stage and elevated upon short-term weight restoration. *Mol Psychiatry.* 1997;2(4):330–334.
7. Hebebrand J, Himmelmann GW, Herzog W, et al. Prediction of low body weight at long-term follow-up in acute anorexia nervosa by low body weight at referral. *Am J Psychiatry.* 1997;154(4):566–569. https://doi.org/10.1176/ajp.154.4.566.
8. Golden NH, Jacobson MS, Sterling WM, Hertz S. Treatment goal weight in adolescents with anorexia nervosa: use of BMI percentiles. *Int J Eat Disord.* 2008;41(4):301–306. https://doi.org/10.1002/eat.20503.
9. Fichter MM, Quadflieg N, Crosby RD, Koch S. Long-term outcome of anorexia nervosa: results from a large clinical longitudinal study. *Int J Eat Disord.* 2017;50(9):1018–1030.
10. Gianini L, Roberto CA, Attia E, et al. Mild, moderate, meaningful? Examining the psychological and functioning correlates of DSM-5 eating disorder severity specifiers. *Int J Eat Disord.* 2017;50(8):906–916.
11. Sternheim L, Danner U, Adan R, Van Elburg A. Drive for activity in patients with anorexia nervosa. *Int J Eat Disord.* 2015;48(1):42–45.
12. Alberti M, Galvani C, El Ghoch M, et al. Assessment of physical activity in anorexia nervosa and treatment outcome. *Med Sci Sports Exerc.* 2013;45(9):1643–1648. https://doi.org/10.1249/MSS.0b013e31828e8f07.
13. Sawyer SM, Whitelaw M, Le Grange D, Yeo M, Hughes EK. Physical and psychological morbidity in adolescents with atypical anorexia nervosa. *Pediatrics.* 2016;137(4). https://doi.org/10.1542/peds.2015-4080.
14. Bulik CM, Marcus MD, Zerwas S, Levine MD, La Via M. The changing "weightscape" of bulimia nervosa. *Am J Psychiatry.* 2012;169(10):1031–1036. https://doi.org/10.1176/appi.ajp.2012.12010147.
15. American Psychiatric Association. *Diagnostic and Statistical Manual of Mental Disorders (DSM-5®).* American Psychiatric Pub; 2013.
16. DerMarderosian D, Chapman HA, Tortolani C, Willis MD. Medical considerations in children and adolescents with eating disorders. *Child Adolesc Psychiatr Clin N Am.* 2018;27(1):1–14. https://doi.org/10.1016/j.chc.2017.08.002.
17. Mehler PS, Winkelman AB, Andersen DM, Gaudiani JL. Nutritional rehabilitation: practical guidelines for refeeding the anorectic patient. *J Nutr Metab.* 2010;2010(article 625782):1–7. https://doi.org/10.1155/2010/625782.
18. Schorr M, Miller KK. The endocrine manifestations of anorexia nervosa: mechanisms and management. *Nat Rev Endocrinol.* 2017;13(3):174.
19. Mainz V, Schulte-Rüther M, Fink GR, Herpertz-Dahlmann B, Konrad K. Structural brain abnormalities in adolescent anorexia nervosa before and after weight recovery and associated hormonal changes. *Psychosom Med.* 2012;74(6):574–582. https://doi.org/10.1097/PSY.0b013e31824ef10e.
20. Paulukat L, Frintrop L, Liesbrock J, et al. Memory impairment is associated with the loss of regular oestrous cycle and plasma oestradiol levels in an activity-based anorexia animal model. *World J Biol Psychiatry.* 2016;17(4):274–284.
21. Swanson SA, Crow SJ, Le Grange D, Swendsen J, Merikangas KR. Prevalence and correlates of eating disorders in adolescents. Results from the national comorbidity survey replication adolescent supplement. *Arch Gen Psychiatry.* 2011;68(7):714–723. https://doi.org/10.1001/archgenpsychiatry.2011.22.
22. Puccio F, Fuller-Tyszkiewicz M, Ong D, Krug I. A systematic review and meta-analysis on the longitudinal relationship between eating pathology and depression. *Int J Eat Disord.* 2016;49(5):439–454. https://doi.org/10.1002/eat.22506.
23. Bühren K, Schwarte R, Fluck F, et al. Comorbid psychiatric disorders in female adolescents with first-onset anorexia nervosa. *Eur Eat Dis Rev.* 2014;22(1):39–44. https://doi.org/10.1002/erv.2254.
24. Mattar L, Thiébaud M-R, Huas C, Cebula C, Godart N. Depression, anxiety and obsessive–compulsive symptoms in relation to nutritional status and outcome in severe anorexia nervosa. *Psychiatry Res.* 2012;200(2–3):513–517.
25. Bühren K, von Ribbeck L, Schwarte R, et al. Body mass index in adolescent anorexia nervosa patients in relation to age, time point and site of admission. *Eur Child Adolesc Psychiatry.* 2013;22(7):395–400. https://doi.org/10.1007/s00787-013-0376-z.

26. Godart N, Berthoz S, Perdereau F, Jeammet P. Comorbidity of anxiety with eating disorders and OCD. *Am J Psychiatry.* 2006;163(2):326; author reply 327-329. https://doi.org/10.1176/appi.ajp.163.2.326.

27. Fennig S, Hadas A. Suicidal behavior and depression in adolescents with eating disorders. *Nord J Psychiatry.* 2010;64(1):32-39. https://doi.org/10.3109/08039480903265751.

28. Kerr-Gaffney J, Harrison A, Tchanturia K. Social anxiety in the eating disorders: a systematic review and meta-analysis. *Psychol Med.* 2018:1-15. https://doi.org/10.1017/S0033291718000752.

29. Cederlöf M, Thornton LM, Baker J, et al. Etiological overlap between obsessive-compulsive disorder and anorexia nervosa: a longitudinal cohort, multigenerational family and twin study. *World Psychiatry.* 2015;14(3):333-338. https://doi.org/10.1002/wps.20251.

30. Brainstorm Consortium, Anttila V, Bulik-Sullivan B, et al. Analysis of shared heritability in common disorders of the brain. *Science.* 2018;360(6395). https://doi.org/10.1126/science.aap8757.

31. Hofer PD, Wahl K, Meyer AH, et al. Obsessive-compulsive disorder and the risk of subsequent mental disorders: a community study of adolescents and young adults. *Depress Anxiety.* 2018;35(4):339-345. https://doi.org/10.1002/da.22733.

32. Westwood H, Tchanturia K. Autism spectrum disorder in anorexia nervosa: an updated literature review. *Curr Psychiatry Rep.* 2017;19(7):41.

32a. Nazar BP, Peynenburg V, Rhind C, et al. An examination of the clinical outcomes of adolescents and young adults with broad autism spectrum traits and autism spectrum disorder and anorexia nervosa: A multi centre study. *Int J Eat Disord.* 2018 Feb;51(2):174-179. https://doi.org/10.1002/eat.22823.

33. Levin RL, Rawana JS. Attention-deficit/hyperactivity disorder and eating disorders across the lifespan: a systematic review of the literature. *Clin Psychol Rev.* 2016;50:22-36. https://doi.org/10.1016/j.cpr.2016.09.010.

34. Nazar BP, Bernardes C, Peachey G, Sergeant J, Mattos P, Treasure J. The risk of eating disorders comorbid with attention-deficit/hyperactivity disorder: a systematic review and meta-analysis. *Int J Eat Disord.* 2016;49(12):1045-1057. https://doi.org/10.1002/eat.22643.

35. Bleck JR, DeBate RD, Olivardia R. The comorbidity of ADHD and eating disorders in a nationally representative sample. *J Behav Health Serv Res.* 2015;42(4):437-451. https://doi.org/10.1007/s11414-014-9422-y.

36. Ziobrowski H, Brewerton TD, Duncan AE. Associations between ADHD and eating disorders in relation to comorbid psychiatric disorders in a nationally representative sample. *Psychiatry Res.* 2018;260:53-59. https://doi.org/10.1016/j.psychres.2017.11.026.

37. Seitz J, Kahraman-Lanzerath B, Legenbauer T, et al. The role of impulsivity, inattention and comorbid ADHD in patients with bulimia nervosa. *PLoS One.* 2013;8(5):e63891. https://doi.org/10.1371/journal.pone.0063891.

38. Kaye WH, Wierenga CE, Bailer UF, Simmons AN, Wagner A, Bischoff-Grethe A. Does a shared neurobiology for foods and drugs of abuse contribute to extremes of food ingestion in anorexia and bulimia nervosa? *Biol Psychiatry.* 2013;73(9):836-842.

39. Nazar BP, Suwwan R, de Sousa Pinna CM, et al. Influence of attention-deficit/hyperactivity disorder on binge eating behaviors and psychiatric comorbidity profile of obese women. *Compr Psychiatry.* 2014;55(3):572-578. https://doi.org/10.1016/j.comppsych.2013.09.015.

40. Smith AR, Zuromski KL, Dodd DR. Eating disorders and suicidality: what we know, what we don't know, and suggestions for future research. *Curr Opin Psychol.* 2017;22:63-67. https://doi.org/10.1016/j.copsyc.2017.08.023.

41. Fichter MM, Quadflieg N. Mortality in eating disorders-results of a large prospective clinical longitudinal study. *Int J Eat Disord.* 2016;49(4):391-401.

42. Kostro K, Lerman JB, Attia E. The current status of suicide and self-injury in eating disorders: a narrative review. *J Eat Disord.* 2014;2(1):19.

43. Brown RC, Heines S, Witt A, et al. The impact of child maltreatment on non-suicidal self-injury: data from a representative sample of the general population.. *B.M.C. Psychiatry.* 2018;18(1):181. https://doi.org/10.1186/s12888-018-1754-3.

CHAPTER 8

Adolescent Obesity and Comorbidity

MARTIN WABITSCH, MD, PHD • STEPHANIE LAVIANI, MSC •
JOHANNES HEBEBRAND, MD • YVONNE MÜHLIG, PHD

In the last decades, an increase in the prevalence rate of obesity in pediatric populations has been observed accompanied by the continuously increasing prevalence of severe obesity especially in adolescents. Due to the increased prevalence in this age group, severe obesity in adolescents has become a serious health concern for which few effective treatments exist.[1-3] Affected adolescents can show a broad spectrum of obesity-related comorbidities which are often underdiagnosed and sometimes even unrecognized. Therefore, these patients require special attention. Especially in severe obesity, comorbidities are often serious and include somatic conditions, psychiatric disorders, and psychosocial consequences. The diagnostic approach toward a young patient with obesity is summarized in Table 8.1.

Health status and physical well-being of the patient can be affected directly (e.g., orthopedic disorders, obstructive sleep apnea [OSA]) or comorbidities can lead to serious sequelae at a later age (hypertension, dyslipidemia, metabolic syndrome; for an overview see Fig. 8.1). Adolescents with severe obesity represent a special risk group and only a small percentage seeks medical attention.[3] Severe obesity in adolescence shows substantial tracking into adulthood with about 90% of affected adolescents staying severely obese as adults. Adolescents with severe obesity experience high morbidity and elevated mortality. Irrespective of whether the disease persists into adulthood, obesity in adolescents has an adverse effect on morbidity and mortality in adulthood.

SOMATIC COMORBIDITIES

Somatic comorbidities of obesity in adolescents include endocrine, metabolic, cardiovascular, musculoskeletal, respiratory, dermatological, gastrointestinal, renal, neurological, and immunological disorders.[4-13] Obesity, glucose intolerance, and hypertension in childhood and adolescence are strongly associated with increased rates of premature death.[1,14] Heart disease,

OSA, hypertension, dyslipidemia, and type 2 diabetes mellitus represent frequent comorbidities. Other less frequent serious conditions include pseudotumor cerebri, steatohepatitis, slipped capital femoral epiphysis, cholelithiasis, polycystic ovary syndrome (PCOS), and early severe degenerative joint disease.

Endocrine, metabolic, and cardiovascular disorders: Overall, obesity is associated with changes in classic endocrine axes (hypothalamic-pituitary-thyroid, hypothalamic-pituitary-gonadal, hypothalamic-pituitary-adrenal [HPA]). Accordingly, various endocrine functions and body weight seem to be closely related. For example, a reduced pituitary release of growth hormone in patients with obesity leads to a diminished concentration in serum. Serum concentrations of growth hormone are inversely correlated with visceral fat depots, which can be ascribed to a postulated reduced lipolytic effect of growth hormone. The relationship between the hypothalamic-pituitary-gonadal axis and body weight is dealt with separately in the context of the pubertal development of children with obesity (see below).

The predisposition to surplus fat depots favors the occurrence of various sequelae like dyslipoproteinemia, also referred to as dyslipidemia, disturbances of glucose regulation, diabetes mellitus type 2 (T2DM), and hypertension, which finally implicate an increased risk of arteriosclerosis. Insulin insensitivity marks a central pathogenetically relevant clinical finding. Elevated blood lipid levels as well as characteristic dyslipidemia (most commonly type 2a or type 2b according to the Fredrickson classification) are induced or enhanced by obesity as early as in childhood. T2DM accounts for a third of all newly diagnosed diabetes mellitus cases in adolescents in the United States. This increased prevalence rate of T2DM is related to the increase of the obesity prevalence in this age group. Cohort studies in Germany showed a 1% prevalence for T2DM and a 3%–6% prevalence for impaired glucose tolerance in adolescents with obesity.[12] Elevated blood

TABLE 8.1
Health Risk and Comorbidity Assessment

Clinical Findings	Possible Comorbidity	Diagnostic Approach
For all forms of obesity	Dyslipidemia Diabetes mellitus type 2 Steatosis hepatis Mental health problems	Cholesterol, HDL/LDL-cholesterol, triglycerides (fasting), liver enzyme (GPT/ALAT), glucose (fasting) Exploration of the patient, screening for mental health problems (e.g., Strengths and Difficulties Questionnaire)
Risk/signs of impaired glucose tolerance and/or BMI >99.5th percentile	Insulin insensitivity Impaired glucose tolerance Diabetes mellitus type 2	Oral glucose tolerance test
Hirsutism Premature adrenarche Menstrual cycle disturbances	Adrenal/ovarian hyperandrogenemia Polycystic ovary syndrome	Exclusion of androgen-producing tumors, AGS
Familial hyperuricemia	Hyperuricemia	Serum uric acid
First- or second-grade relatives with hypercholesterolemia and/or atherosclerosis with sequelae <55 years)	Risk for early onset atherosclerosis and sequelae	Screening: serum lipids, homocysteine in serum, lipoprotein a in serum, consider DNA diagnostics
Snoring Daytime sleepiness Lack of concentration Enuresis nocturna	Obstructive sleep apnea Bronchopathy	Sleep apnea screening, polysomnographic monitoring
Chronic pain in hip/knee joint Genu valgum Pes valgus/planus/transversus Spinal column malposition and/or BMI >99.5th percentile	Epiphysiolysis capitis femoris	Orthopedic evaluation
Abdominal discomfort/pain and/or BMI >99.5th percentile	Cholelithiasis	Abdominal ultrasound
Mental disorders and/or BMI >99.5th percentile	Eating disorders Attention deficit hyperactivity disorder Major depressive disorder Anxiety disorders	Psychological/psychiatric evaluation including use of appropriate psychological questionnaires and tests

pressure levels are commonly found in obese adolescents accompanied by an increased risk of morbidity. A veritable arterial hypertension is not easy to diagnose; monitoring of blood pressure for 24 h is required.

For insulin, cholesterol and triglyceride levels and blood pressure tracking seemingly exists because the relative level of measured values remains more or less constant with growing age. Theoretically, pathologic glucose tolerance, dyslipidemia and/or hypertension in adulthood can already be predicted in childhood. Consequently, a risk assessment of obesity can already be performed in childhood. A clustering of risk factors is well known in obese adults: the combination of hyperinsulinemia, pathologic glucose tolerance, dyslipoproteinemia, hyperuricemia, and hypertension is indicative of the metabolic syndrome.

A familial accumulation of these clinical findings can imply an underlying genetic predisposition which is possibly associated causally with the activity of 1β-hydroxysteroid dehydrogenase type 1 (11β-HSD-1). This enzyme is expressed in omental adipocytes and catalyzes the conversion of cortisone to active cortisol. Patients show pronounced abdominal body fat and enlarged intra-abdominal fat depots. Visceral adipose tissue (VAT) plays a key role in the development of the metabolic syndrome. VAT is characterized by higher cellular density, denser innervation, smaller cells with a higher density of adrenergic receptors, and

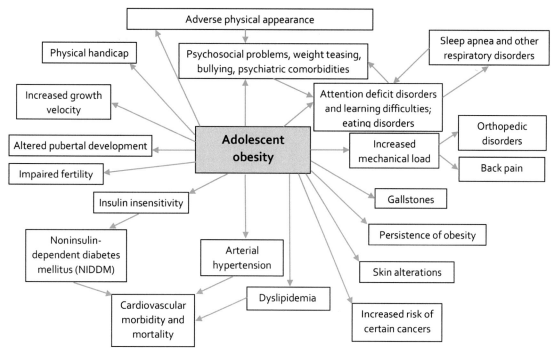

FIG. 8.1 Health risks and comorbidities of adolescent obesity.

increased blood flow, all of which results in a higher metabolic activity. Dependent on the lipolytic activity in the VAT, free fatty acids accumulate in the portal circulation leading to an increase of lipoprotein synthesis and impairment of the hepatic insulin extraction. Since visceral fat increases in size during puberty, these metabolic changes may also appear with increased frequency.

A clustering of risk factors of the metabolic syndrome can be found in obese children already before the onset of puberty. A pronounced manifestation of these risk factors during puberty occurs due to increased pubertal insulin insensitivity. In the United States, the prevalence of the metabolic syndrome is 0.1% in normal weight adolescents, 6.8% in overweight adolescents, and 28.7 in obese adolescents.[15] Obviously, prevalence rates depend on the applied definition and the cut-off values for factors of the metabolic syndrome. The metabolic syndrome underlies the development of cardiovascular disease and T2DM. Adolescents showing signs of a metabolic syndrome should receive regular follow-up care. Apart from behavior modification programs to improve nutrition and to enhance physical activity/reduce physical inactivity, drug use requires further evaluation. It appears sensible to use insulin-sensitizers (e.g., metformin) to treat insulin insensitivity. However, there is a need for more controlled studies in order to make general recommendations.

Pubertal development disorders: A relationship between pubertal development and the amount of energy reservoirs in the body is well known. An early puberty predicts increased body fat content in adulthood. Children with obesity show a premature adrenarche, an accelerated bone age as well as elevated growth rates. Girls experience menarche at an earlier age, whereas interestingly boys attain gonadarche at later age. According to preliminary findings the delayed gonadarche results from a delayed and reduced gonadotropin release. Additionally a pronounced pseudogynecomastia and pseudohypogenitalism represent frequent findings among obese boys. Hyperestrogenemia in the context of obesity as well as a true gynecomastia in obese boys results from the elevated aromatization of steroid hormones due to adiposity. PCOS, a combination of disturbances in the menstrual cycle, hirsutism, and insulin insensitivity, is reported in female obese adolescents and usually improves upon weight loss.

Gastrointestinal disorders: Gastroesophageal reflux disease as well as gastric voiding disorders, which result from increased intra-abdominal pressure, occurs more frequently in obese children compared with normal weight individuals. Obesity in childhood increases the risk of gallstones 10-fold, especially due to repetitive and intermittently successful attempts to lose weight. Signs of steatosis hepatis can be found in up to 25% of obese children and adolescents. Usually, these patients show additional signs of insulin insensitivity or a metabolic syndrome. Elevated liver enzyme levels (particularly alanine aminotransferase) as well as increased liver echogenicity in ultrasound examinations are signs of steatohepatitis. Studies in adults revealed that some patients with steatohepatitis develop a nonalcoholic steatohepatitis (NASH) leading to an increased risk of hepatic cirrhosis or hepatic fibrosis. The diagnosis of NASH requires a biopsy to allow a histological examination. The significance of elevated liver enzymes or sonomorphological changes of the liver in children and adolescents with obesity has not been yet established owing to a lack of studies, thus necessitating further clinical research.

Respiratory disorders: Obese infants and toddlers suffer from obstructive bronchitis more frequently than normal weight individuals. Reports about occurrences of OSA and obstructive snoring (upper airway resistance syndrome) together with nocturnal hypoventilation and hypoxemia in obese adolescents are of great relevance because neurocognitive deficits and impairments in academic achievements can occur in obese adolescents with sleep apnea syndrome. Because the obesity hypoventilation syndrome has been associated with a high mortality rate, an aggressive therapeutic approach is seemingly warranted. Elimination of OSA can be achieved in adolescents by pronounced weight loss. Elimination in adults occurs only very rarely because the underlying instability of the pharyngeal walls and tongue base muscles is not reversible at a later age.

Orthopedic disorders: Apart from more frequent occurrences of strained muscles and factures, the following relevant findings can be observed frequently in obese adolescents: genu valgum and, as precursor of a later gonarthrosis, Blount's disease, which is an aseptic epiphyseal necrosis of the medial proximal tibial epiphysis, mainly occurring in African-Americans, as well as epiphysiolysis capitis femoris. The latter can be latent in severely obese adolescents and leads to dislocation of the femoral head ("tilt deformity"), thus paving the way for the development of coxarthrosis.

Dermatological disorders: Severe forms of panniculus adiposus, striae distensae, and intertriginous skin infections are observed in obese adolescents and may cause psychological distress. Acanthosis nigricans is estimated to occur in up to 25% of obese adolescents and is frequently overlooked upon physical examinations. However, this dermatologic symptom may signal the presence of impaired glucose tolerance or T2DM. Frequent occurrences of acne have been reported in obese female adolescents; hyperhidrosis should also be screened for in both heavy males and females.

PSYCHOLOGICAL PROBLEMS AND PSYCHIATRIC COMORBIDITIES

Adolescent patients are very often exposed to psychosocial discrimination including weight teasing and bullying and adverse social interactions because of their physical appearance. Obese adolescents are perceived significantly more negatively than obese adults. Although having equal intelligence obese patients are viewed as being less intelligent compared with normal weight individuals. Patients suffer from a low self-esteem and distorted self-image resulting in social isolation and sometimes impaired development of social skills. Parents, treatment teams, school, and job centers can face substantial challenges integrating obese adolescents in social life, education, and employment. Social withdrawal and school absenteeism may ensue.

Stigmatization of obese people is widespread and broadly accepted in Western societies. Stigmatization comprises prejudices to character and self-control as well as disadvantages in daily life, e.g., in personal relationships, in medical care, or in working life. Obesity-related comorbidities or health risk factors can be enhanced by discrimination; e.g., unhealthy diet behavior, avoidance of physical activities, and low use of medical care have been associated with experienced discrimination. Obese children and adolescents with stigmatization experiences have an increased risk of depressive disorders, a low self-esteem, and dissatisfaction with their own body as well as a reduced physical and psychological well-being.

Depression is the most frequent psychiatric comorbidity of adolescent obesity.[16] However, depression is only partially related to stigmatization. Overall, depression and obesity are linked via a range of possibly shared etiological mechanisms such as a direct effect of visceral fat mass on mood, chronic low-grade systemic inflammation, vitamin D deficiency, disturbances of the HPA axis and the dopaminergic reward system, and genetic factors. In combination, these factors potentially mediate the relationship of obesity and depression.[16] Another important mental disorder in the context of obesity is social anxiety disorder (SAD; social phobia); patients can become so ashamed of themselves that they systematically avoid social interactions and thus develop symptoms of SAD. Besides stigmatization, the health-related quality of life of adolescents with obesity is substantially reduced due to the multiple impairments in daily life (e.g., mobility, autonomy). High levels of psychological stress represent a risk factor for somatic disorders, e.g., for the development of cardiovascular diseases, T2DM, and unhealthy abdominal fat depots. Not uncommonly, teasing of obese adolescents results in suicidal ideation.

Psychiatric morbidity is particularly elevated in severely obese adolescents.[17] Other than depression, binge eating disorder and atypical eating disorders (e.g., night eating syndrome), other anxiety disorders than SAD, attention deficit disorders with or without hyperactivity (ADHD) or substance use disorders, and addictive-like behaviors (e.g., excessive screen times) are consistently reported.

Discrimination and weight-related stigmatization frequently start in early childhood resulting in a pronounced psychological burden and health problems. Psychosocial problems significantly affect the socioeconomic status of the patient into adulthood. There is an extensive need for information in society about the various causes of obesity and the effects of discriminating obese people. Advice and practical assistance for patients to cope with discrimination and stigmatization as well is required.

REFERENCES

1. Juonala M, Magnussen CG, Berenson GS, et al. Childhood adiposity, adult adiposity, and cardiovascular risk factors. *N Engl J Med.* 2011;365:1876–1885.
2. Lobstein T, Baur L, Uauy R. Obesity in children and young people: a crisis in public health. *Obes Rev.* 2004;5(suppl):4–85.
3. Wabitsch M, Moss A, Reinehr T, et al. Medical and psychosocial implications of adolescent extreme obesity - acceptance and effects of structured care, short: youth with Extreme Obesity Study (YES). *BMC Publ Health.* 2013;13:789.
4. Amin R, Daniels S. Relationship between obesity and sleep-disordered breathing in children: is it a closed loop? *J Pediatr.* 2002;140:641–643.
5. Freedman DS, Mei Z, Srinivasan SR, Berenson GS, Dietz WH. Cardiovascular risk factors and excess adiposity among overweight children and adolescents: the Bogalusa Heart Study. *J Pediatr.* 2007;150:12–17. e12.
6. Han JC, Lawlor DA, Kimm SYS. Childhood obesity. *Lancet.* 2010;375:1737–1748.
7. I'Allemand D, Wiegand S, Reinehr T, et al. Cardiovascular risk in 26,008 European overweight children as established by a multicenter database. *Obesity (Silver Spring).* 2008;16(7):1672–1679.
8. Kelly AS, Barlow SE, Rao G, et al. Severe obesity in children and adolescents: identification, associated health risks, and treatment approaches: a scientific statement from the American Heart Association. *Circulation.* 2013;128(15):1689–1712.
9. Schwimmer JB, Deutsch R, Rauch JB, Behling C, Newbury R, Lavine JE. Obesity, insulin resistance, and other clinicopathological correlates of pediatric nonalcoholic fatty liver disease. *J Pediatr.* 2003;143:500–505.
10. Shah AS, Dolan LM, Khoury PR, Gao Z, Kimball TR, Urbina EM. Severe obesity in adolescents and young adults is associated with subclinical cardiac and vascular changes. *J Clin Endocrinol Metab.* 2015;100(7):2751–2757.
11. Reinehr T, Hinney A, de Sousa G, Austrup F, Hebebrand J, Andler W. Definable somatic disorders in overweight children and adolescents. *J Pediatr.* 2007:618–622. 622 e1-5.
12. Wabitsch M, Hauner H, Hertrampf M, et al. Type II diabetes mellitus and impaired glucose regulation in Caucasian children and adolescents with obesity living in Germany. *Int J Obes Relat Metab Disord.* 2004;28(2):307–313.
13. Weiss R, Dziura J, Burgert TS, et al. Obesity and the metabolic syndrome in children and adolescents. *N Engl J Med.* 2004;350:2362–2374.
14. Twig G, Yaniv G, Levine H, et al. Body-mass index in 2.3 million adolescents and cardiovascular death in adulthood. *N Engl J Med.* 2016;374(25):2430–2440.
15. Cook S, Weitzman M, Auinger P, Nguyen M, Dietz W. Prevalence of a metabolic syndrome phenotype in adolescents. *Arch Pediatr Adolesc Med.* 2003;157:821–827.
16. Mühlig Y, Antel J, Föcker M, Hebebrand J. Are bidirectional associations of obesity and depression already apparent in childhood and adolescence as based on high-quality studies? A systematic review. *Obes Rev.* 2016;17:235–249.
17. Britz B, Siegfried W, Ziegler A, et al. Rates of psychiatric disorders in a clinical study group of adolescents with extreme obesity and in obese adolescents ascertained via a population based study. *Int J Obes Relat Metab Disord.* 2000;24:1707–1714.

CHAPTER 9

Incidence and Prevalence of Eating Disorders Among Children and Adolescents

ANNA KESKI-RAHKONEN, MD, PHD, MPH • YASMINA SILÉN, MD

INTRODUCTION

How many children and adolescents in your area are currently suffering from eating disorders (EDs)? How many of them will be able to access treatment each year? Is there a mismatch between the need for help and available services? These questions are important because eating and feeding disorders are a major source of burden for young people and their caregivers.[1] EDs can also have serious consequences for the growth and maturation of children and adolescents. Understanding the magnitude of the problem helps to plan appropriate, timely, and adequate local treatment and prevention services. This practical need drives descriptive epidemiology. Because reliable biomarkers for EDs are not currently available, case detection is based on diagnostic criteria that evolve over time. The Fifth Diagnostic and Statistical Manual (DSM-5) of 2013 broadened and relaxed the diagnostic definitions of anorexia nervosa (AN) and bulimia nervosa (BN) and established binge eating disorder (BED) as an independent diagnostic category. DSM-5 also provided definitions for other specified feeding or EDs (atypical AN; BN of low frequency and/or limited duration; BED of low frequency and/or limited duration; purging disorder; night eating syndrome) and a new residual category, unspecified feeding or eating disorder. Finally, a new diagnostic category particularly relevant for children, avoidant/restrictive food intake disorder, was added to the DSM-5 diagnostic classification. The upcoming ICD-11 classification is expected to adopt similar definitions. These new diagnostic categories will with time also impact diagnostic options available for children and adolescents (for a more detailed description see chapter "Definition, Symptomatology, and Comorbidity of Adolescent EDs)."

WHAT DOES DESCRIPTIVE EPIDEMIOLOGY AIM TO DO?

The goal of descriptive epidemiology is to estimate how many new-onset cases emerge, and how many are affected currently, over a defined time period, or over their entire life span. The occurrence of new cases over time is called incidence. The accumulation of cases up to the current moment or over time is called prevalence.

The relationship of incidence and prevalence is analogous to a bathtub. Incidence, the onset of new cases, is the incoming flow of water into a bathtub. Prevalence is the pool of cases contained by the bathtub. The relationship of incidence and prevalence in stable populations is easy to understand: prevalence equals incidence multiplied by time. The balance of incoming and outgoing flow determines the water level (current prevalence). Factors that impact current prevalence include mortality and recovery. Neither has an impact on lifetime prevalence (the high water mark in the bathtub), but both can decrease the prevalence of currently symptomatic individuals. A discrepancy between lifetime and current prevalence can therefore imply that the disorder of interest has an excellent prognosis or that it is fatal. Conversely, even if the incidence of the disorder is stable, its prevalence can increase, if mortality is low and the symptoms are longstanding. Increased prevalence can merely reflect a longer duration of acute illness.

To measure unmet need for treatment, one needs to understand how many individuals in the community experience symptoms and how many individuals are in treatment. *Clinical prevalences* estimate how many patients are treated by primary care physicians or mental health specialists or other health professionals in treatment settings. Healthcare and health insurance registries are an excellent resource for obtaining this information. Recently, nationwide healthcare data have become available from several different countries, particularly from Scandinavia.

The *true prevalence* of a psychiatric disorder is much harder to estimate. It refers to the underlying prevalence of the disorder of interest *in the community*: true prevalences include both treated and untreated cases. The best information sources for estimating true prevalences are systematic community-based studies that use rigorous protocols for case definition. Information is gathered by interviewing all participants using structured diagnostic interviews, preferably repeatedly to increase reliability. These procedures can be very costly; an alternative information gathering procedure is a two-stage protocol: a large number of individuals are surveyed with a screening questionnaire; next, screen-positive cases and a subset of negative cases are confirmed with a diagnostic interview.

Prevalences are simple proportions that can be calculated in many different study settings, including cross-sectional studies. For this reason, they are generally readily reported. Incidences are more challenging to address. In community-based studies, a large group of individuals undergo diagnostic assessment. Incidences are usually expressed as rates, calculated as the number of new onset cases divided by person-time at risk (e.g., 100 new onset cases per 100,000 person-years). Even in relatively large cohorts consisting of thousands of individuals, a relatively small number of active cases are usually detected. Therefore, confidence intervals of the estimated incidence rates that tend to be very wide and large fluctuations in the estimates are to be expected.

In the next section, the incidence and prevalence of EDs among children and adolescents are described based on landmark community-based and registry-based studies. Childhood and adolescence can be defined in various different ways: this review will include studies up to an of age 20 years.

INCIDENCE
Community-Based Incidence of Eating Disorders

In an American community–based study of adolescent girls, the incidence of DSM-5 AN was 100 per 100,000 person years, BN was 290 per 100,000 person years, BED was 340 per 100,000 person years, and feeding or eating disorder not elsewhere classified 1400 per 100,000 person years (Stice et al.[20]).

Clinical Incidence of Anorexia Nervosa

Several high-quality studies have addressed the clinical incidence of EDs among youth. They provide a better understanding of how EDs emerge over time.

The incidence of AN among girls rises sharply with age. A Dutch primary care–based study conducted among females in 2005–09 found that the incidence rate of DSM-IV AN was 20 per 100,000 person-years among 10- to 14-year-old girls, but 100 per 100,000 person-years among 15- to 19-year-old girls.[2] Similarly, in the extensive Swedish healthcare registers, the annual incidence of AN among girls rose sharply after the age of 11 years and peaked between the ages 15 and 18 years at around 200 per 100 000 persons, falling thereafter.[3] A recent study based on Danish registry data also found an increase of incidence rates of AN from 6.4 to 12.6 per 100,000 person-years.[4]

In Swedish registers, boys showed a similar peaking of ED incidences between ages 12 and 17 years than did girls; however, the peak incidence among boys was smaller by a factor of 10, 20 per 100,000 person-years.[3]

Clinical Incidence of Bulimia Nervosa

The recorded clinical peak incidences of BN among adolescents are lower by more than a half than those of AN. The incidence rate of BN was 5 per 100,000 person-years among 10- to 14-year-old Dutch girls, but 40 per 100,000 person-years among 15- to 19-year-old girls.[2] In Danish registries, the incidence BN was 4.5 among 11 - to 15-year-old girls, 60 per 100,000 person-years among 16- to 20-year-old women, and 2 per 100,000 person-years among 16- to 20-year-old men.[5] Another Danish registry–based study of BN found a relatively stable incidence rate of 6.3–7.2 per 100,000 person-years.[4]

Despite their extensive coverage, the Swedish registries have not documented the incidence rates of BN. They do, however, include a mixed category, "other EDs," with reported annual incidences of 370 per 100 000 among women in the peak 16- to 17-year-old age group.[3]

Has the True Incidence of EDs Increased Over Time Among Adolescents?

Researchers in different countries have tackled this difficult question. Dutch researchers were able to assess their patients in the 1980, 1990, and 2000s using the same diagnostic procedures. Based on the findings, the incidence rates of DSM-IV AN and BN among adolescents appear to have remained relatively stable over three decades.[2] However, conflicting results have emerged from Swedish registries. There, incidences of

AN and other EDs were tracked from the year 1979; they rose sharply among adolescents between 2000 and 2009.[3] Similarly, in nationwide Danish registries, the incidence of AN doubled between 1995 and 2010 from 10 to 10 per 100 000 person-years.[4] However, after taking into account changes in diagnostic practices and better access to treatment, it is likely that the observed increase has more to do with improved detection than changes in true incidences. Further studies from other countries should confirm and extend these initial findings.

PREVALENCE

Lifetime Prevalence

"Lifetime prevalences" intend to cover the entire life span, but for practical reasons, most lifetime prevalence studies of EDs have been conducted among adolescents and young adults (here, up to the age of 20 years). Key high-quality lifetime prevalence studies are listed in Table 9.1.

Overall lifetime prevalences assessed by different two-stage community-based studies range from 3.0% to 13.1% (Table 9.2). Generally, studies with higher overall prevalences have paid more careful attention to including forms of EDs other than AN and BN.

Lifetime prevalences of EDs among adolescent girls ranged as follows: AN from 0.3% to 2.6% and BN from 0% to 2.6% (Table 9.2). BED was not assessed by all studies, but estimates of lifetime prevalence of BED among adolescent girls ranged from 1.0% to 3.0%. Inclusion criteria and definitions for other specified eating or feeding disorders varied widely, from 0.6% to 15.7% (details in Table 9.2). Comparisons across studies are not possible; every study measured different atypical presentations. The most commonly studied and detected other specified eating or feeding disorders among adolescents were atypical AN, BN of low frequency and/or limited duration, and BED of low frequency and/or limited duration.

Lifetime prevalences of EDs among adolescent boys have been addressed by relatively few studies.[6-8] Based on available studies, EDs affect 1.2%–1.5% of boys. BED is the most common ED among boys, affecting 0.7%–0.8% of them; AN and BN are relatively rare, affecting 0.1%–0.3% and 0.1%–0.5% of boys, respectively (Table 9.2).

Current Prevalence

The number of current cases can be addressed either by measuring point prevalences (the number of persons ill at any given moment) or period prevalences (the number of persons ill within a defined time period.) The most commonly estimated period in ED research is past 12 months. Current prevalences are useful for service planning. They also minimize recall bias. A large discrepancy between current and lifetime prevalences also has prognostic implications: it can mean that the outlook of the illness is favorable or fatal.

Key studies detailing 12-month prevalences of EDs among adolescents are listed in Table 9.3.

They all are based two large and rigorous nationwide community-based datasets. In the National Health and Nutrition Examination Survey, the 12-month prevalence of DSM-IV EDs was 0.2% among girls and 0.1% among boys.[7] The National Comorbidity Survey Replication detected the following 12-month prevalences of EDs among 13- to 18-year-old girls: AN 0.1%, BN 0.9%, and BED 1.4%.[8] Among boys in the same dataset, the 12-month prevalence of AN was 0.2%, BN 0.3%, and BED 0.4%.[8] Based on both studies, current DSM-IV EDs are quite rare among adolescents. However, neither study embraced DSM-5 definitions of EDs.

The most relevant current information source on point prevalences of DSM-5 EDs is based on the Dutch primary care–based study.[6] The overall point prevalence of any DSM-5 ED among youth aged up to 20 years was 3.7% among girls and 0.5% among boys. The point prevalence of AN was 1.2% among girls and 0.1% among boys; BN currently affected 0.6% of girls and 0.1% of boys, whereas BED affected 1.6% of girls and 0.3% of boys. The point prevalence of other specified eating or feeding disorder was 0.3% among girls and 0% among boys; that of unspecified feeding and eating disorder was 0% among both sexes.

Finally, a cross-sectional German study entirely based on self-report conducted among adolescents whose mean age was 13 years found the following point prevalences of DSM-5 EDs: AN was reported by 0.6% of girls and 0% of boys; BN by 0.6% of girls and 0.1% of boys; BED by 0.6% of girls and 0.4% of boys (estimates calculated from figures given in the article).[9] Although new DSM-5 criteria broadened definitions of EDs, and generally increased prevalences, these increases were not always fully consistent because of widely varying base prevalences. Some studies based on DSM-IV criteria[10-12] report higher prevalences than a Dutch DSM-5 primary care–based study that used DSM-5 definitions.[6] The large gaps between the US-based, Dutch and German estimates can partially be explained by different age groups and diagnostic definitions. However, more research is needed on DSM-5 EDs, particularly their subthreshold manifestations.

TABLE 9.1
Lifetime Prevalence of Eating Disorders (EDs) Among Adolescents

Author (year)	N	Age	Setting	Sample Characteristics	Lifetime Prevalence
Merikangas et al.[7]	10,148	13–17 years	USA	The National Comorbidity Survey Replication Adolescent Supplement, face-to-face interviews + parent of each adolescent (questionnaires), CIDI, DSM-IV.	Lifetime DSM-IV prevalence of EDs: Girls 3.8%: 13–14 years 2.4% 15–16 years 2.8% 17–18 years 3.0% Boys 1.5%:
Swanson et al.[8]	10,123	13–18 years	USA	The National Comorbidity Survey Replication Adolescent Supplement, a nationally representative cross-sectional survey of adolescents with face-to-face interviews using CIDI, DSM-IV.	Lifetime DSM-IV prevalence, sexes pooled: Anorexia nervosa (AN) 0.3% Bulimia nervosa (BN) 0.9% BED 1.6% Subthreshold anorexia 0.8% Subthreshold BED 2.5% Lifetime prevalence for girls: AN 0.3% BN 1.3% BED 2.3%, 1.5% subthreshold anorexia 1.5% Subthreshold BED 2.3% Lifetime prevalence for boys: AN 0.3% BN 0.5% BED 0.8% Subthreshold anorexia 0.1% Subthreshold BED 2.6%
Le Grange et al.[19]		13–18 years	USA	Two cross-sectional surveys: National Comorbidity Survey Replication Adolescent Supplement (NCS-A); The National Comorbidity Survey Replication (NCS-R) face-to-face survey CIDI, DSM-IV.	For adolescents, lifetime DSM-IV prevalence of ED not otherwise defined was 4.8% The most prevalent subtype was subthreshold BED
Smink et al.[6]	1584	11–19 years	The Netherlands	Longitudinal study Assessment: Baseline Child Behavior Checklist, Youth Self-Report + DSM-5 CIDI interview.	Lifetime DSM-5 prevalence of AN in girls: AN 1.7% (1.0%–2.9%) BN 0.8% (0.3%–1.7%) BED 2.3% (1.4%–3.6%) Other specified feeding or ED 0.6% (0.2%–1.3%) Unspecified feeding or ED 0.2% (0.0%–0.8%) Any ED: 5.7% (4.2%–7.5%) Lifetime prevalence of AN in boys: AN 0.1% (0.0%–0.8%) BN 0.1% (0.0%–0.8%) BED 0.7% (0.2%–1.6%) Other specified feeding or ED 0.3% (0.0%–1.0%) Unspecified feeding or ED 0% Any ED 1.2% (0.6%–2.3%)

TABLE 9.1
Lifetime Prevalence of Eating Disorders (EDs) Among Adolescents—cont'd

Author (year)	N	Age	Setting	Sample Characteristics	Lifetime Prevalence
Stice et al.[10]	496	12–20 years	USA	Participants were 496 adolescent girls in a large US city recruited from schools. At baseline, participants ranged from 12 to 15 years of age, and they were interviewed annually for 8 years using the Eating Disorder Diagnostic Interview, a semistructured interview, to elicit DSM-IV diagnoses.	Lifetime prevalence by age 20 years in girls: Combined DSM-IV ED prevalence 12% AN 0.6% BN 1.6% BED 1.0% Subthreshold AN 0.6% Subthreshold BN 6.1% Subthreshold BED 4.6% Purging disorder 4.4.%
Stice et al.[20]	496	12–20 years	USA	Participants were 496 adolescent girls in a large US city recruited from schools. At baseline, participants ranged from 12 to 15 years of age, and they were interviewed annually for 8 years using the Eating Disorder Diagnostic Interview, a semistructured interview, to elicit DSM-5 diagnoses.	Lifetime prevalence by age 20 in girls: Combined prevalence of AN, BN, or BED 5.2% Combined prevalence of any DSM-5 ED 13.1% AN 0.8% BN 2.6% BED 3.0% atypical AN 2.8% Subthreshold BN 4.4% Subthreshold BED 3.6% Purging disorder 3.4% for purging disorder
Machado et al.[21]	2028	12–23 years	Portugal	Female students in the 9th to 12th grades, screened by the Eating Disorder Examination. In Stage 2, ED experts interviewed 901 participants using the Eating Disorder Examination using DSM-IV criteria.	All EDs among girls 3.0% AN was 0.4%, BN 0.3%, ED not otherwise defined 2.4%.
Fairweather-Schmidt and Wade[11] Wade and O'Shea[12]	699	12–19 years	Australia	Adolescent female twins interviewed with the Eating Disorder Examination on three occasions spanning 12.70–19.84 years of age.	Lifetime prevalence of DSM-5 EDs among girls: All EDs 10.4%: (95% confidence interval: 8.3%–12.9%) AN, BN, and BED: 5.4% Other specified feeding or ED 5% Lifetime prevalences of individual diagnoses: AN 2.0% BN 1.0% BED 2.4% Atypical AN 1.9% Atypical BN 2.6% Purging disorder 0.6% A further 4.7% had unspecified feeding or ED

Continued

TABLE 9.1
Lifetime Prevalence of Eating Disorders (EDs) Among Adolescents—cont'd

Author (year)	N	Age	Setting	Sample Characteristics	Lifetime Prevalence
Nagl et al.[22]	3021	14–24 years	Germany	Prospective-longitudinal community study adolescents followed up at three assessment waves over 10 years, DSM-IV M-CIDI interview.	Baseline lifetime prevalence for any threshold + subthreshold ED 1.1% Cumulative incidence of all threshold and subthreshold EDs pooled across sexes, 14–17 years old: 3.9% Girls: 8.3% (6.8%–10.1%) Boys: 1.0% (0.6%–1.8%)
Wagner et al.[23]	3613	10–18 years	Austria	A nationwide school-based epidemiological study that used SCOFF for screening and Children's Diagnostic Interview for Mental Disorders for establishing DSM-5 diagnoses.	Lifetime prevalence of all feeding and EDs: 5.5% in girls, 0.6% in boys Prevalences pooled across sexes: AN 1.4% BN 0.3% BED 0.2% Other specified eating or feeding disorder 0.6%
Isomaa et al.[13]	606	15 years	Finland	A self-report questionnaire was administered at schools (half of participants were girls, half boys), questions concerning anorectic and bulimic eating pathology were formulated according to the DSM-IV diagnostic criteria of EDs. The second step consisted of a semistructured interview Rating of Anorexia and Bulimia-Teenager version (RAB-T).	Lifetime DSM-IV prevalence in girls overall EDs (anorexia, bulimia, and their subthreshold forms): 7.0% AN 1.8% BN 0% Anorexia not otherwise specified 4.9% Subclinical EDs 4.9% No boys with AN
Isomaa et al.[24]	595	15–18 years	Finland	Three-year follow-up study of 15-year-old ninth graders described above. A screening questionnaire followed by a semistructured Rating of Anorexia and Bulimia-Teenager interview	Lifetime DSM-IV prevalence for females at age 18 were: AN 2.6% 0.4% for BN 7.7% for AN-NOS 1.3% for BN-NOS 8.5% for subclinical EDs No prevalent cases of DSM-IV EDs were found among the male participants

WHY STUDYING EPIDEMIOLOGY OF EDs IS CHALLENGING

Many different factors make the reliable assessment of the occurrence of EDs challenging. Key sources of variation in estimates of prevalence and incidence of EDs are all related to study design. Changing diagnostic definitions and the age of individuals addressed will impact the estimates. Also, sampling tries to reflect the underlying reality as closely as possible, but various sampling strategies and methods of case detection (in-person

TABLE 9.2
A Comparison of Lifetime Eating Disorders (EDs) in Adolescents Across Different Studies

	Diagnostic classification	ED-All	AN	BN	BED	SAN	SBN	SBED	PD	NES	OSFED	UFED
GIRLS, LIFETIME PREVALENCE												
Stice et al.[20]	DSM-5	13.1	0.8	2.6	3.0	2.8	4.4	3.6	3.4			
Stice et al.[10]	DSM-IV	12.0	0.6	1.6	1.0	0.6	6.1	4.6	4.4			
Fairweather-Schmidt and Wade 2014[11] Wade and O'Shea[12]		10.4	2	1	2.4	1.9	2.6		0.6			4.7
Isomaa et al.[13]	DSM-IV	7.0	1.8	0		4.9						
Smink et al.[6]	DSM-5	5.7	1.7	0.8	2.3	0	0.1	0.2	0.2	0.2	0.6	0.2
Le Grange et al.[19]		4.8									4.8	
Merikangas et al.[7] Swanson et al.[8]	DSM-IV	3.8	0.3	1.3	2.3	1.5		2.3				
Machado et al.[21]		3.0	0.4	0.3	2.4							
Isomaa[24]	DSM-IV		2.6	0.4		7.7	1.3					
BOYS, LIFETIME PREVALENCE												
Smink et al.[6]	DSM-5	1.2	0.1	0.1	0.7	0.3			1		0	1.2
Merikangas et al.[7] Swanson et al.[8]	DSM-IV	1.5	0.3	0.5	0.8	0.1		2.6				1.5

AN, anorexia nervosa; *BED*, binge eating disorder; *BN*, bulimia nervosa; *ED-All*, all eating disorders; *NES*, night eating syndrome; *OSFED*, other specified feeding and eating disorder; *SAN*, subthreshold anorexia nervosa, *SBED*, subthreshold binge eating disorder; *SBN*, subthreshold bulimia nervosa; *UFED*, unspecified feeding and eating disorder.

interviews, telephone interviews, school-based sampling) can also have a major impact on the results. The highest prevalence estimates are generally obtained by studies that only use self-report questionnaires.[14]

Community-based studies seek to estimate the true rates of occurrence, but their major drawback is often low statistical power and very wide confidence intervals for estimates of occurrence. Clinical registry–based studies often have high statistical power, but because access of treatment is usually limited, they capture only

a part of individuals with EDs. A nationally representative sample from the United States revealed that only 20% of adolescent girls and <10% adolescent boys with an ED had sought treatment for their problems.[15] Therefore, the clinical and community-based measures of occurrence are expected to differ.

Systematic data collection is particularly important because it helps to decrease bias. EDs have historically been thought to afflict "skinny, white, affluent girls" (the SWAG stereotype).[16] However, this view could

TABLE 9.3
Twelve-Month Prevalence of Eating Disorders (EDs) Among Adolescents

Author (Year)	N	Age	Setting	Sample Characteristics	Twelve-Month prevalence
Merikangas et al.[7]	3042	8–15 years	USA	National Health and Nutrition Examination Survey, a structured diagnostic interview for DSM-IV mental disorders (provides scant details on ED diagnoses)	Pooled across sexes: 0.1% for EDs: 0.1% for anorexia nervosa (AN) 0.1% for bulimia nervosa (BN) Sex-specific prevalences: 0.1% for boys 0.2% for girls
Kessler et al.[25]	10,148	13–17 years	USA	The National Comorbidity Survey Replication Adolescent Supplement, face-to-face interviews + parent of each adolescent (questionnaires), CIDI, DSM-IV	Pooled across sexes: EDs (AN, BN, binge-eating behavior) 12-month prevalence 2.8%; 30-day prevalence 1.1%
Swanson et al.[8]	10,123	13–18 years	USA	The National Comorbidity Survey Replication Adolescent Supplement, a nationally representative cross-sectional survey of adolescents with face-to-face interviews using CIDI, DSM-IV	Pooled across sexes: AN 0.2% BN 0.6%, Binge eating disorder (BED) 0.9% Girls: AN 0.1% BN 0.9% BED 1.4% Boys: AN 0.2% BN 0.3% BED 0.4%
Taylor et al.[26]	1170	13–17 years	USA	African-American adolescents (n = 1170) interviewed in their homes using CIDI, DSM-IV	12-month prevalence Girls: AN 0% BN 0.43% BED 0.57% Boys: AN 0.15% BN 0.37% BED 0%

result from differential access to care and other systematic biases. For this reason, studies that also include males, minorities, and individuals from socioeconomically disadvantaged backgrounds are particularly important.

CONCLUSION

EDs are a serious and growing concern among adolescents. Overall lifetime prevalence of EDs ranged from 3% to 13% among adolescent girls and from 1.2% to 1.5% among adolescent boys. Current prevalences of EDs ranged from 0.2% to 3.7% among girls and 0.1%–0.5% among boys. More recent studies generally report increasing incidences and lifetime prevalences.

The uncertainty and order-of-magnitude difference in lifetime and current prevalences make comparisons across different studies and settings challenging. In practice, service planning can use lowest and highest estimates of occurrence to create best-case and worst-case scenarios of need for treatment. However, several studies have shown that there is a sizable unmet need for treatment.

Whether unmet need for treatment among adolescents is a pressing concern requiring immediate action depends on the prognosis of the disorder. Comparisons of lifetime and current prevalences show large differences. Mortality rates associated with EDs cannot explain these differences.[17,18] This implies that EDs are ultimately transient illnesses for most sufferers.

In the future, descriptive epidemiology of EDs should move beyond simple cross-sectional studies. A more detailed understanding of how EDs unfold over time will be helpful in optimizing treatment and prevention.

REFERENCES

1. Herpertz-Dahlmann B. Treatment of eating disorders in child and adolescent psychiatry. *Curr Opin Psychiatry.* 2017;30:438–445.
2. Smink FR, van HD, Donker GA, Susser ES, Oldehinkel AJ, Hoek HW. Three decades of eating disorders in Dutch primary care: decreasing incidence of bulimia nervosa but not of anorexia nervosa. *Psychol Med.* 2016;46:1189–1196.
3. Javaras KN, Runfola CD, Thornton LM, et al. Sex- and age-specific incidence of healthcare-register-recorded eating disorders in the complete Swedish 1979-2001 birth cohort. *Int J Eat Disord.* 2015;48:1070–1081.
4. Steinhausen HC, Jensen CM. Time trends in lifetime incidence rates of first-time diagnosed anorexia nervosa and bulimia nervosa across 16 years in a Danish nationwide psychiatric registry study. *Int J Eat Disord.* 2015;48(7):845–850. doi: 10.1002/eat.22402.. Epub 2015 Mar 23. PubMed PMID: 25809026.
5. Zerwas S, Larsen JT, Petersen L, Thornton LM, Mortensen PB, Bulik CM. The incidence of eating disorders in a Danish register study: associations with suicide risk and mortality. *J Psychiatr Res.* 2015;65:16–22. https://doi.org/10.1016/j.jpsychires.2015.03.003. Epub;%2015 Mar 13:16–22.
6. Smink FR, van HD, Oldehinkel AJ, Hoek HW. Prevalence and severity of DSM-5 eating disorders in a community cohort of adolescents. *Int J Eat Disord.* 2014;47:610–619.
7. Merikangas KR, He JP, Burstein M, et al. Lifetime prevalence of mental disorders in U.S. Adolescents: results from the national comorbidity survey replication–adolescent supplement (NCS-a). *J Am Acad Child Adolesc Psychiatry.* 2010;49:980–989.
8. Swanson SA, Crow SJ, Le GD, Swendsen J, Merikangas KR. Prevalence and correlates of eating disorders in adolescents. Results from the national comorbidity survey replication adolescent supplement. *Arch Gen Psychiatry.* 2011;68:714–723.
9. Hammerle F, Huss M, Ernst V, Burger A. Thinking dimensional: prevalence of DSM-5 early adolescent full syndrome, partial and subthreshold eating disorders in a cross-sectional survey in German schools. *BMJ Open.* 2016;6:e010843.
10. Stice E, Marti CN, Shaw H, Jaconis M. An 8-year longitudinal study of the natural history of threshold, subthreshold, and partial eating disorders from a community sample of adolescents. *J Abnorm Psychol.* 2009;118:587–597.
11. Fairweather-Schmidt AK, Wade TD. DSM-5 eating disorders and other specified eating and feeding disorders: is there a meaningful differentiation? *Int J Eat Disord.* 2014;47:524–533.
12. Wade TD, O'Shea A. DSM-5 unspecified feeding and eating disorders in adolescents: what do they look like and are they clinically significant? *Int J Eat Disord.* 2015;48:367–374.
13. Isomaa R, Isomaa AL, Marttunen M, Kaltiala-Heino R, Bjorkqvist K. The prevalence, incidence and development of eating disorders in Finnish adolescents: a two-step 3-year follow-up study. *Eur Eat Disord Rev.* 2009;17:199–207.
14. Lindvall DC, Wisting L. Transitioning from DSM-IV to DSM-5: a systematic review of eating disorder prevalence assessment. *Int J Eat Disord.* 2016;49:975–997.
15. Forrest LN, Smith AR, Swanson SA. Characteristics of seeking treatment among U.S. adolescents with eating disorders. *Int J Eat Disord.* 2017;50:826–833.
16. Sonneville KR, Lipson SK. Disparities in eating disorder diagnosis and treatment according to weight status, race/ethnicity, socioeconomic background, and sex among college students. *Int J Eat Disord.* 2018;10.
17. Arcelus J, Mitchell AJ, Wales J, Nielsen S. Mortality rates in patients with anorexia nervosa and other eating disorders. A meta-analysis of 36 studies. *Arch Gen Psychiatry.* 2011;68:724–731.
18. Ackard DM, Richter S, Egan A, Cronemeyer C. Poor outcome and death among youth, young adults, and midlife adults with eating disorders: an investigation of risk factors by age at assessment. *Int J Eat Disord.* 2014;47:825–835.
19. Le Grange D, Swanson SA, Crow SJ, Merikangas KR. Eating disorder not otherwise specified presentation in the US population. *Int J Eat Disord.* 2012;45:711–718.
20. Stice E, Marti CN, Rohde P. Prevalence, incidence, impairment, and course of the proposed DSM-5 eating disorder diagnoses in an 8-year prospective community study of young women. *J Abnorm Psychol.* 2013;122:445–457.
21. Machado PP, Machado BC, Goncalves S, Hoek HW. The prevalence of eating disorders not otherwise specified. *Int J Eat Disord.* 2007;40:212–217.
22. Nagl M, Jacobi C, Paul M, et al. Prevalence, incidence, and natural course of anorexia and bulimia nervosa among adolescents and young adults. *Eur Child Adolesc Psychiatry.* 2016;25:903–918.
23. Wagner G, Zeiler M, Waldherr K, et al. Mental health problems in Austrian adolescents: a nationwide, two-stage epidemiological study applying DSM-5 criteria. *Eur Child Adolesc Psychiatry.* 2017;26:1483–1499.

24. Isomaa AL, Isomaa R, Marttunen M, Kaltiala-Heino R. Obesity and eating disturbances are common in 15-year-old adolescents. A two-step interview study. *Nord J Psychiatry*. 2010;64:123–129.

25. Kessler RC, Avenevoli S, Costello EJ, et al. Prevalence, persistence, and sociodemographic correlates of DSM-IV disorders in the national comorbidity survey replication adolescent supplement. *Arch Gen Psychiatry*. 2012;69:372–380.

26. Taylor JY, Caldwell CH, Baser RE, Faison N, Jackson JS. Prevalence of eating disorders among blacks in the national survey of American life. *Int J Eat Disord*. 2007;40(suppl):S10–S14. https://doi.org/10.1002/eat.20451:S10–S14.

CHAPTER 10

Development, Tracking, Distribution, and Time Trends in Body Weight During Childhood

LISE G. BJERREGAARD, MSC, PHD • JENNIFER L. BAKER, PHD • THORKILD I.A. SØRENSEN, MD

NATURAL COURSE OF WEIGHT GAIN AND DEVELOPMENT OF OBESITY

Treatment or prevention of abnormal body weight development during childhood requires knowledge about the natural course of body development. The body fat content is ~13% at birth and increases to ~28% by the end of the first year of life. This is followed by a fall in the adipose tissue mass and percentage of body fat over the next 6–10 years due to relatively higher increase in lean body mass during growth. During early puberty, the percentage body fat increases a second time. In girls, this increase in body fat continues until adulthood. In boys, the amount of body fat remains constant during the pubertal growth spurt in the 11th–15th year of life. Hereafter it increases a third time.[1]

Although body mass index (BMI; kg/m^2) is only a proxy for body fat, it is generally accepted as a valid indirect measure of adiposity. Changes in BMI parallel those of body fat. BMI increases rapidly during infancy, after which it declines. Beginning at around age 6 years, BMI rises for a second time. This increase is likely due to alterations in the amount of body fat rather than lean mass and is termed the "adiposity rebound." An early adiposity rebound is associated with an increased risk of obesity. Children who later develop obesity have an adiposity rebound that occurs around age 3 years.[2]

TRACKING OF BMI DURING CHILDHOOD AND THROUGH ADULTHOOD

Tracking of BMI is defined as the maintenance of an individual's relative position compared with a reference population over time, and it applies across the whole range of BMI values.[3] Thus, it implies a higher relative risk of overweight and obesity among individuals with a relatively high BMI at an earlier age and vice versa for underweight.

Tracking by Age

Childhood and adulthood BMI are positively associated in men and women.[4–6] The strength is heavily dependent on the time interval between body size assessments.[4] The longer time interval with increasing adult age makes it more likely that individual body size changes for various reasons, implying that the position in the overall distribution of the population changes whereby the correlation with childhood BMI weakens. Thus, correlations between BMI at 7 years and adult BMI are moderate at around 18–19 years of age (r = 0.55) and steadily decline to rather weak levels at 60–69 years of age (r ≈ 0.26).[5] Correspondingly, the correlations between BMI at 35 years and BMI in preceding ages increases from ≈0.15 at age 2 years to ≈0.5 at age 10 years to ≈0.7 at age 18 years.[6]

Changes in Tracking Over Birth Cohorts

The societal and environmental changes that occurred during the last decades, resulting in a pronounced upward shift especially at the upper end of the BMI distribution over time, may influence the tracking of BMI. In Copenhagen, Denmark, correlations between BMIs at childhood ages (7 and 13 years) increased across birth cohorts from 1930 to 1969,[7] but correlations between child BMI and adult BMI were stable across birth cohorts.[5]

PREVALENCE AND INCIDENCE OF OVERWEIGHT AND OBESITY IN CHILDREN AND ADOLESCENTS

Prevalence by Sex and Age

Using the age- and sex-specific WHO growth reference for children, mean BMI and prevalence of underweight, overweight and obesity were recently estimated among children aged 5–19 years (Table 10.1).[8] The global averages of the prevalence of obesity reflect a wide range

TABLE 10.1
Body Mass Index (BMI) Categories and Global Prevalence of Underweight, Overweight, and Obesity in Children Aged 5–19 Years[a]

BMI Category	PREVALENCE (%)	
	Girls	Boys
Moderate and severe underweight	8.4	12.4
Mild underweight	17.5	19.2
Healthy weight	56.6	49.2
Overweight not obese	11.8	11.4
Obesity	5.6	7.8

[a]Adapted from: NCD Risk Factor Collaboration (NCD-RisC). Worldwide trends in body-mass index, underweight, overweight, and obesity from 1975 to 2016: a pooled analysis of 2416 population-based measurement studies in 128.9 million children, adolescents, and adults. Lancet. 2017;390:2627–2642. Numbers downloaded from: http://ncdrisc.org/data-downloads-adiposity-ado.html, weighted by population sizes.

of prevalence levels, from <2% in several countries in Africa and Asia up to 30% in some of the Pacific islands. These overall high levels constitute a serious public health problem with around 50 million girls and 75 million boys classified as obese in 2016.[8]

Changes in Prevalence over Time

Mean BMI and the prevalence and severity of overweight and obesity among children and adolescents increased significantly in most global regions and countries during the last four decades and more so in regions with low levels of obesity.[8–10] However, the prevalence levels and mean BMI in boys and girls have now plateaued in many high-income countries, albeit at high levels, whereas it is still increasing in parts of Africa, Asia, the Caribbean, Oceania, and Central and South America.[8]

Since the interwar period, the obesity epidemic among schoolchildren in Copenhagen evolved in two phases of increasing and stable prevalence.[9,10] Australian schoolchildren showed a similar pattern.[11] The changes over time were not concordant with the continuous economic growth in Denmark, but occurred by birth cohorts,[9,10] suggesting that some, so far unknown, changes in early life conditions initiated these increases in obesity prevalence.

Incidence of Overweight and Obesity

The incidence of overweight and obesity, defined as newly developed overweight and obesity within a specified time period, implies that there has been a departure from the tracking of body weight. Several studies have reported on the incidence of overweight and obesity among children and adolescents from different countries.[7,12–17] Differences in the definitions of overweight and obesity and the ages of the children influence the results.[7,12–17] The incidence of overweight[14,16] and obesity[12,16,17] was slightly higher among boys than among girls, and the incidence rates declined with increasing age.[12,17] Not surprisingly, the incidence of obesity was higher in children who were already overweight.[12,13,17]

The increase in prevalence of childhood obesity may be due to increases in incidence and/or decreases in remission and hence an increase in the persistence or duration of obesity. Among Danish children the early development of the obesity epidemic was due to an increase in both incidence and persistence.[7] The respective contributions of differences in incidence and persistence to the trends in more recent years and in other age groups need further studies.

PREVALENCE OF UNDERWEIGHT IN CHILDREN AND ADOLESCENTS

Globally, approximately 10% of children aged 5–19 years are moderately to severely underweight (Table 10.1). The worldwide prevalence of moderate to severe underweight decreased slightly from 1975 to 2016; it fell from 9% to 8% among girls and from 15% to 12% among boys.[8] The decline was smaller than the increase in the prevalence of obesity in most regions. Consequently, the mean value of BMI moved upwards and the distribution became more right skewed. The numbers of moderately and severely underweight children peaked in the year 2000 and subsequently decreased to 75 million girls and 117 million boys in 2016.[8]

PERSISTENCE OF OVERWEIGHT AND OBESITY

Heavy children often remain overweight or obese as adults, but the likelihood of persistence strongly depends, as expected, on the degree of childhood overweight or obesity[4,18] and the age of the children and the adults.[5] A review reported a relative risk of 2–10 for an overweight child to stay overweight as adult compared with a normal weight child.[4] Even though the positive predictive values are high, the sensitivity values are not; thus, although many overweight children are also overweight or obese in adulthood, most overweight and obese adults were not overweight or obese as children, so the proportion of overweight or obese in both childhood and adulthood is relatively small.[5,18]

Birth weight shows a weak positive relation to childhood obesity. However, a Danish study showed that the birth weight distribution and its association with overweight did not change during the early rise in the prevalence of childhood obesity.[19] In addition, both high infant weight and early weight gain strongly relate to later childhood obesity and the strength of this association is consistent across birth cohorts from different settings and eras.[20]

Determinants of Persistence of Overweight and Obesity

The risk that overweight and obesity persists into adulthood varies greatly and depends on several factors. The risk of persistence is higher with more severe overweight and obesity in childhood, and when the child has at least one obese parent, and the risk is lower at late than at young adult ages.[4,5,21] Moreover, a recent study found that among obese adolescents, the most rapid weight gain had occurred between 2 and 6 years of age with a further rise in BMI thereafter,[22] which is in agreement with the association between early onset of adiposity rebound and later obesity.[2] Further, genetic, epigenetic, and continued environmental influences may operate. However, the parent-offspring association has not changed during the early phases of the obesity epidemic, indicating that there may not be, as often presumed, a strong synergy between genetic risk and environmental influences.[23]

CONCLUSIONS

The prevalence of overweight and obesity in children increased during the last decades in most of the global regions. Although the levels stabilize in Western countries, they are doing so at high levels. The causes of childhood overweight and obesity, and hence the reasons for the changes in prevalence, are largely unknown. Heavy children often remain overweight as adults, but the likelihood depends on several factors and varies considerably. The epidemic of childhood overweight and obesity together with a still very large number of underweight children constitutes major global health problems to which there currently is no obvious solution.

REFERENCES

1. Wabitsch M. Molecular and biologic factors with emphasis on adipose tissue development. In: Burniat W, Cole TJ, Lissau I, Poskitt EME, eds. *Child and Adolescent Obesity. Causes and Consequences, Prevention and Management.* Cambridge: University Press; 2002:50–68.

2. Rolland-Cachera MF, Deheeger M, Maillot M, Bellisle F. Early adiposity rebound: causes and consequences for obesity in children and adults. *Int J Obes.* 2006;30:S11.

3. Twisk JW. The problem of evaluating the magnitude of tracking coefficients. *Eur J Epidemiol.* 2003;18:1025–1026.

4. Singh AS, Mulder C, Twisk JW, van Mechelen W, Chinapaw MJ. Tracking of childhood overweight into adulthood: a systematic review of the literature. *Obes Rev.* 2008;9:474–488.

5. Aarestrup J, Bjerregaard LG, Gamborg M, et al. Tracking of body mass index from 7 to 69 years of age. *Int J Obes.* 2016;40:1376–1383.

6. Guo SS, Roche AF, Chumlea WC, Gardner JD, Siervogel RM. The predictive value of childhood body mass index values for overweight at age 35 y. *Am J Clin Nutr.* 1994;59:810–819.

7. Andersen LG, Baker JL, Sørensen TIA. Contributions of incidence and persistence to the prevalence of childhood obesity during the emerging epidemic in Denmark. *PLoS One.* 2012;7:e42521.

8. NCD Risk Factor Collaboration (NCD-RisC). Worldwide trends in body-mass index, underweight, overweight, and obesity from 1975 to 2016: a pooled analysis of 2416 population-based measurement studies in 128.9 million children, adolescents, and adults. *Lancet.* 2017;390:2627–2642.

9. Bua J, Olsen LW, Sørensen TIA. Secular trends in childhood obesity in Denmark during 50 years in relation to economic growth. *Obesity.* 2007;15:977–985.

10. Olsen LW, Baker JL, Holst C, Sørensen TIA. Birth cohort effect on the obesity epidemic in Denmark. *Epidemiology.* 2006;17:292–295.

11. Olds TS, Harten NR. One hundred years of growth: the evolution of height, mass, and body composition in Australian children, 1899-1999. *Hum Biol.* 2001;73:727–738.

12. Kim J, Must A, Fitzmaurice GM, et al. Incidence and remission rates of overweight among children aged 5 to 13 years in a district-wide school surveillance system. *Am J Public Health.* 2005;95:1588–1594.

13. Robbins JM, Khan KS, Lisi LM, Robbins SW, Michel SH, Torcato BR. Overweight among young children in the Philadelphia health care centers: incidence and prevalence. *Arch Pediatr Adolesc Med.* 2007;161:17–20.

14. Plachta-Danielzik S, Landsberg B, Johannsen M, Lange D, Muller MJ. Determinants of the prevalence and incidence of overweight in children and adolescents. *Public Health Nutr.* 2010;13:1870–1881.

15. Do LM, Tran TK, Eriksson B, Petzold M, Ascher H. Prevalence and incidence of overweight and obesity among Vietnamese preschool children: a longitudinal cohort study. *BMC Pediatr.* 2017;17:150.

16. Jalali-Farahani S, Amiri P, Abbasi B, et al. Maternal characteristics and incidence of overweight/obesity in children: a 13-year follow-up study in an Eastern Mediterranean population. *Matern Child Health J.* 2017;21:1211–1220.

17. Cunningham SA, Kramer MR, Narayan KM. Incidence of childhood obesity in the United States. *N Engl J Med.* 2014;370:403–411.

18. Sørensen TIA, Sonne-Holm S. Risk in childhood of development of severe adult obesity: retrospective, population-based case-cohort study. *Am J Epidemiol.* 1988;127:104–113.

19. Rugholm S, Baker JL, Olsen LW, Schack-Nielsen L, Bua J, Sørensen TIA. Stability of the association between birth weight and childhood overweight during the development of the obesity epidemic. *Obes Res.* 2005;13:2187–2194.

20. Druet C, Stettler N, Sharp S, et al. Prediction of childhood obesity by infancy weight gain: an individual-level meta-analysis. *Paediatr Perinat Epidemiol.* 2012;26:19–26.

21. Whitaker RC, Wright JA, Pepe MS, Seidel KD, Dietz WH. Predicting obesity in young adulthood from childhood and parental obesity. *N Engl J Med.* 1997;337:869–873.

22. Geserick M, Vogel M, Gausche R, et al. Acceleration of BMI in Early Childhood and Risk of Sustained Obesity. *N Engl J Med.* 2018;379:1303–1312.

23. Ajslev TA, Angquist L, Silventoinen K, Baker JL, Sørensen TIA. Stable intergenerational associations of childhood overweight during the development of the obesity epidemic. *Obesity.* 2015;23:1279–1287.

CHAPTER 11

Genetics of Eating and Weight Disorders

ANKE HINNEY, PHD • JOHANNA GIURANNA, MSC

INTRODUCTION

Monogenic forms of obesity are mostly the result of mutations in genes of the leptinergic-melanocortineric system.[1] The absence or reduced function of a gene product in this system can lead to early-onset extreme obesity. However, these variants are infrequent to rare and do not explain a large part of the high heritability of body mass index (BMI). For eating disorders, monogenic forms have not been described. Heritability estimates derived from twin studies suggest that genetic variation accounts for 50%–70% of the variance in human BMI. Twin studies for anorexia nervosa (AN), bulimia nervosa (BN), and binge eating disorder (BED) have also provided evidence for substantial heritability for the respective eating disorders.[2] The largest part of the heritability for eating and weight disorders is attributable to polygenic factors, which have become detectable by GWAS.[3–6] Such GWASs or metaanalyses thereof have been conducted for BMI, obesity, fat mass, fat-free mass, and AN. The variants (alleles) predisposing to an elevated BMI or high fat mass are identified more frequently in subjects with obesity. In AN, only a single locus has been detected; it is a matter of time until the analysis of larger sample sizes will entail the identification of further loci.[3,4,6] The respective alleles can be identified and validated as BMI/obesity or AN risk alleles by statistical analyses only with sample sizes being crucial for achievement of significant results.[1]

GWASs have proven extremely successful for complex disorders.[3–6] Major technological advances have made single nucleotide polymorphism (SNP)-based GWAS feasible and led to the identification of currently more than 50,000 loci for numerous disorders and phenotypes (http://www.ebi.ac.uk/gwas/). Within a brief period of time, GWAS revolutionized the molecular genetic analyses of complex phenotypes. Assuming an average number of 1,000,000 analyzed SNPs per individual, Bonferroni correction for multiple testing results in the P-value threshold of $p \leq 5 \times 10^{-8}$, which has been accepted as the gold standard to circumvent the problem of multiple testing.[7] Unfortunately, even upon availability of large total sample sizes in the hundreds of thousands, a large number of potentially truly associated SNPs cannot be identified due to this stringent threshold.[8] On the positive side, almost all SNPs with a $p \leq 5 \times 10^{-8}$ continue to be associated with the phenotype in question upon enlargement of the original sample size.

"Polygene" is a term used for an etiologically relevant gene in a chromosomal locus that harbors intragenic or extragenic interindividual sequence variations accounting for a small fraction of the variation of a specific quantitative trait. GWAS based on SNPs are used to detect polygenic loci. Such a polygenic locus usually encompasses more than one gene. As such, the detection of the relevant gene(s) in a locus detected via GWAS remains a complex and time-consuming task. The additive effect of such polygenes has been shown to explain almost 25% of the variance of body height.[5] For most phenotypes, however, the explained variance is at or below 5%. The explained variance crucially depends on sample size, heritability, and the genetic architecture of the respective phenotype.

A GWAS is followed-up by extensive analyses with the aim to detect the underlying gene. As a first guess the gene closest to the GWAS lead SNP (the SNP with the lowest P-value in the region) is usually regarded as a candidate gene for the analyzed trait. For obesity, only 2 of 97 GWAS hits[3] were located in the coding regions of genes. An example for the long road from a GWAS hit to the functionally relevant target gene is the fat mass and obesity-associated (*FTO*) locus. The first BMI/obesity GWAS in 2007 identified a chromosomal region that harbors the *FTO* gene.[9] It is currently still not known whether *FTO* is the gene underlying the association signal. Recent data provide impressive evidence for a major importance of genes downstream of *FTO*.[10]

MAJOR FINDINGS
Obesity
More than 700 polygenic loci relevant for body weight regulation have been identified in the most recent metaanalysis of GWAS for BMI, the results of which have preliminarily published in a non-peer reviewed article. This recent update of previous GWAS metaanalyses of the Genetic Investigation of ANthropometric Traits consortium (GIANT; http://portals.broadinstitu te.org/collaboration/giant/index.php/GIANT_consor tium) combined the analysis of N~700,000 individuals. A total of 716 near-independent SNPs associated with BMI, upon use of a very strict genome-wide significance threshold of $p < 1 \times 10^{-8}$, were identified; 554 of these were novel. These genome-wide significant SNPs explained ~5% of the variance of BMI in an independent sample.[5] The interindividual heterogeneity is pronounced and implies that a specific set of polygenic variants predisposing to obesity in any one individual will rarely overlap with those of an independent obese subject.[1,11]

The largest GIANT GWAS for BMI, that was published as a peer-reviewed article, comprised 339,224 individuals and identified 97 BMI-associated loci, 41 of which had been detected in previous GWAS. These loci accounted for ~2.7% of the BMI variation. Based on the central expression of most of the genes in the respective loci, a major role of the central nervous system was postulated. The mean additive effect of the lead SNP risk alleles at the 97 BMI loci in 8164 individuals of European descent averaged 0.1 BMI units (kg/m²). Therefore, homozygous and heterozygous carriers of a body height in the range of 160–180 cm weigh 512–648 g and 256–324 g, respectively, more than an individual without any such allele with the mean effect size. The number of weight-increasing alleles is correlated with BMI. Mean BMI was 1.8 kg/m² higher in the 145 people carrying the greatest number of BMI-increasing alleles (>104), relative to those carrying the mean number of these alleles in the sample. This amounts to 4.6–5.8 kg for a person 160–180 cm tall.[3]

A more recent GWAS for BMI in Japanese subjects (n = 173,430) revealed a total of 112 new BMI loci. The annotation of associated variants with cell type–specific regulatory marks showed an enrichment of variants in CD19+ cells. Genetic correlations between BMI and lymphocyte count were also described implicating lymphocytes in body weight regulation.[4]

Anorexia Nervosa
The first GWAS for AN to pick up a significant locus included a total of 3495 patients with AN and 10,982 controls.[6] The single genome-wide significant locus was identified on chromosome 12 (lead SNP: rs4622308). Interestingly, the respective chromosomal region comprises previously reported hits for diabetes mellitus type 1 and autoimmune disorders.[6]

In 2017, a GWAS focusing on low frequency and rare variants (exome chip) was performed in 2158 cases with AN from nine populations of European origin and 15,485 controls. None of the low-frequency/rare variants showed genome-wide associations with AN.[12] The absence of an association of infrequent variants with AN might be explained by the small number of analyzed individuals in combination with small effect sizes. Alternatively, a major effect of genetic variation outside of the exome currently cannot be excluded.[12]

Composite Phenotype, Cross-Trait, and Look-Up Studies
For BMI/obesity the metaanalyses of GWAS have proven successful. Data were additionally used either for (1) composite phenotypes which comprise a number of obesity- and BMI-related traits or (2) traits/disorders, for which deviations from a normal BMI distribution had been described on clinical terms (e.g., eating disorders, attention deficit hyperactivity disorder, bipolar disorder, schizophrenia, Alzheimer's disease; i.e., "cross-phenotype, cross-disorder, cross-trait" analyses). Such cross-phenotype analyses can also be performed without a clear-cut *a priori* hypothesis. The current major findings are summarized in the following paragraphs.

Composite Phenotype Analyses
Recently, large metaanalyses of GWAS for single anthropometric traits (BMI, height, weight, waist and hip circumference, waist-to-hip ratio) were used for combined analyses. Six novel loci were detected with an effect on body shape as a composite phenotype that is represented by a combination of six anthropometric traits. These results underscore the value of using multiple traits to define complex phenotypes.[13]

Cross-Trait Analyses
A method (cross-trait Linkage Disequilibrium SCore regression; LDSC) to estimate genetic correlations from GWAS summary statistics had been established.

Initially, LDSC was used to estimate 276 genetic correlations of 24 traits including obesity, AN, and educational attainment. A negative genetic correlation between BMI and AN was observed. Hence, a substantial subgroup of alleles associated with lower BMI/leanness overlaps with the SNP-based genetic predisposition to AN.[14] Other negative genetic correlations were found between AN and serum fasting insulin and glucose levels and triglycerides and low-density lipoproteins. Positive LDSC genetic correlations were reported between AN and schizophrenia, neuroticism, educational attainment, and high-density lipoprotein cholesterol. Thus, AN is genetically related to both mental phenotypes and metabolic traits.[6]

The extent of shared genetic contributions has also been analyzed for 23 psychiatric and neurological brain disorders (n = 842,820), 11 quantitative and 4 dichotomous traits of interest (n = 722,125). For psychiatric disorders, substantial sharing of common variant risk was shown, whereby many of the neurological disorders seemed more distinct from each other. Little evidence was detected for sharing of common genetic risk between neurological and psychiatric disorders. Overlapping genetic predispositions between brain disorders (e.g., major depressive disorder and neuroticism personality score) and anthropometric measures (e.g., BMI, height) were also detected.[15] For educational attainment a GWAS (discovery: 293,723 individuals, replication: 111,349 individuals) recently identified 74 genome-wide significant loci associated with the number of completed years of schooling. There was a negative correlation between genetic variation associated with school attainment and BMI, so that a subset of SNPs associated with an increased school attainment are also associated with lower BMI.[16]

Although previously undetermined genetic correlations between different traits/disorders have now become detectable, the precise genetic variants that underlie such correlations have remained elusive. This drawback was recently overcome by introduction of a new method that combines the advantage of a cross-trait analysis by summary statistics with the localization of the hits gained by the combined analysis. Turley et al.[17] introduced multitrait analysis of GWAS (MTAG). The method can be used for joint analyses of summary statistics from GWAS of different traits, even including overlapping samples. For some tested traits (depressive symptoms, neuroticism, and subjective well-being), the number of identified loci increased considerably. MTAG provides the opportunity to prioritize SNPs for functional analyses, as SNPs relevant for both traits are depicted.[17] Thus these SNPs and their surrounding genomic regions can be analyzed in functional *in vitro* studies.

Look-Up Studies

Complementary to these approaches that use GWAS summary statistics, a number of look-ups have been performed: GWAS hits for one trait (e.g., BMI/obesity) were looked-up in GWAS data for related traits (e.g., AN) and vice versa, to identify shared genetic variants. Thus, the look-up of the 1000 SNPs with the lowest *P*-values in a GWAS for AN (no genome-wide significant SNP in the respective study)[18] in the GWAS for BMI[19] revealed three genomic regions seemingly relevant for both. Risk alleles were the same for AN and lower BMI. Special attention was drawn to a locus on chromosome 10 because the SNP allele associations with lower BMI were mainly driven by females. Additionally, in mice hypothalamic expression of the gene C-Terminal Binding Protein 2 (*CTBP2*) was altered by fasting and overfeeding in opposite directions.[20] The most recent GWAS for BMI[5] revealed that all SNPs identified in the look-up of AN SNPs have now become genome-wide significantly associated with lower BMI. Hence, the approach was successful to identify "true" BMI GWAS hits among the SNPs that did not reach genome-wide significant association in smaller study groups (unpublished data). Another example for a successful look-up was based on a cross-disorder analysis for Alzheimer's disease and obesity which identified a SNP (rs10838725) at the locus CUGBP, elav-like family member 1 gene *(CELF1)* that is genome-wide significant for both traits.[21]

CONCLUSION

Molecular genetic studies have identified a small number of major genes for human obesity. The underlying rare to infrequent mutations have a profound impact on the development of an extremely high body weight. However, the genetic predisposition to obesity is mainly polygenic. The contribution of each single polygene to the development of eating and weight disorders is small. The identification and confirmation of loci associated with these disorders requires the analysis of thousands of individuals.

More than 700 polygenic loci for body weight regulation have currently been reported.[4,22] Variation in genes expressed in the central nervous system plays a prominent role in BMI variation.[3] As the role of the brain in behavior and energy balance is pivotal, this is not surprising. Another study revealed evidence for the relevance of lymphocytes in body weight regulation.[4]

Only 5% of the heritability of BMI variation is explained by GWAS so far.[5] Effect sizes of the currently detected polygenes are mostly very small. Undoubtedly, sample sizes need to be further enlarged (over one million subjects) to detect further signals. For AN the first GWAS hit was detected[6]; increments in total available sample size will also lead to the identification of more polygenic loci for this eating disorder.

Cross-trait/-disorder analyses have revealed genetic loci that had been overlooked in single-trait analyses. Advances in statistical analyses (e.g., MTAG[17]) will speed up the detection of additional variants. The methods will be useful for both weight and eating disorders.

Recently a large-scale study revealed evidence for an interplay between genetic factors for BMI and dietary patterns. In 8828 women from the Nurses' Health Study and 5218 men from the Health Professionals Follow-up Study, a genetic predisposition score was calculated based on 77 SNPs associated with BMI. Three different dietary patterns were assessed (Alternate Healthy Eating Index 2010: AHEI-2010, Dietary Approach to Stop Hypertension: DASH, and Alternate Mediterranean Diet: AMED). Surprisingly, during a 20-year follow-up, genetic association with BMI changes was attenuated with increasing adherence to a healthy diet (AHEI-2010) in both study groups. The higher the genetic loading, or the more BMI increasing alleles the participants harbored, the higher the weight reduction. The study implied that better adherence to healthy dietary patterns might attenuate the genetic predisposition to weight gain. Even more strikingly, individuals with the highest genetic risk for obesity profited most.[23]

OUTLOOK

Recent advances in technology and statistical analyses along with considerable increments in proband numbers led to the identification of a substantial number of variants involved in body weight regulation; the first genome-wide locus for AN was also recently detected. The genetic makeup of an individual likely has an effect on weight loss upon adherence to a healthy diet.[23] As the costs of the detailed genetic analyses have rapidly decreased during the last years, it is conceivable that genetic data will be integrated into routine medical checkups. Future analysis of genetic mechanisms in weight and eating disorders will substantiate our understanding of the mechanisms leading to eating and weight disorders and hopefully lead to improved therapeutic approaches.

ACKNOWLEDGMENTS

This work was supported by grants from the Bundesministerium für Bildung und Forschung (NGFNplus 01GS0820), the Deutsche Forschungsgemeinschaft (HE 1446/4-1, HI 865/2-1), and the European Union (FP7 n245009 NeuroFast).

REFERENCES

1. Hebebrand J, Hinney A, Knoll N, Volckmar AL, Scherag A. Molecular genetic aspects of weight regulation. *Dtsch Arztebl Int.* 2013;110(19):338–344.
2. Mayhew AJ, Pigeyre M, Couturier J, Meyre D. An evolutionary genetic perspective of eating disorders. *Neuroendocrinology.* 2018;106(3):292–306.
3. Locke AE, Kahali B, Berndt SI, et al. Genetic studies of body mass index yield new insights for obesity biology. *Nature.* 2015;518(7538):197–206.
4. Akiyama M, Okada Y, Kanai M, et al. Genome-wide association study identifies 112 new loci for body mass index in the Japanese population. *Nat Genet.* 2017;49(10):1458–1467.
5. Yengo L, Sidorenko J, Kemper KE, et al. Meta-analysis of genome-wide association studies for height and body mass index in ~700,000 individuals of European ancestry. *Biorxiv.* 2018. https://doi.org/10.1101/274654.
6. Duncan L, Yilmaz Z, Gaspar H, et al. Significant locus and metabolic genetic correlations revealed in genome-wide association study of anorexia nervosa. *Am J Psychiatry.* 2017;174(9):850–858.
7. Dudbridge F, Gusnanto A. Estimation of significance thresholds for genomewide association scans. *Genet Epidemiol.* 2008;32(3):227–234.
8. Stahl EA, Wegmann D, Trynka G, et al. Bayesian inference analyses of the polygenic architecture of rheumatoid arthritis. *Nat Genet.* 2012;44(5):483–489.
9. Frayling TM, Timpson NJ, Weedon MN, et al. A common variant in the FTO gene is associated with body mass index and predisposes to childhood and adult obesity. *Science.* 2007;316(5826):889–894.
10. Claussnitzer M, Dankel SN, Kim KH, et al. FTO obesity variant circuitry and adipocyte browning in humans. *N Engl J Med.* 2015;373(10):895–907.
11. Walley AJ, Asher JE, Froguel P. The genetic contribution to non-syndromic human obesity. *Nat Rev Genet.* 2009;10(7):431–442.
12. Huckins LM, Hatzikotoulas K, Southam L, et al. Investigation of common, low-frequency and rare genomewide variation in anorexia nervosa. *Mol Psychiatry.* 2017;23(5):1169–1180.
13. Ried JS, Jeff MJ, Chu AY, et al. A principal component meta-analysis on multiple anthropometric traits identifies novel loci for body shape. *Nat Commun.* 2016;7:13357.
14. Bulik-Sullivan B, Finucane HK, Anttila V, et al. An atlas of genetic correlations across human diseases and traits. *Nat Genet.* 2015;47(11):1236–1241.

15. Anttila V, Bulik-Sullivan B, Finucane HK, et al. Analysis of shared heritability in common disorders of the brain. *BioRxiv.* 2016. https://doi.org/10.1101/048991.

16. Okbay A, Beauchamp JP, Fontana MA, et al. Genome-wide association study identifies 74 loci associated with educational attainment. *Nature.* 2016;533(7604):539–542.

17. Turley P, Walters RK, Maghzian O, et al. Multi-trait analysis of genome-wide association summary statistics using MTAG. *Nat Genet.* 2018;50(2):229–237.

18. Boraska V, Franklin CS, Floyd JA, et al. A genome-wide association study of anorexia nervosa. *Mol Psychiatry.* 2014;19(10):1085–1094.

19. Speliotes EK, Willer CJ, Berndt SI, et al. Association analyses of 249,796 individuals reveal 18 new loci associated with body mass index. *Nat Genet.* 2010;42(11):937–948.

20. Hinney A, Kesselmeier M, Jall S, et al. Evidence for three genetic loci involved in both anorexia nervosa risk and variation of body mass index. *Mol Psychiatry.* 2017;22(2):192–201.

21. Hinney A, Albayrak O, Antel J, et al. Genetic variation at the CELF1 (CUGBP, elav-like family member 1 gene) locus is genome-wide associated with Alzheimer's disease and obesity. *Am J Med Genet B Neuropsychiatr Genet.* 2014;165B(4):283–293.

22. Yazdi FT, Clee SM, Meyre D. Obesity genetics in mouse and human: back and forth, and back again. *PeerJ.* 2015;3:e856.

23. Wang T, Heianza Y, Sun D, et al. Improving adherence to healthy dietary patterns, genetic risk, and long term weight gain: gene-diet interaction analysis in two prospective cohort studies. *BMJ.* 2018;360:j5644.

CHAPTER 12

Influence of Hormones on the Development of Eating Disorders

KATHERINE A. THOMPSON, MA • ALEXANDRA J. MILLER, BS • JESSICA H. BAKER, PHD

INTRODUCTION

This chapter discusses the role of reproductive and appetite hormones in the etiology of eating disorders (EDs). We focus on the reproductive hormones estrogen and progesterone and the appetite hormones leptin and ghrelin in adult female populations, given that research to date has focused here. Although other hormones have been examined,[1] more research is needed about their functions in EDs and obesity during childhood and adolescence. We describe the child and adolescent literature where available.

REPRODUCTIVE HORMONES

Reproductive hormones act on human behavior in an organizational-activational manner. Organizational effects occur by shaping the growth and patterns of neural circuits during development (i.e., in utero and during adolescence) and are considered stable and permanent. Activational effects occur by stimulating, regulating, or inhibiting behaviors associated with the presence or absence of the hormones within the existing circuits and can be less permanent since they influence behavior only after the neural circuits in the brain are developed.

Estradiol and Progesterone

Early data regarding the link between estradiol (primary estrogen–based hormone) and eating behaviors showed that ovariectomized animals experienced significant increases in food intake, meal size, and body weight,[2] which were reversed upon estradiol administration.[3] Thus, estradiol has an inhibiting effect on food intake. In contrast, progesterone (primary progestogen steroid) does not have a direct effect on eating behaviors: ovariectomized animals show no changes in food intake with progesterone administration.[4]

Eating disorders

Research examining the role of reproductive hormones in the etiology of EDs has generally explored connections at the symptom level. Initial studies that examined whether ED symptoms fluctuate over the menstrual cycle indicated that binge eating and emotional eating are higher during the midluteal and premenstrual phases of the cycle compared with the follicular and ovulatory phases. Additionally, psychological symptoms including body dissatisfaction and weight preoccupation fluctuate during the menstrual cycle, with the highest levels during the premenstrual and menstrual phases.[4]

There are also significant associations between hormone concentrations and ED symptoms. In women with bulimia nervosa (BN) binge eating and purging behaviors increase when estradiol concentrations diminish.[5] Similarly, animal models show an increase in the consumption of highly palatable foods in ovariectomized rats compared with nonovariectomized rats.[6] There are also negative associations between decreased estradiol and psychological symptoms of EDs in humans including body dissatisfaction, weight/shape concerns, drive for thinness, and preoccupation with weight.[4]

In regard to progesterone, a positive relationship has been observed with binge eating in women with BN[5] and with body dissatisfaction and drive for thinness in young adults.[4] Progesterone also has indirect effects on ED symptoms when considered in the presence of estradiol simultaneously: emotional eating increases when *both* progesterone and estradiol levels are elevated. However, the independent effect of progesterone is not significant.[7]

Some have also explored hormone administration as a supplement to standard ED treatments. For

Eating Disorders and Obesity in Children and Adolescents. https://doi.org/10.1016/B978-0-323-54852-6.00012-4

example, physiological doses of estradiol improve bone mass density in adolescent girls with anorexia nervosa (AN).[8] Additionally, a 3-month administration of an estradiol-based oral contraceptive among women with BN showed a reduction in compensatory behaviors, meal-related hunger, and gastric distention[9]—although conclusions are limited given this was not a randomized trial. Estradiol and progesterone may serve a beneficial function for ED treatments.

Obesity

Estradiol can be linked to obesity indirectly via eating behaviors and through direct effects on adiposity. A review of the literature described that estrogen levels are higher in nonobese compared with obese premenopausal women as well as an association between diminished levels of estrogens during menopause and increased total obesity.[10,11] Although menopause is markedly distinct from childhood, menopause provides a quasi-experimental design to examine the influence of changing reproductive hormones on obesity that may extrapolate to adolescence. Once puberty is transversed, adolescent estrogen levels may have a direct impact on obesity. Indeed, estradiol administration in animals increases carbohydrate and lipid metabolism, thus the effect of estrogen on obesity could be a result of metabolic capacity and stimulation.[12] Regarding progesterone, animal models indicate that progesterone interacts with estrogen to effect obesity such that progesterone administration negates the metabolic effects of estrogen by decreasing the capacity for carbohydrate and lipid metabolism. Thus, increased concentrations of progesterone result in a metabolic state that is similar to metabolic syndrome—in which fat concentrations increase and the body is unable to process them.[12]

Taken together, estradiol appears to have a direct, activational effect on ED symptoms and obesity. Specifically, *lower* levels of estradiol are associated with more binge eating, increased ED symptoms, and increased body fat. Progesterone primarily assumes a moderating role such that increasing levels of progesterone may counteract the protective effect of increasing estradiol. Progesterone additionally limits metabolic capacity increasing the likelihood of obesity.

APPETITE HORMONES
Leptin

Leptin is an appetite suppressant, which regulates satiety and increases energy expenditure. Following a meal, leptin secretion increases, signaling fullness.

Eating disorders

Leptin concentrations are lower in individuals with AN and BN compared with healthy controls. One explanation for decreased leptin in AN is the direct link between leptin and body mass index (BMI): decreased leptin levels are a consequence of the low BMIs characteristic of individuals with AN. Corroborating this, food deprivation for several days or weeks results in a significant decline in leptin levels,[13] and leptin concentrations increase once body weight is restored in AN.[1] However, leptin administration in rats with activity-based AN suppresses hyperactivity, suggesting that decreased leptin may have an etiological role in excessive exercise often observed in AN.[14] Moreover, leptin might influence AN outcome and relapse, such that *higher* leptin levels at discharge from inpatient treatment increase risk, albeit inconsistently,[15] for a poorer treatment outcome.[16] Regarding BN, decreased leptin may contribute to binge eating and decreased metabolic rates,[1] whereas children and adolescents who experience loss of control eating episodes have higher fasting leptin levels than those who do not.[17]

Obesity

Obese adolescents exhibit higher levels of leptin relative to nonobese adolescents. Despite leptin's influence on decreasing caloric intake and increasing energy expenditure, increasing leptin fails to prevent progression of obesity. Consequently, obesity is thought to be, in part, the result of leptin resistance. For example, high levels of leptin in children at increased risk for adult obesity (i.e., the child was overweight and/or had overweight parents) predicts future weight gain.[18] Furthermore, leptin administration is ineffective for weight loss in obese individuals.[19] Thus, leptin resistance may promote and maintain obesity regardless of age.

Ghrelin

Ghrelin acts as an appetite stimulant and rises before a meal, reduces feelings of satiety, increases caloric intake, and decreases after meals in healthy adults. Conversely, some data show that children's ghrelin levels remain stable in response to meals,[20] whereas others indicate ghrelin decreases after eating, staying constant over the next 2 h.[21]

Eating disorders

Adolescent females with AN have significantly higher levels of ghrelin than healthy controls. This may be a consequence of both ghrelin's reliance on energy stores and meal status since ghrelin levels tend to normalize once body weight is restored.[1] Further, ghrelin levels increase when individuals intentionally eat less,[22] and food restriction and losing weight by dieting have been linked to rises in ghrelin.[23] However, individuals with AN may have a reduced sensitivity to ghrelin signals such that individuals with AN do not experience an increase in appetite, hunger, or GH receptor response upon ghrelin administration as compared with constitutionally thin or normal weight individuals.[1] Although a small pilot study observed increased food intake after administration of ghrelin in AN,[24] the small sample size and lack of randomization hamper the conclusions that can be drawn.

Associations between ghrelin and BN are less consistent. However, the ghrelin response may be blunted in individuals with BN compared with healthy controls such that it fails to decrease as expected following a standardized meal.[25] This suggests that ghrelin may play a role in binge episodes due to deficiencies in postmeal satiety. Testing this hypothesis, Monteleone et al.[26] presented individuals with BN and healthy controls a meal—who were allowed to smell and chew the food but not swallow it—and found that individuals with BN had greater ghrelin increases than controls and binge-purge frequency was positively associated to this increase.

Obesity

Obese children and adults have diminished concentrations of ghrelin compared with nonobese individuals. For obese children specifically, this diminishment of ghrelin persists after weight loss.[27] Interestingly, animal studies suggest that mice with a ghrelin deficiency administered high-fat diets at a young age develop a resistance to obesity.[28] A ghrelin "vaccine" created to elicit antibodies against ghrelin tested on diet-induced obese mice demonstrated reductions in weight gain by decreasing body fat accumulation and increasing energy expenditure.[29] Thus, low ghrelin levels may play a protective role in obesity—in converse, high levels may elevate risk.

Taken together, it is uncertain whether leptin and ghrelin are involved in the etiology of an ED. In particular, decreased leptin levels may be a consequence of reduced body fat percentage and malnutrition characteristics of AN. However, both leptin and ghrelin may contribute to ED maintenance and/or relapse. Leptin and ghrelin may also play an indirect role in etiology via reproductive hormones. Estradiol attenuates the potency of ghrelin such that exogenous ghrelin administration is less potent in intact female rats compared with ovariectomized rats, whereas leptin sensitivity is impaired in ovariectomized rats.[30] Thus, changes in estradiol that occur with EDs could influence the

production of and sensitivity to appetite hormones. In contrast, both seem to have a direct role in obesity: obesity is thought to be in part due to leptin resistance, whereas ghrelin-deficient animals develop a resistance to obesity.

PUBERTY

Eating Disorders

Puberty is a risk period for the onset of an ED and is a period of dramatic hormonal changes. For example, not only do estrogen and progesterone increase, leptin plays a crucial role in pubertal onset by informing the brain the amount of fat required for the onset of puberty. A preponderance of data indicates that puberty is associated with ED onset, and one mechanism explaining this link is reproductive hormones.[31] Following organizational-activational effects, it is theorized that the genetic effects for EDs that organize during the prenatal period become activated during puberty via reproductive hormones to increase risk for EDs in girls. In line with this, the heritability of ED symptoms among girls before puberty is roughly 0% yet increases to more than 50% during and after puberty.[31] Estradiol may be an important moderator for these effects as estradiol increases markedly during puberty and regulates several genes that have been linked to EDs. Thus, puberty and the changes in estradiol that occur during puberty may activate the prenatally organized genetic risk for an ED in adolescents with a genetic vulnerability.

Obesity

Approximately, 50% of adult body weight is gained during the pubertal transition between childhood and adolescence. During puberty girls experience an increase in percent body fat and fat mass due to interactions between estradiol and growth hormones. There is also an increase and redistribution of adipose tissue thought to be due to increasing estrogen.[10] Thus, pubertal timing may be important in the development of obesity. For example, age of menarche is inversely related to BMI among girls suggesting that experiencing early-onset menarche (<11 years) increased the risk for having a BMI>75th percentile by more than 1.75 times.[32] Importantly, however, obesity can also lead to early-onset puberty. Taken together with observations of the association between reproductive hormones and obesity, it is possible that puberty is a period of risk for obesity and that once puberty is complete reproductive hormones play an important role in etiology.

CONCLUSION

The adult female literature indicates reproductive hormones and puberty play a role in the etiology of EDs and obesity, whereas the direct influence of appetite hormones is less clear. Although studies of children and adolescence are limited, we conclude the following: reproductive hormones, estradiol in particular, (1) activate the genetic risk for EDs at puberty,[31] (2) cause transient changes in ED symptoms across the menstrual cycle, (3) slow down metabolism, and (4) may increase fat mass and decrease lean mass concentrations during puberty and play a causal role in obesity once puberty is complete. Regarding leptin and ghrelin, (1) differences observed between individuals with an ED or obesity and healthy controls may be a consequence of the disorder, (2) changes in leptin and ghrelin may impact maintenance and relapse in EDs, (3) leptin resistance is involved in obesity, whereas ghrelin deficiency is protective, and (4) the impact of appetite hormones on an ED may be mediated through reproductive hormones.

REFERENCES

1. Culbert KM, Racine SE, Klump KL. Hormonal factors and disturbances in eating disorders. *Curr Psychiatry Rep.* 2016;18(7):65.
2. Wade GN. Some effects of ovarian hormones on food intake and body weight in female rats. *J Comp Physiol Psychol.* 1975;88(1):183–193.
3. Geary N, Asarian L. Cyclic estradiol treatment normalizes body weight and test meal size in ovariectomized rats. *Physiol Behav.* 1999;67(1):141–147.
4. Baker JH, Girdler SS, Bulik CM. The role of reproductive hormones in the development and maintenance of eating disorders. *Expert Rev Obstet Gynecol.* 2012;7(6):573–583.
5. Edler C, Lipson SF, Keel PK. Ovarian hormones and binge eating in bulimia nervosa. *Psychol Med.* 2007;37(1):131–141.
6. Klump KL, Suisman JL, Culbert KM, Kashy DA, Keel PK, Sisk CL. The effects of ovariectomy on binge eating proneness in adult female rats. *Horm Behav.* 2011;59(4):585–593.
7. Klump KL, Keel PK, Racine SE, et al. The interactive effects of estrogen and progesterone on changes in emotional eating across the menstrual cycle. *J Abnorm Psychol.* 2013;122(1):131–137.
8. Misra M, Katzman D, Miller KK, et al. Physiologic estrogen replacement increases bone density in adolescent girls with anorexia nervosa. *J Bone Miner Res.* 2011;26(10):2430–2438.
9. Naessén S, Carlström K, Byström B, Pierre Y, Hirschberg AL. Effects of an antiandrogenic oral contraceptive on appetite and eating behavior in bulimic women. *Psychoneuroendocrinology.* 2007;32(5):548–554.
10. Leeners B, Geary N, Tobler PN, Asarian L. Ovarian hormones and obesity. *Hum Reprod Update.* 2017;28:1–15.
11. Mayes JS, Watson GH. Direct effects of sex steroid hormones on adipose tissues and obesity. *Obes Rev.* 2004;5(4):197–216.
12. Campbell SE, Febbraio MA. Effects of ovarian hormones on exercise metabolism. *Curr Opin Clin Nutr Metab Care.* 2001;4(6):515–520.
13. Wolfe BE, Jimerson DC, Orlova C, Mantzoros CS. Effect of dieting on plasma leptin, soluble leptin receptor, adiponectin and resistin levels in healthy volunteers. *Clin Endocrinol.* 2004;61(3):332–338.
14. Exner C, Hebebrand J, Remschmidt H, et al. Leptin suppresses semi-starvation induced hyperactivity in rats: implications for anorexia nervosa. *Mol Psychiatry.* 2000;5(5):476–481.
15. Seitz J, Bühren K, Biemann R, et al. Leptin levels in patients with anorexia nervosa following day/inpatient treatment do not predict weight 1 year post-referral. *Eur Child Adolesc Psychiatry.* 2016;25(9):1019–1025.
16. Holtkamp K, Hebebrand J, Mika C, Heer M, Heussen N, Herpertz-Dahlmann B. High serum leptin levels subsequent to weight gain predict renewed weight loss in patients with anorexia nervosa. *Psychoneuroendocrinology.* 2004;29(6):791–797.
17. Miller R, Tanofsky-Kraff M, Shomaker LB, et al. Serum leptin and loss of control eating in children and adolescents. *Int J Obes.* 2014;38(3):397–403.
18. Fleisch AF, Agarwal N, Roberts MD, et al. Influence of serum leptin on weight and body fat growth in children at high risk for adult obesity. *J Clin Endocrinol Metab.* 2007;92(3):948–954.
19. Heymsfield SB, Greenberg AS, Fujioka K, et al. Recombinant leptin for weight loss in obese and lean adults: a randomized, controlled, dose-escalation trial. *J Am Med Assoc.* 1999;282(16):1568–1575.
20. Lomenick JP, Clasey JL, Anderson JW. Meal-related changes in ghrelin, peptide YY, and appetite in normal weight and overweight children. *Obesity.* 2008;16(3):547–552.
21. Maffeis C, Bonadonna RC, Consolaro A, et al. Ghrelin, insulin sensitivity and postprandial glucose disposal in overweight and obese children. *Eur J Endocrinol.* 2006;154(1):61–68.
22. Schur EA, Cummings DE, Callahan HS, Foster-Schubert KE. Association of cognitive restraint with ghrelin, leptin, and insulin levels in subjects who are not weight-reduced. *Physiol Behav.* 2008;93(4–5):706–712.
23. Leidy HJ, Gardner JK, Frye BR, et al. Circulating ghrelin is sensitive to changes in body weight during a diet and exercise program in normal-weight young women. *J Clin Endocrinol Metab.* 2004;89(6):2659–2664.
24. Hotta M, Ohwada R, Akamizu T, Shibasaki T, Takano K, Kangawa K. Ghrelin increases hunger and food intake in patients with restricting-type anorexia nervosa: a pilot study. *Endocr J.* 2009;56(9):1119–1128.

25. Kojima S, Nakahara T, Nagai N, et al. Altered ghrelin and peptide YY responses to meals in bulimia nervosa. *Clin Endocrinol.* 2005;62(1):74–78.

26. Monteleone P, Serritella C, Scognamiglio P, Maj M. Enhanced ghrelin secretion in the cephalic phase of food ingestion in women with bulimia nervosa. *Psychoneuroendocrinology.* 2010;35(2):284–288.

27. Soriano-Guillén L, Barrios V, Chowen JA, et al. Ghrelin levels from fetal life through early adulthood: relationship with endocrine and metabolic and anthropometric measures. *J Pediatr.* 2004;144(1):30–35.

28. Wortley KE, del Rincon JP, Murray JD, et al. Absence of ghrelin protects against early-onset obesity. *J Clin Invest.* 2005;115(12):3573–3578.

29. Azegami T, Yuki Y, Sawada S, et al. Nanogel-based nasal ghrelin vaccine prevents obesity. *Mucosal Immunol.* 2017;10(5):1351–1360.

30. Brown LM, Clegg DJ. Central effects of estradiol in the regulation of food intake, body weight, and adiposity. *J Steroid Biochem Mol Biol.* 2010;122(1–3):65–73.

31. Klump KL. Puberty as a critical risk period for eating disorders: a review of human and animal studies. *Horm Behav.* 2013;64(2):399–410.

32. Ahmed ML, Ong KK, Dunger DB. Childhood obesity and the timing of puberty. *Trends Endocrinol Metab.* 2009;20(5):237–242.

CHAPTER 13

Endocrine Mechanisms in Obesity

KATRIN FISCHER, PHD • TIMO D. MÜLLER, PHD

INTRODUCTION

The German physician Julius Robert von Mayer (1814–78) enunciated in 1841 the law of conservation of energy. According to Mayer's law, to which we today refer to as the first law of thermodynamics, the energy of a closed system can neither be created nor destroyed; it can merely be transformed from one state into another. Mayer's law can be illustrated by the engine of a car, which transforms chemically bound energy (fuel) into kinetic energy (movement) and thermal energy (heat). The car is, however, like humans and all other individuals, an open rather than a closed system and as such requires external supply of energy to maintain its function. Applied to human metabolism, Mayer's law means that a stable body weight can only be maintained, if energy intake matches energy expenditure. Any prolonged deviation from this equilibrium will result in either weight gain or weight loss. Unfortunately, while Mayer's law is easy to understand in theory, it is challenging to assess its implications for body weight regulation. In order to maintain our body weight in a certain (ideal) range, our body needs to define the desired body weight; this set point then not only has to be defended against episodes of over- and undernutrition, it also has to change with age, in particular from childhood to adolescence. In childhood and adolescence, energy is required for growth, thus adding a dimension to energy regulation during these developmental stages.

The neuroendocrine regulation of food intake is a complex process that is not only regulated by a variety of endocrine factors. Our sensation of hunger and satiety is further influenced by environmental, psychological, and cultural factors, like the time of the day, mood, stress, cultural eating habits, and the accessibility and smell of food. To defend a certain body weight set point, energy intake and expenditure constantly need to be adjusted based on acute changes of the bodies energy demand. To adapt to these changes, energy intake must be regulated through factors that acutely regulate caloric intake. However, importantly, long-term information about the energy stored as fat also needs to be considered. In light of this notion, it seems obvious that the systemic regulation of energy metabolism requires a highly sophisticated endocrine system that depends on constant signal integration and on the multidirectional cross-talk of key metabolic organs. A remarkable achievement of our brain is thus that it constantly integrates information about the nutritional status of the gastrointestinal (GI) tract and the adipose tissue and then modulates energy intake and expenditure to defend a certain body weight set point. The aim of this chapter is to discuss the key endocrine mechanisms implicated in the regulation of systemic energy balance. The chapter complements Chapter 3 (Appetite regulation) and thus puts a focus on selected key peripheral endocrine signals affecting energy metabolism.

The most basic role of the GI tract is the mechanical and enzymatic digestion of food to promote intestinal nutrient absorption. The GI tract represents the largest endocrine organ of the body and is, together with its adjacent organs, the liver and the pancreas, specialized to produce and secrete a variety of hormones with auto-, para-, and endocrine actions to modulate gastric acid secretion (gastrin, secretin), gut motility (GLP-1, GLP-2, PYY, CCK, motilin, ghrelin), gastric emptying (amylin, CCK, OXM, GLP-1), pancreatic enzyme activity (CCK, PYY), and the regulation of glucose metabolism (GLP-1, GIP, glucagon, insulin, amylin, somatostatin, ghrelin). Many of these signal the energy status to the brain and either directly or indirectly affect energy intake and/or expenditure. Some of these endocrine factors can be separated into acute (short-term) or chronic (long-term) regulators of food intake and adiposity. The short-term regulators of food intake (like ghrelin, CCK, GLP-1, PYY) are secreted in either response or anticipation of incoming nutrients

Eating Disorders and Obesity in Children and Adolescents. https://doi.org/10.1016/B978-0-323-54852-6.00013-6

and inform the brain about the acute fuel status of the GI tract. The brain responds to these signals by either acutely stimulating or inhibiting food intake. In contrast, the long-term regulators of systems metabolism (like leptin, adiponectin, insulin, and amylin) are constantly (tonically) secreted into the circulation. The blood concentrations of these factors change in positive (leptin, amylin, insulin) or negative (adiponectin) proportion to body fat and inform the brain about the amount of energy stored as fat. Under nonpathological conditions, the decrease or increase in body fat is thus transmitted via these circulating adiposity signals to the brain, which responds to changes in body fat by, e.g., modulating the sensitivity to short-term satiety/hunger signals to either stimulate or inhibit food intake, to increase/decrease resting energy expenditure and physical activity, thereby defending the body weight set point.

LEPTIN

Discovered in 1994 by positional cloning of the mouse obese (ob) gene,[1] leptin has like no other hormone pioneered our understanding of how peripheral endocrine signals integrate into the complex central network that regulates systems metabolism. The discovery of leptin has not only established the white adipose tissue as an endocrine organ, it has also revolutionized our understanding of how this organ can be targeted pharmacologically. Soon after its discovery, leptin was shown to correct obesity in leptin-deficient ob/ob mice.[2-4] Remarkably, those early studies not only already demonstrated that the anorexigenic effect of leptin is mediated via its action on the central nervous system (CNS)[3] but also showed that leptin improves insulin sensitivity, notably even prior to the much-applauded weight loss.[2,5] Based on these data, leptin received a lot of attention as the long-desired pharmacological silver bullet to fight the ever-rising obesity and diabetes pandemic. Indeed, exogenous supplementation of leptin is effective to correct obesity and insulin resistance in individuals with hypoleptinemia, such as in ob/ob mice,[2-4] congenitally leptin-deficient humans,[6] and individuals with lipodystrophy.[7] Unfortunately, leptin supplementation proved ineffective to improve obesity under conditions of hyperleptinemia.[8] Such leptin resistance is observed in the most common form of obesity, which is of polygenic nature and does not result from a rare loss-of-function mutation in a single key metabolic gene. Notably, while the mechanistic underpinnings of leptin resistance are still subjects of intense scientific investigation, there is evidence indicating that dietary fat and

sugar are detrimental to leptin sensitivity and entail leptin resistance even before the onset of obesity and hyperleptinemia.[9] Nevertheless, several pharmacotherapies have been demonstrated to improve leptin resistance. These include treatment of obese leptin-resistant rodents with celastrol[10] or withaferin A,[11] or adjunct administration of leptin with either amylin,[12] FGF21, exendin-4,[13] or a GLP-1/glucagon dual-agonist.[14]

Leptin acts on the hypothalamic pro-opiomelanocortin (POMC) neurons to decrease food intake and to increase energy expenditure (see Chapter 3 for more details). Beyond its action on the melanocortinergic system, leptin exerts a variety of effects outside the control of food intake. These effects include the regulation of glucose metabolism, hematopoiesis, angiogenesis, inflammation, and reproduction.[9] In line with this notion, the hypoleptinemia that is typically observed in patients with anorexia nervosa (AN) plays a causal role in multiple key features of this eating disorder, including the typically observed amenorrhea, hyperactivity, and activation of the hypothalamus-pituitary-adrenal axis.[15] All of these acute hallmarks of AN are leptin-related and normalize upon body weight restoration.[15]

GHRELIN

The stomach-derived peptide hormone ghrelin was discovered in 1999 as an endogenous ligand of the growth hormone secretagogue receptor 1a (GHS-R1a).[16] Initially identified as a growth hormone secretagogue, ghrelin was soon later found to act on the hypothalamus to stimulate food intake and to decrease energy expenditure.[17] In the arcuate nucleus (ARC), the key feeding center of the hypothalamus, GHS-R1a is coexpressed with agouti-related peptide (AgRP) and neuropeptide Y (NPY), two key orexigenic neuropeptides which promote a positive energy balance by stimulating food intake while decreasing energy expenditure (see Chapter 3). Ghrelin's orexigenic effect resides in its ability to stimulate AgRP/NPY neuronal activity,[18] and ghrelin fails to stimulate food intake in mice lacking these neurons.[19]

As of today, ghrelin is the only peripheral hormone capable of stimulating food intake and adiposity while decreasing energy expenditure and lipid utilization.[20] In line with its role as a hunger hormone, plasma levels of ghrelin rise preprandially and peak directly at meal initiation followed by a postprandial decrease within the first hour after a meal.[21] Circulating levels of ghrelin are inversely correlated to body weight and are thus increased in patients with AN and decline upon body weight restoration.[20] Patients with AN have also higher plasma levels of ghrelin when compared with BMI-matched lean women, suggesting that impaired ghrelin sensitivity might play a causal role in the pathogenesis of AN.[20]

Ghrelin is predominantly produced and secreted from X/A-like cells in the oxyntic glands of the gastric mucosa. In order to bind and activate GHS-R1a, ghrelin requires the attachment (acylation) of a fatty acid (preferably C8 or C10) to its third amino acid residue, which is a serine.[16] Acylation of ghrelin is achieved by the ghrelin-o-acyltransferase (GOAT), which is the only endogenous enzyme capable to acylate ghrelin in vivo.[22] Notably, GOAT uses preferably dietary lipids as substrate for ghrelin acylation, suggesting that acylated ghrelin, beyond its role as a hunger hormone, also acts as a lipid sensor that informs the brain about incoming lipids.[23]

INSULIN

Insulin is produced and secreted by the pancreatic β-cells in response to elevated levels of blood glucose. While the most glorified role of insulin is its ability to lower blood glucose under conditions of hyperglycemia, insulin was the first peripheral hormone demonstrated to act on the brain to regulate food intake and adiposity. In line with this notion, despite glucose-dependent fluctuations of insulin secretion, circulating levels of insulin increase in proportion to body fat[24] and insulin enters the CNS in direct proportion to its concentration in the plasma.[25] When administered directly into the brain of baboons, insulin decreases food intake and body weight[26] and ameliorates hyperphagia in rats made diabetic by administration of streptozotocin.[27] Collectively, these data suggest that insulin, beyond its glucoregulatory action, acts as a peripheral adiposity signal that informs the brain about the amount of fat stored in the body and that the brain in response to increased levels of insulin decreases food intake in order to lower body weight. Further supporting this hypothesis, receptors for insulin are expressed in the ARC and dorsomedial hypothalamus (DMH), two key areas implicated in the regulation of food intake, and insulin supposably promotes its anorectic action via the hypothalamic melanocortinergic system.[28]

GLUCAGON

Cleaved from proglucagon in the pancreatic α-cells by the prohormone convertase 2, glucagon is secreted into the general circulation under conditions of hypoglycemia. In its classical function, glucagon increases levels of blood glucose by stimulating hepatic gluconeogenesis and glycogenolysis, while at the same time inhibiting glycolysis and glycogenesis.[29] For decades, this glucocentric view of glucagon has overshadowed that glucagon is a multifaceted hormone with pleiotropic action well beyond glucose buffering. In line with this notion, glucagon decreases body weight in rodents[30] and humans[31] by inhibiting food intake[30] and by increasing energy expenditure and brown fat thermogenesis.[32] In line with its role as an anorexigenic hormone, glucagon inhibits gastric motility and stimulates lipolysis while at the same time inhibiting de novo lipogenesis.[29] Glucagon's effect on food intake is mediated via the liver-vagus-hypothalamus axis. Accordingly, glucagon is secreted from the α-cells into the hepatic portal vein[33] and infusion of glucagon into the portal vein decreases food intake at concentrations 10 times lower as compared with infusion of glucagon into the general circulation via the vena cava.[34] In line with this notion, glucagon fails to affect food intake when the hepatic branch of the abdominal vagus is disconnected.[35] The hepatic branch of the abdominal vagus seems to transmit the glucagon signal to the area postrema (AP) and the nucleus tractus solitaries (NTS), and glucagon fails to inhibit food intake upon lesion of these regions.[36] Notably, the ability of glucagon to decrease body weight makes glucagon an attractive target for the treatment of obesity. However, glucagon's pharmacological potential to decrease body weight is hampered by its diabetogenic liability.

A revolutionary concept was thus to combine the thermogenic and lipolytic effect of glucagon together with the anorectic and antidiabetic effect of GLP-1 in a single molecule of enhanced potency and sustained action.[14,37] The basic idea behind this approach was the assumption that the anorectic effect of GLP-1 would synergize with glucagon's thermogenic and lipolytic nature to decrease body weight while the diabetogenic effect of glucagon would at the same time be restrained by GLP-1 agonism. This concept turned out to carry high pharmacological potential for the treatment of obesity,[38] and several pharmaceutical companies subsequently adopted this concept with the result that several of such GLP-1/glucagon dual-agonists are currently in clinical evaluation.[29]

AMYLIN

Amylin, also known as islet amyloid polypeptide (IAPP), is a 37-amino-acid hormone that is cosecreted with insulin from the pancreatic β-cells. Like insulin, amylin is to a certain extent tonically secreted into the circulation and its plasma concentration increases in proportion to body fat. Circulating levels of amylin are accordingly higher in obese compared with lean individuals[39] and are largely absent in individuals with type 1 diabetes.[40] In the pancreas, amylin inhibits the release of glucagon and thus decreases blood glucose via inhibition of hepatic glucose production.[41] Beyond its paracrine action in the pancreas, amylin decreases GI motility and peripheral or central administration of amylin decreases body weight through inhibition of food intake,[42] while pharmacological or genetic disruption of amylin signaling has the opposite effect.[43] Amylin's effects on food intake are mediated via the AP. In line with this notion, peripheral administration of amylin increases acute neuronal activation in this region and amylin's anorexigenic effect can be blocked by lesion of the AP.[44] Pramlintide, a synthetic amylin receptor agonist is approved by the US Food and Drug Administration (FDA) for the treatment of obesity and diabetes, and adjunct administration of amylin and leptin has been demonstrated to restore leptin resistance in diet-induced obese rodents and in obese humans.[12]

GLUCAGON-LIKE PEPTIDE 1

The glucagon-like peptide (GLP-1) is primarily produced and secreted from enteroendocrine L-cells of the small intestine in response to nutrient stimuli.[45] As an incretin, GLP-1 directly acts on the pancreatic β-cells to enhance glucose stimulation of insulin secretion.[45] Beyond its classical role as an insulin secretagogue, GLP-1 exerts a remarkable variety of metabolic effects. In rodents, GLP-1 enhances survival of pancreatic β-cells by stimulating proliferation and by decreasing apoptosis of the β-cells.[45] GLP-1 further increases insulin sensitivity in skeletal muscle,[46,47] decreases hepatic glucose production via inhibition of glucagon secretion,[48,49] slows down gastric emptying,[50] improves cardiac performance,[51,52] and acts on the brain to decrease body weight via inhibition of food intake.[53-55] The peripheral glycemic effect of GLP-1 agonism is thereby independent of its central anorexigenic effect, as demonstrated in CNS-specific GLP-1R KO mice, in which the glycemic but not the anorectic effect of GLP-1 is preserved.[54] While the ability of GLP-1 agonism to improve glucose metabolism and to decrease body weight is confirmed by numerous preclinical and clinical studies, the pharmacological potential of native GLP-1 is hampered by a very short half-life, which is in humans less than 5 min when injected into the general circulation.[56] The short half-life of native GLP-1 is

due to the action of the dipeptidyl peptidase IV (DPP-IV), which cleaves the N-terminal alanin 2 residue to yield an inactive GLP-1$_{9-37}$ or GLP-1$_{9-36}$ amide.[57-59] Over the last years, several biochemically optimized GLP-1 analogues with enhanced potency and sustained action relative to native GLP-1 have been developed. The most prominent ones include exenatide (Byetta; AstraZeneca), lixisenatide (Lyxumia, Sanofi), liraglutide (Victoza; Novo Nordisk), dulaglutide (Trulicity; Eli Lilly & Co), and albiglutide (Tanzeum, GlasxoSmith-Kline). Saxenda (Liraglutide 3 mg) was further recently approved by the FDA and the European Medicines Agency (EMA) for the treatment of obesity, and the placebo-subtracted weight loss achieved by Saxenda is typically in the range of 5%–10%.[60]

CHOLECYSTOKININ

Secreted from the I-cells of the small intestine in response to nutrient (especially fat) stimuli, cholecystokinin (CCK) was the first gut peptide identified to affect food intake.[61] Accordingly, upon peripheral administration to either rats or humans, CCK dose-dependently decreases food intake via a decrease in meal size.[61-63] CCK inhibition of food intake is mediated through the CCK1 receptor. Ablation of CCK1R in rodents accordingly abolishes the anorexigenic effect of CCK,[64] while pharmacological inhibition of CCK1R signaling increases food intake in a variety of species including rodents, nonhuman primates and humans.[65-67] CCK-induced inhibition of food intake seems to involve signaling of CCK via efferent vagal neurons to the NTS and AP, from where the satiety signal is then transmitted to the hypothalamus.[68,69]

FIBROBLAST GROWTH FACTOR 21

Fibroblast growth factor 21 (FGF21) is primarily produced in hepatocytes,[70] from where it is secreted into the circulation during states of enhanced fatty acid oxidation, such as during fasting or after feeding a ketogenic diet.[71] Under conditions of fasting, FGF21 increases blood glucose via stimulation of hepatic glucose production. In adipocytes, FGF21 further increases glucose uptake by stimulating the expression of GLUT1.[72] When injected into the general circulation, FGF21 decreases body weight by increasing energy expenditure, notably without affecting food intake.[13] In line with this notion, mice overexpressing FGF21 are protected from diet-induced obesity.[72] FGF21 regulation of energy expenditure seems to include FGF21 signaling in both the CNS and peripheral tissues. In line with this notion, peripheral administration of FGF21 has been shown to increase energy expenditure via activation of the AMP kinase (AMPK) in the adipose tissue.[73] The receptor for FGF21 is, however, also expressed in key hypothalamic neurons like the ARC or the ventromedial hypothalamus,[74] and several lines of evidence indicate that FGF21 induction of energy expenditure is, at least in part, centrally mediated.[75]

In summary, the regulation of systemic energy balance is a complex neuroendocrine process that is orchestrated by the brain and depends on a constant signal integration and the multidirectional crosstalk of brain with key peripheral organs. In concert, a plethora of endocrine factors signal the gastrointestinal energy status to the brain, which responds to these signals with changing our sensation to food intake to defend a certain body weight set point.

REFERENCES

1. Zhang Y, Proenca R, Maffei M, Barone M, Leopold L, Friedman JM. Positional cloning of the mouse obese gene and its human homologue. *Nature*. 1994;372(6505):425–432.
2. Pelleymounter MA, Cullen MJ, Baker MB, et al. Effects of the obese gene product on body weight regulation in ob/ob mice. *Science*. 1995;269(5223):540–543.
3. Campfield LA, Smith FJ, Guisez Y, Devos R, Burn P. Recombinant mouse OB protein: evidence for a peripheral signal linking adiposity and central neural networks. *Science*. 1995;269(5223):546–549.
4. Halaas JL, Gajiwala KS, Maffei M, et al. Weight-reducing effects of the plasma protein encoded by the obese gene. *Science*. 1995;269(5223):543–546.
5. Hedbacker K, Birsoy K, Wysocki RW, et al. Antidiabetic effects of IGFBP2, a leptin-regulated gene. *Cell Metab*. 2010;11(1):11–22.
6. Montague CT, Farooqi IS, Whitehead JP, et al. Congenital leptin deficiency is associated with severe early-onset obesity in humans. *Nature*. 1997;387(6636):903–908.
7. Oral EA, Simha V, Ruiz E, et al. Leptin-replacement therapy for lipodystrophy. *N Engl J Med*. 2002;346(8):570–578.
8. Heymsfield SB, Greenberg AS, Fujioka K, et al. Recombinant leptin for weight loss in obese and lean adults: a randomized, controlled, dose-escalation trial. *J Am Med Assoc*. 1999;282(16):1568–1575.
9. Dagogo-Jack S. *Leptin - Regulation and Clinical Applications*. Springer Cham Heidelberg New York Dordrecht London; 2015.
10. Liu J, Lee J, Salazar Hernandez MA, Mazitschek R, Ozcan U. Treatment of obesity with celastrol. *Cell*. 2015;161(5):999–1011.
11. Lee J, Liu J, Feng X, et al. Withaferin A is a leptin sensitizer with strong antidiabetic properties in mice. *Nat Med*. 2016;22(9):1023–1032.
12. Roth JD, Roland BL, Cole RL, et al. Leptin responsiveness restored by amylin agonism in diet-induced obesity: evidence from nonclinical and clinical studies. *Proc Natl Acad Sci USA*. 2008;105(20):7257–7262.
13. Muller TD, Sullivan LM, Habegger K, et al. Restoration of leptin responsiveness in diet-induced obese mice using an optimized leptin analog in combination with exendin-4 or FGF21. *J Pept Sci*. 2012;18(6):383–393.
14. Clemmensen C, Chabenne J, Finan B, et al. GLP-1/glucagon coagonism restores leptin responsiveness in obese mice chronically maintained on an obesogenic diet. *Diabetes*. 2014;63(4):1422–1427.
15. Muller TD, Focker M, Holtkamp K, Herpertz-Dahlmann B, Hebebrand J. Leptin-mediated neuroendocrine alterations in anorexia nervosa: somatic and behavioral implications. *Child Adolesc Psychiatr Clin N Am*. 2009;18(1):117–129.
16. Kojima M, Hosoda H, Date Y, Nakazato M, Matsuo H, Kangawa K. Ghrelin is a growth-hormone-releasing acylated peptide from stomach. *Nature*. 1999;402(6762):656–660.
17. Tschop M, Smiley DL, Heiman ML. Ghrelin induces adiposity in rodents. *Nature*. 2000;407(6806):908–913.
18. Cowley MA, Smith RG, Diano S, et al. The distribution and mechanism of action of ghrelin in the CNS demonstrates a novel hypothalamic circuit regulating energy homeostasis. *Neuron*. 2003;37(4):649–661.
19. Chen HY, Trumbauer ME, Chen AS, et al. Orexigenic action of peripheral ghrelin is mediated by neuropeptide Y and agouti-related protein. *Endocrinology*. 2004;145(6):2607–2612.
20. Muller TD, Nogueiras R, Andermann ML, et al. Ghrelin. *Mol Metab*. 2015;4(6):437–460.
21. Cummings DE, Purnell JQ, Frayo RS, Schmidova K, Wisse BE, Weigle DS. A prandial rise in plasma ghrelin levels suggests a role in meal initiation in humans. *Diabetes*. 2001;50(8):1714–1719.
22. Yang J, Zhao TJ, Goldstein JL, Brown MS. Inhibition of ghrelin O-acyltransferase (GOAT) by octanoylated pentapeptides. *Proc Natl Acad Sci U S A*. 2008;105(31):10750–10755.
23. Kirchner H, Gutierrez JA, Solenberg PJ, et al. GOAT links dietary lipids with the endocrine control of energy balance. *Nat Med*. 2009;15(7):741–745.
24. Bagdade JD, Bierman EL, Porte Jr D. The significance of basal insulin levels in the evaluation of the insulin response to glucose in diabetic and nondiabetic subjects. *J Clin Invest*. 1967;46(10):1549–1557.
25. Baura GD, Foster DM, Porte Jr D, et al. Saturable transport of insulin from plasma into the central nervous system of dogs in vivo. A mechanism for regulated insulin delivery to the brain. *J Clin Invest*. 1993;92(4):1824–1830.
26. Woods SC, Lotter EC, McKay LD, Porte Jr D. Chronic intracerebroventricular infusion of insulin reduces food intake and body weight of baboons. *Nature*. 1979;282(5738):503–505.

27. Sipols AJ, Baskin DG, Schwartz MW. Effect of intracerebroventricular insulin infusion on diabetic hyperphagia and hypothalamic neuropeptide gene expression. *Diabetes*. 1995;44(2):147–151.

28. Barsh GS, Schwartz MW. Genetic approaches to studying energy balance: perception and integration. *Nat Rev Genet*. 2002;3(8):589–600.

29. Muller TD, Finan B, Clemmensen C, DiMarchi RD, Tschop MH. The new biology and pharmacology of glucagon. *Physiol Rev*. 2017;97(2):721–766.

30. de Castro JM, Paullin SK, DeLugas GM. Insulin and glucagon as determinants of body weight set point and microregulation in rats. *J Comp Physiol Psychol*. 1978;92(3): 571–579.

31. Penick SB, Hinkle Jr LE. Depression of food intake induced in healthy subjects by glucagon. *N Engl J Med*. 1961;264:893–897.

32. Kuroshima A, Yahata T. Thermogenic responses of brown adipocytes to noradrenaline and glucagon in heat-acclimated and cold-acclimated rats. *Jpn J Physiol*. 1979;29(6):683–690.

33. Langhans W, Pantel K, Muller-Schell W, Eggenberger E, Scharrer E. Hepatic handling of pancreatic glucagon and glucose during meals in rats. *Am J Physiol*. 1984;247(5 Pt 2):R827–R832.

34. Geary N, Le Sauter J, Noh U. Glucagon acts in the liver to control spontaneous meal size in rats. *Am J physiol*. 1993;264(1 Pt 2):R116–R122.

35. Geary N, Smith GP. Selective hepatic vagotomy blocks pancreatic glucagon's satiety effect. *Physiol Behav*. 1983;31(3):391–394.

36. Weatherford SC, Ritter S. Lesion of vagal afferent terminals impairs glucagon-induced suppression of food intake. *Physiol Behav*. 1988;43(5):645–650.

37. Day JW, Ottaway N, Patterson JT, et al. A new glucagon and GLP-1 co-agonist eliminates obesity in rodents. *Nat Chem Biol*. 2009;5(10):749–757.

38. Tschop MH, Finan B, Clemmensen C, et al. Unimolecular polypharmacy for treatment of diabetes and obesity. *Cell Metab*. 2016;24(1):51–62.

39. Reda TK, Geliebter A, Pi-Sunyer FX. Amylin, food intake, and obesity. *Obes Res*. 2002;10(10):1087–1091.

40. Ogawa A, Harris V, McCorkle SK, Unger RH, Luskey KL. Amylin secretion from the rat pancreas and its selective loss after streptozotocin treatment. *J Clin Invest*. 1990;85(3):973–976.

41. Castillo MJ, Scheen AJ, Lefebvre PJ. Amylin/islet amyloid polypeptide: biochemistry, physiology, patho-physiology. *Diabete Metab*. 1995;21(1):3–25.

42. Lutz TA, Del Prete E, Scharrer E. Reduction of food intake in rats by intraperitoneal injection of low doses of amylin. *Physiol Behav*. 1994;55(5):891–895.

43. Rushing PA, Hagan MM, Seeley RJ, et al. Inhibition of central amylin signaling increases food intake and body adiposity in rats. *Endocrinology*. 2001;142(11): 5035.

44. Lutz TA, Senn M, Althaus J, Del Prete E, Ehrensperger F, Scharrer E. Lesion of the area postrema/nucleus of the solitary tract (AP/NTS) attenuates the anorectic effects of amylin and calcitonin gene-related peptide (CGRP) in rats. *Peptides*. 1998;19(2):309–317.

45. Drucker DJ. The biology of incretin hormones. *Cell Metab*. 2006;3(3):153–165.

46. Gonzalez N, Acitores A, Sancho V, Valverde I, Villanueva-Penacarrillo ML. Effect of GLP-1 on glucose transport and its cell signalling in human myocytes. *Regul Pept*. 2005;126(3):203–211.

47. Idris I, Patiag D, Gray S, Donnelly R. Exendin-4 increases insulin sensitivity via a PI-3-kinase-dependent mechanism: contrasting effects of GLP-1. *Biochem Pharmacol*. 2002;63(5):993–996.

48. Prigeon RL, Quddusi S, Paty B, D'Alessio DA. Suppression of glucose production by GLP-1 independent of islet hormones: a novel extrapancreatic effect. *Am J Physiol Endocrinol Metab*. 2003;285(4):E701–E707.

49. Valverde I, Morales M, Clemente F, et al. Glucagon-like peptide 1: a potent glycogenic hormone. *FEBS Lett*. 1994;349(2):313–316.

50. Willms B, Werner J, Holst JJ, Orskov C, Creutzfeldt W, Nauck MA. Gastric emptying, glucose responses, and insulin secretion after a liquid test meal: effects of exogenous glucagon-like peptide-1 (GLP-1)-(7-36) amide in type 2 (noninsulin-dependent) diabetic patients. *J Clin Endocrinol Metab*. 1996;81(1):327–332.

51. Sonne DP, Engstrom T, Treiman M. Protective effects of GLP-1 analogues exendin-4 and GLP-1(9-36) amide against ischemia-reperfusion injury in rat heart. *Regul Pept*. 2008;146(1–3):243–249.

52. Timmers L, Henriques JP, de Kleijn DP, et al. Exenatide reduces infarct size and improves cardiac function in a porcine model of ischemia and reperfusion injury. *J Am Coll Cardiol*. 2009;53(6):501–510.

53. Burmeister MA, Ayala JE, Smouse H, et al. The hypothalamic glucagon-like peptide 1 receptor is sufficient but not necessary for the regulation of energy balance and glucose homeostasis in mice. *Diabetes*. 2017;66(2):372–384.

54. Sisley S, Gutierrez-Aguilar R, Scott M, D'Alessio DA, Sandoval DA, Seeley RJ. Neuronal GLP1R mediates liraglutide's anorectic but not glucose-lowering effect. *J Clin Invest*. 2014;124(6):2456–2463.

55. Sisley S, Smith K, Sandoval DA, Seeley RJ. Differences in acute anorectic effects of long-acting GLP-1 receptor agonists in rats. *Peptides*. 2014;58:1–6.

56. Hui H, Farilla L, Merkel P, Perfetti R. The short half-life of glucagon-like peptide-1 in plasma does not reflect its long-lasting beneficial effects. *Eur J Endocrinol*. 2002;146(6):863–869.

57. Deacon CF, Johnsen AH, Holst JJ. Degradation of glucagon-like peptide-1 by human plasma in vitro yields an N-terminally truncated peptide that is a major endogenous metabolite in vivo. *J Clin Endocrinol Metab*. 1995;80(3):952–957.

58. Kieffer TJ, McIntosh CH, Pederson RA. Degradation of glucose-dependent insulinotropic polypeptide and truncated glucagon-like peptide 1 in vitro and in vivo by dipeptidyl peptidase IV. *Endocrinology*. 1995;136(8):3585–3596.

59. Mentlein R, Gallwitz B, Schmidt WE. Dipeptidyl-peptidase IV hydrolyses gastric inhibitory polypeptide, glucagon-like peptide-1(7-36)amide, peptide histidine methionine and is responsible for their degradation in human serum. *Eur J Biochem*. 1993;214(3):829–835.

60. Pi-Sunyer X, Astrup A, Fujioka K, et al. A randomized, controlled trial of 3.0 mg of liraglutide in weight management. *N Engl J Med*. 2015;373(1):11–22.

61. Gibbs J, Young RC, Smith GP. Cholecystokinin decreases food intake in rats. *J Comp Physiol Psychol*. 1973;84(3):488–495.

62. Kissileff HR, Pi-Sunyer FX, Thornton J, Smith GP. C-terminal octapeptide of cholecystokinin decreases food intake in man. *Am J Clin Nutr*. 1981;34(2):154–160.

63. Muurahainen N, Kissileff HR, Derogatis AJ, Pi-Sunyer FX. Effects of cholecystokinin-octapeptide (CCK-8) on food intake and gastric emptying in man. *Physiol Behav*. 1988;44(4–5):645–649.

64. Kopin AS, Mathes WF, McBride EW, et al. The cholecystokinin-A receptor mediates inhibition of food intake yet is not essential for the maintenance of body weight. *J Clin Invest*. 1999;103(3):383–391.

65. Beglinger C, Degen L, Matzinger D, D'Amato M, Drewe J. Loxiglumide, a CCK-A receptor antagonist, stimulates calorie intake and hunger feelings in humans. *Am J Physiol Regul Integr Comp Physiol*. 2001;280(4):R1149–R1154.

66. Hewson G, Leighton GE, Hill RG, Hughes J. The cholecystokinin receptor antagonist L364,718 increases food intake in the rat by attenuation of the action of endogenous cholecystokinin. *Br J Pharmacol*. 1988;93(1):79–84.

67. Moran TH, Ameglio PJ, Peyton HJ, Schwartz GJ, McHugh PR. Blockade of type A, but not type B, CCK receptors postpones satiety in rhesus monkeys. *Am J Physiol*. 1993;265(3 Pt 2):R620–R624.

68. Moran TH, Baldessarini AR, Salorio CF, Lowery T, Schwartz GJ. Vagal afferent and efferent contributions to the inhibition of food intake by cholecystokinin. *Am J Physiol*. 1997;272(4 Pt 2):R1245–R1251.

69. Moran TH, Robinson PH, Goldrich MS, McHugh PR. Two brain cholecystokinin receptors: implications for behavioral actions. *Brain Res*. 1986;362(1):175–179.

70. Nishimura T, Nakatake Y, Konishi M, Itoh N. Identification of a novel FGF, FGF-21, preferentially expressed in the liver. *Biochim Biophys Acta*. 2000;1492(1):203–206.

71. Badman MK, Koester A, Flier JS, Kharitonenkov A, Maratos-Flier E. Fibroblast growth factor 21-deficient mice demonstrate impaired adaptation to ketosis. *Endocrinology*. 2009;150(11):4931–4940.

72. Kharitonenkov A, Shiyanova TL, Koester A, et al. FGF-21 as a novel metabolic regulator. *J Clin Invest*. 2005;115(6):1627–1635.

73. Chau MD, Gao J, Yang Q, Wu Z, Gromada J. Fibroblast growth factor 21 regulates energy metabolism by activating the AMPK-SIRT1-PGC-1alpha pathway. *Proc Natl Acad Sci USA*. 2010;107(28):12553–12558.

74. Matsuo A, Tooyama I, Isobe S, et al. Immunohistochemical localization in the rat brain of an epitope corresponding to the fibroblast growth factor receptor-1. *Neuroscience*. 1994;60(1):49–66.

75. Sarruf DA, Thaler JP, Morton GJ, et al. Fibroblast growth factor 21 action in the brain increases energy expenditure and insulin sensitivity in obese rats. *Diabetes*. 2010;59(7):1817–1824.

Microbiome and Inflammation in Eating Disorders

JOCHEN SEITZ, MD • JOHN BAINES, PHD • BEATE HERPERTZ-DAHLMANN, MD

INTRODUCTION

There are roughly as many gut microbial cells we carry as total eukaryotic cells in the human body,[1] each human has a mix of about 500 different microbial species in his or her gut out of a pool of >1000 species.[2] The combined genetic information of those gut microorganisms is about 150 times greater than that of the human genome. Gut microbes constantly interact with dietary factors and host cells. They break down dietary components; influence metabolism, hormone release, and inflammatory processes; and educate our immune system.[3] Recently, compelling evidence emerged that malnutrition and starvation-induced dysfunction of the gut microbiome and its interaction with the brain ("gut-brain axis") play an important role in the emergence and development of somatic and psychological symptoms in anorexia nervosa (AN) and thus influence the course and outcome of this debilitating disease.[4–7] Here we review different mechanisms of interaction of the gut microbiome with the host and their relevance for AN and then summarize gut microbiome findings in AN and potential consequences for future research and treatment (Fig. 14.1).

METABOLISM AND BODY WEIGHT

Recent studies have demonstrated the important links between the gut microbiome and the regulation of body weight.[8,9] This is not surprising, as gut microbes can metabolize many more substrates than human cells, in turn furnishing the host with their often-essential products, fulfilling important symbiotic functions. Certain species thus also allow to extract more energy from the same amount of food than others, effectively linking the gut microbiome to body weight development. For example, bacteroidetes species was correlated with body mass index in over-, normal,

and underweight participants.[10] They were decreased in acute patients with AN[5,7,10] and normalized during weight rehabilitation of AN patients. The causal role of the gut microbiome in weight regulation is best shown in stool transplantation studies. Mouse models intriguingly showed that the transfer of stool samples from obese to germ-free (GF) mice, bred and born under sterile conditions, leads to obesity.[8] In contrast, the transfer of bacterial species from children with kwashiorkor to GF mice produced significant weight loss and signs of malnutrition.[9] One week of oral antibiotics significantly improved the nutritional status of underfed Malawian children.[11] Transferring stool from bariatric surgery patients to GF mice resulted in significantly less fat mass than colonization with the gut microbiome from obese controls.[12] As AN patients show a significant alteration of the gut microbiome (dysbiosis, see below), an effect on metabolism and weight gain seems more than likely. Interestingly, Mack et al.[7] could show conspicuously different gut microbiome alterations between the restrictive and binge-purging subtype of AN—while patients with restrictive AN are also known to need a markedly increased amount of calories for an equivalent weight gain compared with patients with binge-purge AN.[13]

HORMONES

Although the exact mechanisms are not known, specific changes in hormone levels correlate with the presence of certain gut microbiota. The gut microbiome has been shown to produce hormones, to react to changing hormonal levels of the host and even to regulate host hormone level secretion.[3] Estrogen, e.g., enhances bacterial growth and decreases bacterial virulence in cultured bacteria,[14] while leptin was positively correlated with *Bifidobacterium* and *Lactobacillus* in rats.[15] GF

Eating Disorders and Obesity in Children and Adolescents. https://doi.org/10.1016/B978-0-323-54852-6.00014-8

rats showed a 25% higher TSH level,[16] while ghrelin was positively correlated with Bacteroidetes and Prevotella species and negatively correlated with *Bifidobacterium* and *Lactobacillus* in rats.[15] AN patients suffer from amenorrhea and thus have long-standing estrogen deficits, they also show marked leptin and thyroxin deficiencies, while ghrelin and cortisol are found to be increased,[17] making bidirectional interactions with the gut microbiome likely.

GUT PERMEABILITY AND INFLAMMATION

Increased cortisol as found in acute AN patients in serum, urinary, and salivary samples[18] has been shown to increase intestinal permeability in human studies and animal models alike.[19] In humans, even relatively small stressful situations (public speaking) were sufficient to increase cortisol levels and gut permeability,[20] potentially via activation of mast cells, carrying high-affinity corticotropin-releasing hormone receptors.[19] Thus, in AN, the elevated stress and cortisol levels could contribute to an increased gut permeability. Furthermore, two previous studies revealed a significant intestinal dysbiosis in AN, which was only partially alleviated with weight gain, e.g., lower abundances of Bacteroidetes and carbohydrate utilizing taxa as well as higher abundances of Firmicutes and Verrucobacteria.[5,7] The latter are mucin-degrading and protein-fermenting taxa and are thought to feed on intestinal wall mucins and thus further contribute to increased intestinal wall permeability and even a "leaky gut." This leaky gut has been shown in an animal model of AN especially in the large intestine[21] and is thought to increase translocation of bacteria, their subcomponents, and bacterial products across the intestinal wall barrier, potentially triggering further immune responses and inflammation.[4,7,21] Gut microbe derived–short chain fatty acid and biotransformed bile acid have, e.g., been shown to act as ligands to specific cell signaling receptors influencing the immune system.[22] Indeed, a recent metaanalysis

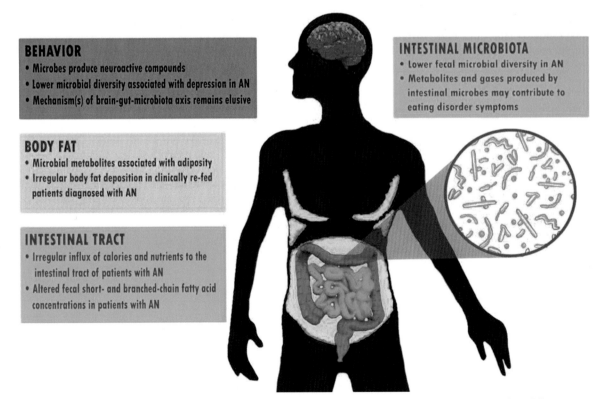

BEHAVIOR
• Microbes produce neuroactive compounds
• Lower microbial diversity associated with depression in AN
• Mechanism(s) of brain-gut-microbiota axis remains elusive

BODY FAT
• Microbial metabolites associated with adiposity
• Irregular body fat deposition in clinically re-fed patients diagnosed with AN

INTESTINAL TRACT
• Irregular influx of calories and nutrients to the intestinal tract of patients with AN
• Altered fecal short- and branched-chain fatty acid concentrations in patients with AN

INTESTINAL MICROBIOTA
• Lower fecal microbial diversity in AN
• Metabolites and gases produced by intestinal microbes may contribute to eating disorder symptoms

FIG. 14.1 Microbiome interactions in AN. (From Glenny EM, Bulik-Sullivan EC, Tang Q, Bulik CM, Carroll IM. Eating disorders and the intestinal microbiota: mechanisms of energy homeostasis and behavioral influence. *Curr Psychiatry Rep.* 2017;19:51.)

showed proinflammatory markers like Il-6 and TNF-α to be significantly increased in AN patients,[23] evidencing a chronic low-grade inflammatory state. An earlier metaanalysis[24] had also shown proinflammatory IL-1β to be significantly increased, which remained significant only for restrictive subtype AN in the more comprehensive second analysis. Thus, gut dysbiosis could contribute to increased gut permeability and chronic inflammation in AN.

IMMUNOLOGY AND AUTOANTIBODIES

One of the possible molecular mechanisms linking the gut microbiome with the brain and specifically with the regulation of feeding was demonstrated by the group of Fetissov[25]: microbiota-induced humoral immune response resulted in antibodies cross-reactive with anorexigenic and orexigenic hormones, such as α-melanocyte-stimulating hormone (α-MSH) and ghrelin, respectively. Indeed, a specific bacterial protein ClpB produced by Enterobacteriaceae was recently identified as an antigen-mimetic of α-MSH, and they found significant correlations between the plasma levels of α-MSH-reactive autoantibodies and psychological traits in patients with eating disorders (EDs), including AN.[26] A small study reported increased plasma levels of ClpB in patients with EDs with a strong correlation to α-MSH autoantibodies.[27] The mechanism of action of autoantibodies, such as α-MSH-reactive IgG, may involve peptide protection from degradation in circulation preserving its physiological activity, as was shown for ghrelin.[28] Also, autoimmune diseases in general are increased in AN as, e.g., shown by a large Finnish population cohort study, with lifetime odds ratios for endocrinal autoimmune diseases increased to 2.4, gastrointestinal diseases in general increased to 1.8, and specifically Crohn's disease increased to 3.9.[29] This further links autoantibody production with AN, potentially also instigated by a leaky gut and increased humoral antigen presentation after traversing the intestinal wall. Interestingly, a recent case study of a young patient with comorbid AN and Crohn's disease showed a significant improvement after anti-TNF-α therapy.[30]

GUT-BRAIN INTERACTION

The gut microbiome also has important consequences for the brain and its function, starting in early development. This becomes evident, when studying GF mice, e.g., with respect to serotonin metabolism: hippocampal levels of main serotonin metabolites 5-hydroxyindoleacetitic acid (5-HIAA) and 5-hydroxytryptamine (5-HT) were significantly increased without contact to a normal gut microbiome during growth.[31] Interestingly, 5-HIAA levels were found to be reduced in the CSF of patients with acute AN, while increased levels were found in recovered AN patients.[32] The gut microbiome furthermore influences peripheral serotonin secretion by altering number and functioning of enterochromaffin cells in the gut wall, increasing gut peristalsis and reducing transit time, but also entering the bloodstream. Serotonin also plays an important role in mood and anxiety disorders, often comorbid in AN. GF mice also show altered brain-derived neurotropic factor (BDNF) in the hippocampus, a nerve growth factor influencing neuron growth and protection as well as synapse formation and connectivity, further evidencing the importance of gut microbiota for normal brain development and function. Antibiotics use was shown to reduce hippocampal BDNF and altering anxiety levels.[33] Patients with AN also show reduced levels of BDNF in the acute state, which seems to recover upon weight rehabilitation.[34] The brain of adolescent AN patients also shows a marked loss in volume of gray and white matter, linked to deficits in neuropsychological functioning and a negative outcome.[35] In the animal models of AN, a striking reduction of astrocytes[36] and reduced cell neogenesis have been shown by our group. Interestingly, the eradication of the gut microbiome with antibiotics has been also been reported to affect neuropsychological functioning and reduce brain cell neogenesis[37] in mice, and supplementation with psychobiotics was able to reverse these changes. However, the extent of the gut microbiome–associated brain changes in AN patients has yet to be analyzed in detail.

GUT MICROBIOME ALTERATIONS IN ANOREXIA NERVOSA

Several studies have so far analyzed the gut microbiome in AN show mixed results.[4,38] The groups of Armougoum,[39] Million,[10] Borgo,[40] Kleiman,[5] Morita[41] and Mack[7] analyzed cross-sectional samples in 9–55 acutely ill AN patients each, while Kleiman[5] and Mack[7] also performed longitudinal gut microbiome analysis in 10 and 44 patients, respectively, all using stool sample analyses. Kleiman[5] found reduced microbial richness (a measure of α-diversity, the number of different organisms in a sample) in acute and recovered patients with AN compared with controls which were not significant in Mack's[7] and Borgo's[40] samples. However, Mack[7] showed a significant increase in richness with weight gain, while Kleiman[5] showed a similar trend. Importantly, the number of observed species correlated with eating disorder symptom severity and depressive symptoms.[5] β-Diversity (a measure of similarity of the microbiome between two different individuals) was increased compared with HC in Mack's[7] and Kleiman's[5] samples showing stronger heterogeneity in AN. Bβ-Diversity decreased during weight gain; however, AN patients' gut microbiome after weight gain still more resembled their own gut microbiome in the acute state than that of HC, evidencing persisting alterations even after weight gain. Increased Firmicutes and decreased Bacteroidetes were observed by Mack[7] and as a trend by Kleiman,[5] low Roseburia species by Mack,[7] Borgo[40] and Armougom,[39] Borgo[40] and Mack[7] also found increased levels of the archaeon *Methanobrevibacter smithii*. Increased Firmicutes could be partly responsible for the leaky gut mentioned above, due to their mucin-degrading properties. This is further underpinned by an increased amount of branched chain fatty acids shown by Mack[7] and a trend by Morita,[41] which are fermentation products of this protein digestion. They are known to negatively impact appetite by furthering the release of PYY, a gastric peptide, and to also increase depressive symptoms.[42]

CONSEQUENCES FOR RESEARCH AND THERAPY

Thus, the gut microbiome might become an essential research and therapeutic target for the treatment of AN and weight rehabilitation to influence food utilization, appetite, and gastrointestinal symptoms as well as neuropsychological functioning and behavior. Moreover, current refeeding practices in AN potentially contribute to a poor outcome. AN patients often maintain a vegetarian or vegan diet low in fat and high in protein and fiber. After admission diet is often quickly changed to a high-caloric diet rich in fat and carbohydrates. Some patients are given oral liquid supplements. Most of these are based on cow's milk, e.g., an animal-based food product which might increase the growth of inflammation-inducing bacteria.[4] David et al.[43] showed how a purely animal-based diet quickly changed the gut microbiome in healthy participants within days. Thus, we may even induce an iatrogenic worsening of the course of AN by negatively affecting the gut microbiome. These interactions need to be researched. Furthermore, a selective stimulation of the growth of certain bacterial strains by the administration of psychobiotics ("live bacteria, which when applied in adequate amounts, confer mental health benefits"[44]), prebiotics, dietary fibers favoring the growth of these bacteria, and other nutritional interventions are

increasingly of interest, as preclinical trials continue to show health benefits.[45] This emerging evidence of preclinical studies encourages the investigation of psychobiotics in mental disorders (e.g., Kelly et al.[46]). A systematic review of 10 RCTs provides initial support for the use of psychobiotics in reducing human anxiety and depression.[47] The authors concluded that there was preliminary evidence for the detection of psychological benefits from psychobiotics, although there were methodological limitations (such as using different strains of bacteria).

Selective psychobiotics, prebiotics, and other nutritional interventions might thus become important additions to AN therapy by altering gut microbiome and gut-brain interaction via several therapeutic approaches. Firstly, one could try to induce more energy retrieval aided by gut bacteria from the same amount of food, effectively increasing weight gain without increasing food volume. Secondly, gut permeability and inflammation could be reduced via favoring specific gut microbiome known for their antiinflammatory properties,[48] e.g., by prebiotics. And finally, psychobiotics could potentially help reduce depressive and anxious symptoms[47] as well as increase cognitive functioning as recently shown by Bagga et al.[49] using Lactobacilli and Bifidobacteria.

REFERENCES

1. Sender R, Fuchs S, Milo R. Revised estimates for the number of human and bacteria cells in the body. *PLoS Biol.* 2016;14(8):e1002533. https://doi.org/10.1371/journal.pbio.1002533.
2. Clavel T, Lagkouvardos I, Hiergeist A. Microbiome sequencing: challenges and opportunities for molecular medicine. *Expert Rev Mol Diagn.* 2016;16(7):795–805. https://doi.org/10.1080/14737159.2016.1184574.
3. Neuman H, Debelius JW, Knight R, Koren O. Microbial endocrinology: the interplay between the microbiota and the endocrine system. *FEMS Microbiol Rev.* 2015;39(4):509–521. https://doi.org/10.1093/femsre/fuu010.
4. Herpertz-Dahlmann B, Seitz J, Baines J. Food matters: how the microbiome and gut–brain interaction might impact the development and course of anorexia nervosa. *Eur Child Adolesc Psychiatry.* 2017;26(9):1031–1041.
5. Kleiman SC, Watson HJ, Bulik-Sullivan EC, et al. The intestinal microbiota in acute anorexia nervosa and during renourishment: relationship to depression, anxiety, and eating disorder psychopathology. *Psychosom Med.* 2015;77(9):969.
6. Carr J, Kleiman SC, Bulik CM, Bulik-Sullivan EC, Carroll IM. Can attention to the intestinal microbiota improve understanding and treatment of anorexia nervosa? *Expert Rev Gastroenterol Hepatol.* 2016;10(5):565–569. https://doi.org/10.1586/17474124.2016.1166953.

7. Mack I, Cuntz U, Grämer C, et al. Weight gain in anorexia nervosa does not ameliorate the faecal microbiota, branched chain fatty acid profiles, and gastrointestinal complaints. *Sci Rep*. 2016;6:26752.

8. Ridaura VK, Faith JJ, Rey FE, et al. Gut microbiota from twins discordant for obesity modulate metabolism in mice. *Science*. 2013;341(6150):1241214.

9. Smith MI, Yatsunenko T, Manary MJ, et al. Gut microbiomes of Malawian twin pairs discordant for kwashiorkor. *Science*. 2013;339(6119):548–554. https://doi.org/10.1126/science.1229000.

10. Million M, Angelakis E, Maraninchi M, et al. Correlation between body mass index and gut concentrations of *Lactobacillus reuteri, Bifidobacterium animalis, Methanobrevibacter smithii and Escherichia coli*. 2005 *Int J Obes*. 2013;37(11):1460–1466. https://doi.org/10.1038/ijo.2013.20.

11. Trehan I, Goldbach HS, LaGrone LN, et al. Antibiotics as part of the management of severe acute malnutrition. *N Engl J Med*. 2013;368(5):425–435. https://doi.org/10.1056/NEJMoa1202851.

12. Tremaroli V, Karlsson F, Werling M, et al. Roux-en-Y gastric bypass and vertical banded gastroplasty induce long-term changes on the human gut microbiome contributing to fat mass regulation. *Cell Metab*. 2015;22(2):228–238.

13. Marzola E, Nasser JA, Hashim SA, Shih P-AB, Kaye WH. Nutritional rehabilitation in anorexia nervosa: review of the literature and implications for treatment. *BMC Psychiatry*. 2013;13:290. https://doi.org/10.1186/1471-244X-13-290.

14. Roshchina V. Evolutionary considerations of neurotransmitters in microbial, plant, and animal cells. In: Lyte M, Fitzgerald P, eds. *Microbial Endocrinology: Interkingdom Signaling in Infectious Disease and Health*. New York: Springer; 2010:17–52.

15. Queipo-Ortuño MI, Seoane LM, Murri M, et al. Gut microbiota composition in male rat models under different nutritional status and physical activity and its association with serum leptin and ghrelin levels. *PLoS One*. 2013;8(5):e65465. https://doi.org/10.1371/journal.pone.0065465.

16. Wostmann B. Morphology and physiology, endocrinology and biochemistry. In: Wostmann BS, ed. *Germfree and Gnotobiotic Animal Models*. Boca Raton, Florida: CRC Press,; 1996:43–71.

17. Herpertz-Dahlmann B. Adolescent eating disorders: update on definitions, symptomatology, epidemiology, and comorbidity. *Child Adolesc Psychiatr Clin N Am*. 2015;24(1):177–196. https://doi.org/10.1016/j.chc.2014.08.003.

18. Schorr M, Miller KK. The endocrine manifestations of anorexia nervosa: mechanisms and management. *Nat Rev Endocrinol*. 2017;13(3):174–186. https://doi.org/10.1038/nrendo.2016.175.

19. Petra AI, Panagiotidou S, Stewart JM, Conti P, Theoharides TC. Spectrum of mast cell activation disorders. *Expert Rev Clin Immunol*. 2014;10(6):729–739. https://doi.org/10.1586/1744666X.2014.906302.

20. Vanuytsel T, van Wanrooy S, Vanheel H, et al. Psychological stress and corticotropin-releasing hormone increase intestinal permeability in humans by a mast cell-dependent mechanism. *Gut*. 2014;63(8):1293–1299. https://doi.org/10.1136/gutjnl-2013-305690.

21. Jesus P, Ouelaa W, Francois M, et al. Alteration of intestinal barrier function during activity-based anorexia in mice. *Clin Nutr Edinb Scotl*. 2014;33(6):1046–1053. https://doi.org/10.1016/j.clnu.2013.11.006.

22. Rizzetto L, Fava F, Tuohy KM, Selmi C. Connecting the immune system, systemic chronic inflammation and the gut microbiome: the role of sex. *J Autoimmun*. 2018;92:12–34.

23. Dalton B, Bartholdy S, Robinson L, et al. A meta-analysis of cytokine concentrations in eating disorders. *J Psychiatr Res*. 2018;103:252–264.

24. Solmi M, Veronese N, Favaro A, et al. Inflammatory cytokines and anorexia nervosa: a meta-analysis of cross-sectional and longitudinal studies. *Psychoneuroendocrinology*. 2015;51:237–252.

25. Fetissov SO. Role of the gut microbiota in host appetite control: bacterial growth to animal feeding behaviour. *Nat Rev Endocrinol*. 2017;13(1):11.

26. Tennoune N, Chan P, Breton J, et al. Bacterial ClpB heat-shock protein, an antigen-mimetic of the anorexigenic peptide alpha-MSH, at the origin of eating disorders. *Transl Psychiatry*. 2014;4:e458. https://doi.org/10.1038/tp.2014.98.

27. Breton J, Legrand R, Akkermann K, et al. Elevated plasma concentrations of bacterial ClpB protein in patients with eating disorders. *Int J Eat Disord*. 2016;49(8):805–808.

28. François M, Barde S, Legrand R, et al. High-fat diet increases ghrelin-expressing cells in stomach, contributing to obesity. *Nutr Burbank Los Angel Cty Calif*. 2016;32(6):709–715. https://doi.org/10.1016/j.nut.2015.12.034.

29. Raevuori A, Haukka J, Vaarala O, et al. The increased risk for autoimmune diseases in patients with eating disorders. *PLoS One*. 2014;9(8):e104845. https://doi.org/10.1371/journal.pone.0104845.

30. Solmi M, Santonastaso P, Caccaro R, Favaro A. A case of anorexia nervosa with comorbid Crohn's disease: beneficial effects of anti-TNF-α therapy? *Int J Eat Disord*. 2013;46(6):639–641. https://doi.org/10.1002/eat.22153.

31. Clarke G, Grenham S, Scully P, et al. The microbiome-gut-brain axis during early life regulates the hippocampal serotonergic system in a sex-dependent manner. *Mol Psychiatry*. 2013;18(6):666–673. https://doi.org/10.1038/mp.2012.77.

32. Kaye WH, Wierenga CE, Bailer UF, Simmons AN, |Wagner A, Bischoff-Grethe A. Does a shared neurobiology for foods and drugs of abuse contribute to extremes of food ingestion in anorexia and bulimia nervosa? *Biol Psychiatry*. 2013;73(9):836–842. https://doi.org/10.1016/j.biopsych.2013.01.002.

33. Desbonnet L, Clarke G, Traplin A, et al. Gut microbiota depletion from early adolescence in mice: implications for brain and behaviour. *Brain Behav Immun*. 2015;48:165–173. https://doi.org/10.1016/j.bbi.2015.04.004.

34. Zwipp J, Hass J, Schober I, et al. Serum brain-derived neurotrophic factor and cognitive functioning in underweight, weight-recovered and partially weight-recovered females with anorexia nervosa. *Prog Neuro-Psychopharmacol Biol Psychiatry*. 2014;54:163–169. https://doi.org/10.1016/j.pnpbp.2014.05.006.

35. Seitz J, Walter M, Mainz V, Herpertz-Dahlmann B, Konrad K, Polier G von. Brain volume reduction predicts weight development in adolescent patients with anorexia nervosa. *J Psychiatr Res*. 2015;68:228–237. https://doi.org/10.1016/j.jpsychires.2015.06.019.

36. Frintrop L, Liesbrock J, Paulukat L, et al. Reduced astrocyte density underlying brain volume reduction in activity-based anorexia rats. *World J Biol Psychiatry*. 2018;19(3):225–235. https://doi.org/10.1080/15622975.2016.1273552.

37. Möhle L, Mattei D, Heimesaat MM, et al. Ly6Chi monocytes provide a link between antibiotic-induced changes in gut microbiota and adult hippocampal neurogenesis. *Cell Rep*. 2016;15(9):1945–1956.

38. Mack I, Penders J, Cook J, Dugmore J, Mazurak N, Enck P. Is the impact of starvation on the gut microbiota specific or unspecific to anorexia nervosa? A narrative review based on a systematic literature search. *Curr Neuropharmacol*. 2018;16(8):1131–1149.

39. Armougom F, Henry M, Vialettes B, Raccah D, Raoult D. Monitoring bacterial community of human gut microbiota reveals an increase in Lactobacillus in obese patients and Methanogens in anorexic patients. *PLoS One*. 2009;4(9):e7125.

40. Borgo F, Riva A, Benetti A, et al. Microbiota in anorexia nervosa: the triangle between bacterial species, metabolites and psychological tests. *PLoS One*. 2017;12(6):e0179739.

41. Morita C, Tsuji H, Hata T, et al. Gut dysbiosis in patients with anorexia nervosa. *PLoS One*. 2015;10(12):e0145274.

42. Holzer P, Farzi A. Neuropeptides and the microbiota-gut-brain axis. *Adv Exp Med Biol*. 2014;817:195–219. https://doi.org/10.1007/978-1-4939-0897-4_9.

43. David LA, Maurice CF, Carmody RN, et al. Diet rapidly and reproducibly alters the human gut microbiome. *Nature*. 2014;505(7484):559–563. https://doi.org/10.1038/nature12820.

44. Dinan TG, Stanton C, Cryan JF. Psychobiotics: a novel class of psychotropic. *Biol Psychiatry*. 2013;74(10):720–726.

45. Kelly JR, Kennedy PJ, Cryan JF, Dinan TG, Clarke G, Hyland NP. Breaking down the barriers: the gut microbiome, intestinal permeability and stress-related psychiatric disorders. *Front Cell Neurosci*. 2015;9:392.

46. Kelly JR, Allen AP, Temko A, et al. Lost in translation? The potential psychobiotic *Lactobacillus rhamnosus* (JB-1) fails to modulate stress or cognitive performance in healthy male subjects. *Brain Behav Immun*. 2017;61:50–59. https://doi.org/10.1016/j.bbi.2016.11.018.

47. Pirbaglou M, Katz J, de Souza RJ, Stearns JC, Motamed M, Ritvo P. Probiotic supplementation can positively affect anxiety and depressive symptoms: a systematic review of randomized controlled trials. *Nutr Res NY N*. 2016;36(9):889–898. https://doi.org/10.1016/j.nutres.2016.06.009.

48. Lam YY, Maguire S, Palacios T, Caterson ID. Are the gut bacteria telling us to eat or not to eat? Reviewing the role of gut microbiota in the etiology, disease progression and treatment of eating disorders. *Nutrients*. 2017;9(6). https://doi.org/10.3390/nu9060602.

49. Bagga D, Reichert JL, Koschutnig K, et al. Probiotics drive gut microbiome triggering emotional brain signatures. *Gut Microb*. 2018 (just-accepted):00–00.

CHAPTER 15

Eating Disordered Mothers and Their Children: Intergenerational Effects

NADIA MICALI, MD, PHD, MRCPSYCH • MARIA G. MARTINI, MD, MSC • MANUELA BARONA, MSC • ELINE TOMBEUR, MSC

INTRODUCTION

The past 20 years have seen an increased interest in the study of the intergenerational effects of maternal eating disorders (EDs). This is not only due to an increased recognition of the effects of parental psychiatric disorders on their offspring but also due to the impetus provided by large population-based and register studies with enough power to enable answering research questions requiring large enough samples.

In 2005, Bulik et al. suggested a cycle of risk model for the development of anorexia nervosa (AN), whereby the effect of maternal AN on the offspring (and on the offspring own risk for AN) via perinatal complications is conceptualized as being shaped by environmental factors, genetic factors, and environmental factors that are genetically driven (such as pregnancy nutrition and weight gain—in utero, and appearance focus and restrictive eating—during childhood/adolescence).[1] In 2009, we proposed a risk model for the effects of maternal EDs on child development that aimed to encompass all EDs and focus on perinatal risk factors in particular, zooming in on the in utero period. We proposed that specific maternal genetic and environmental, epigenetic and endocrine mechanisms that alter fetal development might be relevant to the adverse outcomes seen in the children of ED mothers.[2] This model has been tested in part in our longitudinal work.[3–5] Nevertheless, the likely effect of maternal EDs on offspring phenotype is likely a result of the interplay of genetic (maternal and child) and environmental (prenatal, in utero, and postnatal) factors that shape the offspring phenotype via developmental pathways across several areas (see Fig. 15.1).

Understanding the effects of maternal EDs on child development across domains and ages can help identify both risk and resilience factors that might be targeted for effective therapeutic and preventative strategies, given the limited therapies available for EDs.

THE EFFECT OF MATERNAL EDs ON COGNITIVE AND PSYCHOLOGICAL DEVELOPMENT

The number of studies investigating the impact of maternal EDs on the psychological development of their offspring remains sparse to this day; however, the literature available suggests that a maternal ED can have an impact on the child's cognitive, social, and emotional development.

Temperament

Temperament is understood as the way children respond to the world around them, how they regulate their emotions and how comfortable they are with new situations, both social and others.[6] It represents the earliest appearance of the child's individual differences in emotional reactivity. Furthermore, temperament has been used in developmental psychology as a proxy for negative emotionality and has been associated with childhood psychiatric disorders later in life.[7,8] Maternal depression and anxiety have been shown to affect childhood temperament (greater fussiness). Furthermore, interpersonal difficulties have been found in patients with EDs, which could affect the way mothers with EDs respond to their child's cues, and in turn affect temperament.

Mothers with EDs have been shown to be more likely to describe their infant as having a difficult temperament. Compared with women with no history or current EDs, they tend to rate their children as having high levels of difficult temperament[9]; and perceive them as having greater negative effect, that is, demonstrating more sadness, irritability, and crying compared with controls.[10] In a more recent large longitudinal study, we found that mothers with EDs were more likely to perceive their children as having a "difficult temperament" characterized by the child being less happy and active than other children of their age, more

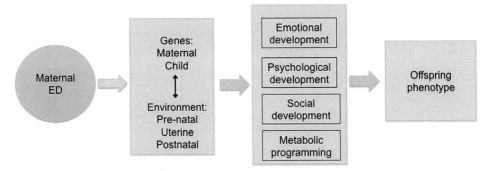

FIG. 15.1 Effects of maternal eating disorder (ED) on offspring phenotype.

restless and as having more tantrums and as being less cautious and guarded than other children of their age.[11] Many studies, however, including our own, have relied on maternal reports rather than direct observations and therefore should be considered with caution. Although it is possible that children of mothers with EDs are objectively more difficult, we should not discard the possibility that mothers with EDs perceive their children as being difficult. This could be due to their own preoccupation with the disorder, or due to difficulties processing their children's emotional cues. However, even if the latter is true, this maternal perception of a difficult temperament might have an impact on how they respond to their child's needs, and in turn affect their child's temperament and later development. Interestingly, in our recent study [11] on childhood psychopathology in children of mothers with EDs, we found that child temperament partially mediated the effect of maternal bulimia nervosa (BN) on childhood psychopathology at the age of 7 years (pointing to a shared genetic and environmental effect). For maternal AN, however, the effect of the EDs on childhood psychopathology was completely mediated by temperament. Lastly, as temperament has been found to have a genetic influence,[7] we cannot discard the hypothesis that children of mothers with EDs have a genetic predisposition to a difficult temperament, which in itself predisposes to later psychopathology.

Cognitive Development/Neuropsychological Profile

The last 15 years have seen an increase in research focusing on thinking styles that might be associated with ED presentations.[12] The study of neuropsychology aims to understand behaviors related directly to brain function and uses psychological, neurological, cognitive, and behavioral principles and techniques to evaluate neurocognitive, behavioral, and emotional profiles.

Different neuropsychological characteristics have been described in EDs, including alterations in attention, visuospatial ability, memory, social cognition, and executive functions, encompassing set shifting and central coherence.[12–14] The study of neuropsychological factors in mental health has greatly developed in the last decades, and in EDs there has been a shift on trying to understand whether some of the neuropsychological characteristics seen during active illness might be (1) correlates of EDs, (2) a result of severe illness with important medical complications that affect brain structure and function (scars), or (3) endophenotypes/intermediate phenotypes, i.e., markers of disorder that might lie on the pathways between genetic/biological risk and actual phenotypical manifestations.[15]

Our investigation has focused on cognitive development and neuropsychological profiles in children of women with EDs, with a double aim, firstly to understand the impact of maternal EDs on child development; secondly (studying children of mothers with EDs prior to ED onset), as an ideal model to understand endophenotypes/intermediate phenotypes of EDs. Our studies have shown that specific cognitive and neuropsychological differences might be present in the offspring of mothers with EDs.[3,16–18] In a study carried out by Kothari et al.[17] on children from a population-based study aged 8–10 years, when compared with children of mothers with no psychiatric disorders, children of mothers with lifetime BN displayed poorer visuospatial functioning; children of mothers with lifetime AN had higher full-scale and performance IQ, increased working memory (WM) capacity, better visuospatial functioning, and decreased attentional control. We were also able to study early cognitive development (18 months and 4 years) in a subset of these children, showing that children of women with lifetime AN had difficulties with social understanding, poorer motor skills, planning, and abstract reasoning.[16] In a smaller ongoing longitudinal study of children born to mothers with EDs by our group,[3] we recently found that infants (1 year old) of mothers with EDs had poorer language and motor development compared with healthy control mothers. Interestingly, after studying differential outcomes based on active versus past EDs, we found that child cognitive difficulties were associated both with maternal active EDs and past EDs. Overall these findings highlight early developmental difficulties in motor and cognitive development in offspring of EDs mothers. The study of later cognitive characteristics suggests a more specific pattern of strengths and difficulties across several domains of cognition, for example, higher IQ, better visuospatial performance and WM in children of mothers with lifetime AN, and poorer visuospatial functioning in children of mothers with lifetime BN.

Only one study to date has investigated social cognition in children of mothers with EDs in middle childhood and early adolescence, with some evidence of differences between at-risk offspring and controls. In particular, differential facial emotion processing, poorer recognition of fear, and higher scores on the social communication disorders checklist were present in children of mothers with binge eating and purging behaviors, the latter one also present in children of mothers with lifetime binge eating disorder (BED).[18] These very preliminary findings hint to a link between social communication difficulties and bulimic/bing eating type phenotypes; however, replication is needed.

Psychopathology

The effect of maternal psychiatric disorders on their offspring's mental health has been well documented, both for homotypic and heterotypic transmissions, establishing that children of parents with psychiatric disorders are at higher risk of developing psychopathology themselves.[19,20] Children of mothers with depression, for example, have been shown to be at risk for emotional disorders themselves (homotypic transmission); however, they are also at higher risk for other internalizing and externalizing difficulties (heterotypic transmission).[19] Understanding the risk model for the development of psychopathology in children of mothers with mental health difficulties can allow not only an understanding of possible mechanisms of intergenerational transmission but also the potential shared risk between different psychiatric disorders. While the risk of psychiatric disorders in the offspring of parents with other psychiatric disorders has been widely studied, EDs lag behind.

Although relatively sparse, studies examining associations between maternal EDs and childhood psychopathology have identified higher levels of psychological and emotional difficulties as well as general psychopathology in children of mothers with EDs. There is evidence in clinical cohorts of higher levels of emotional problems in offspring of mothers with EDs.[21] Our work in large longitudinal cohort studies has identified a higher risk for emotional and behavioral disorders in offspring of EDs mothers at an early age (3.5 years). Specifically, we identified associations between maternal ED type (AN vs. BN) and child psychopathology (emotional vs. behavioral problems), as well as gender differences.[22] Emotional difficulties were found in both girls and boys of mothers with AN, while more hyperactivity and peer difficulties were found in both girls and boys of mothers with BN. This study also aimed to understand risk mechanisms and highlighted a mediating role for maternal anxiety and depression in the postpartum. These findings were confirmed and extended in a later study when the same children were aged 7, 10, and 13 years,[23] where we found that maternal EDs (both AN and BN) strongly predicted emotional and anxiety disorders. In a recent longitudinal study, we [11] showed that maternal EDs were associated with childhood psychopathology in girls and boys at the age of 7 years, both emotional and behavioral problems. Disorder and gender-specific findings across studies point to an effect of maternal lifetime AN on emotional disorders, in particular anxiety, across ages, while maternal BN seems to be associated with hyperactivity, conduct, and peer problems.[11]

These findings support those of smaller clinical studies. In a longitudinal study using the Child Behavior Checklist, Cimino and colleagues[24] found that children of women with EDs had higher levels of emotional adaptive, internalizing, as well as externalizing problems compared with children of healthy mothers. Furthermore, the results showed that the latter tends to increase with age. Similarly, in a recent small study, mothers with EDs reported higher levels of behavioral problems in their children compared with control mothers.[25]

Overall, the literature shows that a maternal lifetime history of ED may have a negative impact on children's cognitive, psychological development, and psychopathology. Recent studies on genetic and heritability factors in EDs and related behaviors have identified important genetic correlations between these and other psychiatric disorders, i.e., AN and obsessive compulsive disorder (OCD),[26] binge eating, and ADHD symptoms in females.[27] However less is known on cognition and neuropsychological characteristics in offspring of mothers with EDs prior to the onset of psychopathology, these might be an important focus of study in at-risk offspring, helping future prevention and early intervention.

THE EFFECT OF MATERNAL EDs ON CHILDHOOD FEEDING AND EATING

Given its relevance, the effect of maternal EDs on children's feeding and eating has been the focus of a relatively large body of literature. The accomplishment of adequate feeding is a complex task, involving relational aspects as well as biological and psychological ones, hence maternal psychopathology as well as interpersonal difficulties can impact on child feeding and eating development.[28,29] Feeding difficulties starting in infancy often persist into school age as well as later in life, with effects on all aspect of child and adolescent development,[30,31] including mental health. Moreover, children with feeding and eating problems can be an important source of stress for parents, which can exacerbate existing difficulties, such as depression or anxiety.

The effects of maternal EDs on childhood feeding and eating have been shown in a series of clinical and population-based studies. We will review below the available evidence starting form infancy into later life.

In infancy, breastfeeding practices have been shown to differ in mothers with EDs (AN, BN, BED, EDNOS) versus controls; in particular mothers with EDs started to breastfeed their infants as often as controls; however, they were more likely to interrupt breastfeeding early.[32] On the other hand, we found that mothers with EDs were more likely to breastfeed, particularly those with BN.[33] Mothers with EDs were also more likely to encounter difficulties with infant feeding and growth in the first year of life. Infants of women with AN were at higher risk for feeding difficulties between age 0 and 6 months, while infants of mothers with BN were significantly more likely to be overweight and to have faster growth rates at age 9 months compared with controls. Although feeding difficulties can be common during the first few months of the infant's life, mothers with AN reported early-onset persistent feeding problems, difficulties in domains such as slow feeding, small quantities feeding, and no established feeding routine (for infants aged 1 and 6 months).[33,34] On the other hand, infants of women with BN had higher levels of refusal to take solids in comparison with controls.[33] It is important to note that a direct link has been found between increased risk for feeding difficulties

and maternal lifetime ED as well as active ED symptomatology in pregnancy, but this association was also mediated by maternal distress (i.e., depression and anxiety).[35] Furthermore, feeding difficulties at 6 months were significantly related to anxiety and depression symptomatology at 8 months postpartum.[35] Blisset and Meyer[36] found similar results, with some gender specificity, showing that maternal eating psychopathology predicted maternal report of food refusal in girls but not in boys. They also showed that unhealthy maladaptive cognitive features, such as defectiveness or shame beliefs, were significantly associated with food refusal in girls.[36] However, contrasting results have also been found, as Whelan and Cooper,[37] did not find child gender differences in the effect of maternal ED, nor did gender moderate the relationship between feeding difficulties and maternal ED.

There is a well-known relationship between specific parenting styles in women with EDs and feeding problems in their offspring. During both mealtime and play, negative expressed emotions and intrusive behaviors were found to be more frequent among mothers with EDs.[38] In the same study, infants of mothers with EDs tended to weigh less compared with controls, while no differences in weight between the two groups were found at birth. Mealtime interaction between offspring (ages 1–4 years) and mothers with EDs was also investigated by Waugh and Bulik,[39] who found that mothers with EDs made fewer positive comments about food and eating compared with healthy controls. Differences between ED diagnoses and their impact on infant feeding problems are worth noting. While mothers with BN or BED are more likely to report higher levels of restrictive feeding styles compared with controls,[40] mothers with a history of AN are less likely to use pressuring feeding strategies.[41]

Thus, maternal EDs can influence nutritional intake but also the dietary patterns in infants. Indeed, comparing dietary patterns of children of mothers with EDs with the diet of children of healthy controls, Easter et al.[42] found that across a four-time period (ages 3, 4, 7, and 9 years), children of mothers with EDs showed increased levels of a "health-conscious/vegetarian" dietary pattern, diet characterized by high content of vegetarian foods, nuts, salad, rice, pasta, and fruits. Furthermore, they also showed less adherence to the "traditional" dietary pattern which consisted of a typical British meal with "meat and two vegetables dinner" across all four-time points. Energy intake was higher among BN and AN + BN offspring, and this intake increased significantly over time for children of mothers with BN. In another study,[32] it was found that mothers with BN and BED were less likely to use "homemade traditional food" than "commercial jarred baby food" when compared with mothers without EDs. However, in women with BED the associations were significant only before controlling for relevant confounders.

In summary, these findings indicate that mothers with EDs tend to experience difficulties in feeding their children both in infancy and childhood. Although studies on breastfeeding yield mixed results, women with EDs often report difficulties with this. As the infant develops, difficulties such as slow feeding, small quantities feeding, not having established a feeding routine emerged as common among mothers with EDs. Restricting parental feeding styles, negative expressed emotions, and intrusive behaviors also appeared to be more frequent in mothers with EDs compared with controls.

THE EFFECT OF MATERNAL EDs ON EDs IN CHILDREN

Very few studies have investigated the specific risk for EDs in children of parents with EDs. Studies of first-degree relatives have highlighted higher prevalence of AN in first-degree relatives of AN patients[43]; and of AN and BN in first-degree relatives of AN and BN patients in a case-control study.[44]

A more recent large patient register–based linkage study based in Sweden found that a diagnosed ED in either parent and in mothers was independently associated with a diagnosed ED in their female child, with twofold increased hazard ratios.[45]

Although this initial evidence is very important, given that the two large studies cited above focused on diagnosed disorders, it remains to be determined whether the increased risk of offspring disorder is a pure increase in risk versus increased recognition and access to healthcare among children who have a parent with an ED. It also remains to be determined what the risk pathways might be.

CONCLUSIONS

Maternal EDs have an impact on child psychological, cognitive, and eating development and might affect the development of EDs in the offspring. Despite this evidence, little is know on specific risk mechanisms and how genetic and environmental factors affect risk. No available literature has focused on resilience, and why some children of parents with EDs do not develop psychiatric pathology. The latter has important implications for therapeutic targets and prevention.

REFERENCES

1. Bulik CM, Reba L, Siega-Riz A-M, Reichborn-Kjennerud T. Anorexia nervosa: definition, epidemiology, and cycle of risk. *Int J Eat Disord*. 2005;37(S1):S2–S9.
2. Micali N, Treasure J. Biological effects of a maternal ED on pregnancy and foetal development: a review. *Eur Eat Disord Rev*. 2009;17(6):448–454.
3. Barona M, Taborelli E, Corfield F, et al. Neurobehavioural and cognitive development in infants born to mothers with eating disorders. *J Child Psychol Psychiatry*. 2017;58(8):931–938.
4. Easter A, Taborelli E, Bye A, et al. Perinatal hypothalamic-pituitary-adrenal axis regulation among women with eating disorders and their infants. *Psychoneuroendocrinology*. 2017;76:127–134.
5. Micali N, Al Essimii H, Field AE, Treasure J. Pregnancy loss of control over eating: a longitudinal study of maternal and child outcomes. *Am J Clin Nutr*. 2018;108(1):101–107.
6. Chess S, Thomas A. Temperament and the parent-child interaction. *Pediatr Ann*. 1977;6(9):574–582.
7. Rettew DC, McKee L. Temperament and its role in developmental psychopathology. *Harv Rev Psychiatry*. 2005;13(1):14–27.
8. Wichstrøm L, Penelo E, Rensvik Viddal K, de la Osa N, Ezpeleta L. Explaining the relationship between temperament and symptoms of psychiatric disorders from preschool to middle childhood: hybrid fixed and random effects models of Norwegian and Spanish children. *J Child Psychol Psychiatry*. 2018;59(3):285–295.
9. Zerwas S, Von Holle A, Torgersen L, Reichborn-Kjennerud T, Stoltenberg C, Bulik CM. Maternal eating disorders and infant temperament: findings from the Norwegian mother and child cohort study. *Int J Eat Disord*. 2012;45(4):546–555.
10. Agras S, Hammer L, McNicholas F. A prospective study of the influence of eating-disordered mothers on their children. *Int J Eat Disord*. 1999;25(3):253–262.
11. Barona M, Nybo Andersen AM, Micali N. Childhood psychopathology in children of women with eating disorders. *Acta Psychiatr Scand*. 2016;134(4):295–304.
12. Jáuregui-Lobera I. Neuropsychology of eating disorders: 1995–2012. *Neuropsychiatric Dis Treat*. 2013;9:415–430.
13. Kanakam N, Raoult C, Collier D, Treasure J. Set shifting and central coherence as neurocognitive endophenotypes in eating disorders: a preliminary investigation in twins. *World J Biol Psychiatry*. 2013;14(6):464–475.
14. Lopez C, Tchanturia K, Stahl D, Treasure J. Central coherence in eating disorders: a systematic review. *Psychol Med*. 2008;38.
15. Micali N, Dahlgren CL. All that glisters is not an endophenotype: rethinking endophenotypes in anorexia nervosa. *Eur Child Adolesc Psychiatry*. 2016;25(11):1149–1150.
16. Kothari R, Rosinska M, Treasure J, Micali N. The early cognitive development of children at high risk of developing an eating disorder. *Eur Eat Disord Rev*. 2014;22(2):152–156.

17. Kothari R, Solmi F, Treasure J, Micali N. The neuropsychological profile of children at high risk of developing an eating disorder. *Psychol Med.* 2013;43(7):1543–1554.

18. Kothari R, Barona M, Treasure J, Micali N. Social cognition in children at familial high-risk of developing an eating disorder. *Front Behav Neurosci.* 2015;9:208.

19. McLaughlin KA, Gadermann AM, Hwang I, et al. Parent psychopathology and offspring mental disorders: results from the WHO World Mental Health Surveys. *Br J Psychiatry.* 2012;200(4):290–299.

20. Dean K, Stevens H, Mortensen PB, Murray RM, Walsh E, Pedersen CB. Full spectrum of psychiatric outcomes among offspring with parental history of mental disorder. *Arch Gen Psychiatry.* 2010;67(8):822–829.

21. Stein A, Woolley H, Cooper S, Winterbottom J, Fairburn CG, Cortina-Borja M. Eating habits and attitudes among 10-year-old children of mothers with eating disorders: longitudinal study. *Br J Psychiatry.* 2006;189:324–329.

22. Micali N, Stahl D, Treasure J, Simonoff E. Childhood psychopathology in children of women with eating disorders: understanding risk mechanisms. *J Child Psychol Psychiatry.* 2014;55(2):124–134.

23. Micali N, De Stavola B, Ploubidis GB, Simonoff E, Treasure J. The effects of maternal eating disorders on offspring childhood and early adolescent psychiatric disorders. *Int J Eat Disord.* 2014;47(4):385–393.

24. Cimino C, Paciello S. A six-year prospective study on children of mothers with eating disorders: the role of paternal psychological profiles. *Eur Eat Disord Rev.* 2013;21(3):238–246.

25. Sadeh-Sharvit S, Levy-Shiff R, Arnow KD, Lock JD. The interactions of mothers with eating disorders with their toddlers: identifying broader risk factors. *Am J Bioeth.* 2016;18(4):418–428.

26. Duncan L, Yilmaz Z, Gaspar H, et al. Significant locus and metabolic genetic correlations revealed in genome-wide association study of anorexia nervosa. *Am J Psychiatry.* 2017;174(9):850–858.

27. Capusan AJ, Yao S, Kuja-Halkola R, et al. Genetic and environmental aspects in the association between attention-deficit hyperactivity disorder symptoms and binge-eating behavior in adults: a twin study. *Psychol Med.* 2017;47(16):2866–2878.

28. Chatoor I, Ganiban J, Colin V, Plummer N, Harmon RJ. Attachment and feeding problems: a reexamination of nonorganic failure to thrive and attachment insecurity. *J Am Acad Child Adolesc Psychiatry.* 1998;37(11):1217–1224.

29. Lindberg L, Bohlin G, Hagekull B, Palmérus K. Interactions between mothers and infants showing food refusal. *Infant Ment Health J.* 1996;17(4):334–347.

30. Patel P, Wheatcroft R, Park RJ, Stein A. The children of mothers with eating disorders. *Clin Child Fam Psychol Rev.* 2002;5(1):1–19.

31. Drewett RF, Corbett SS, Wright CM. Physical and emotional development, appetite and body image in adolescents who failed to thrive as infants. *J Child Psychol Psychiatry.* 2006;47(5):524–531.

32. Torgersen L, Ystrom E, Haugen M, et al. Breastfeeding practice in mothers with eating disorders. *Matern Child Nutr.* 2010;6(3):243–252.

33. Micali N, Simonoff E, Treasure J. Infant feeding and weight in the first year of life in babies of women with eating disorders. *J Pediatr.* 2009;154(1):55–60. e51.

34. Micali N, Simonoff E, Stahl D, Treasure J. Maternal eating disorders and infant feeding difficulties: maternal and child mediators in a longitudinal general population study. *J Child Psychol Psychiatry.* 2011;52(7):800–807.

35. Micali N, Simonoff E, Elberling H, Rask CU, Olsen EM, Skovgaard AM. Eating patterns in a population-based sample of children aged 5 to 7 years: association with psychopathology and parentally perceived impairment. *J Dev Behav Pediatr.* 2011;32(8):572–580.

36. Blissett J, Meyer C. The mediating role of eating psychopathology in the relationship between unhealthy core beliefs and feeding difficulties in a nonclinical group. *Int J Eat Disord.* 2006;39(8):763–771.

37. Whelan E, Cooper PJ. The association between childhood feeding problems and maternal eating disorder: a community study. *Psychol Med.* 2000;30(1):69–77.

38. Stein A, Woolley H, Cooper SD, Fairburn CG. An observational study of mothers with eating disorders and their infants. *J Child Psychol Psychiatry.* 1994;35(4):733–748.

39. Waugh E, Bulik CM. Offspring of women with eating disorders. *Int J Eat Disord.* 1999;25(2):123–133.

40. Reba-Harrelson L, Von Holle A, Hamer RM, Torgersen L, Reichborn-Kjennerud T, Bulik CM. Patterns of maternal feeding and child eating associated with eating disorders in the Norwegian Mother and Child Cohort Study (MoBa). *Eat Behav.* 2010;11(1):54–61.

41. de Barse LM, Tharner A, Micali N, et al. Does maternal history of eating disorders predict mothers' feeding practices and preschoolers' emotional eating? *Appetite.* 2015;85:1–7.

42. Easter A, Naumann U, Northstone K, Schmidt U, Treasure J, Micali N. A longitudinal investigation of nutrition and dietary patterns in children of mothers with eating disorders. *J Pediatr.* 2013;163(1):173–178.e171.

43. Steinhausen HC, Jakobsen H, Helenius D, Munk-Jorgensen P, Strober M. A nation-wide study of the family aggregation and risk factors in anorexia nervosa over three generations. *Int J Eat Disord.* 2015;48(1):1–8.

44. Strober M, Freeman R, Lampert C, Diamond J, Kaye W. Controlled family study of anorexia nervosa and bulimia nervosa: evidence of shared liability and transmission of partial syndromes. *Am J Psychiatry.* 2000;157(3):393–401.

45. Bould H, Sovio U, Koupil I, et al. Do eating disorders in parents predict eating disorders in children? Evidence from a Swedish cohort. *Acta Psychiatr Scand.* 2015;132(1):51–59.

CHAPTER 16

An Addiction Perspective on Eating Disorders and Obesity

ADRIAN MEULE, PHD

INTRODUCTION

The assumption that certain foods or nutrients such as sugar can be addictive is widely held in the general population. In studies from the United Kingdom,[1-3] more than 90% of participants thought that some people are addicted to certain foods and about 25% indicated that they perceived themselves as being "food addicted." These self-perceptions, however, seem to be easily influenced by media reports: when the researchers provided participants with a bogus newspaper article that claimed that "food addiction is real," more than 50% indicated that they perceived themselves to be addicted to some foods.

Given the widespread availability of and easy accessibility to processed, high-calorie foods, and the high prevalence rates of obesity in the past decades, many people (including scientists) assume that a potential addiction to certain foods is a phenomenon of the 21st century. In actuality, the first scientific papers that introduced an addiction perspective on eating even date back to the end of the 19th and the beginning of the 20th century.[4] Nevertheless, both media reports about and scientific investigations of "food addiction" have risen sharply in the past 5–10 years.

The reasons for this interest in the topic can be found in the apparent parallels between substance use and overeating. For example, substance use is often preceded by a strong desire to consume the substance. Such cravings can be found for both drugs of abuse (e.g., alcohol, tobacco, caffeine, illegal drugs) and foods (including nonalcoholic beverages), and it appears that behavioral aspects as well as cognitive and neural mechanisms of craving experiences are largely similar across different substances (including food).[5-7] Other parallels between substance use and overeating include loss of control over consumption and unsuccessful attempts to reduce consumption.

However, these are not the only symptoms of addictive behavior. Therefore, it is inevitable to address the scientific definitions of addiction to be able to evaluate the concept of "food addiction" properly.

DEFINITIONS OF ADDICTION

According to the American Society of Addiction Medicine, addiction is a primary, chronic disease of brain reward, motivation, memory, and related circuitry. Dysfunction in these circuits leads to characteristic biological, psychological, social, and spiritual manifestations. This is reflected in an individual pathologically pursuing reward and/or relief by substance use and other behaviors. It is characterized by inability to consistently abstain, impairment in behavioral control, craving, diminished recognition of significant problems with one's behaviors and interpersonal relationships, and a dysfunctional emotional response. Like other chronic diseases, addiction often involves cycles of relapse and remission. Without treatment or engagement in recovery activities, addiction is progressive and can result in disability or premature death (www.asam.org/quality-practice/definition-of-addiction).

Similar (but not equivalent) to this definition, the current version of the Diagnostic and Statistical Manual of Mental Disorders (DSM-5) specifies 11 symptoms of substance use disorder:

1. Taking the substance in larger amounts or over a longer period than intended
2. Having a desire or unsuccessful efforts to cut down or control substance use
3. Spending much time to obtain or use the substance or recover from its effects
4. Having substance cravings
5. Failing to fulfill major role obligations because of substance use

6. Continuing substance use despite social or inter-personal problems
7. Reducing important activities because of substance use
8. Using the substance in situations that can be physically hazardous
9. Continuing substance use despite physical or psychological problems
10. Developing tolerance to the effects of the substance
11. Having withdrawal symptoms after cessation of substance use

In addition, gambling disorder has been included in DSM-5 as a non–substance-related, addictive disorder.[8] Given this inclusion of both substance-related and behavioral addictions in DSM-5, it has also been suggested that when considering overeating from an addiction perspective, a conceptualization as "eating addiction" (in terms of a behavioral addiction) may be more appropriate than a conceptualization as "food addiction" (in terms of a substance-related disorder).[9]

MEASURING ADDICTION-LIKE EATING IN HUMANS

Several approaches have been developed to assess "food addiction" or "eating addiction" in humans. These are based on self-identification of addiction-like eating with single questions, interview techniques, and standardized questionnaires (Table 16.1). The great majority of studies has used the Yale Food Addiction Scale (YFAS), which was originally designed by "translating" the seven symptoms of substance dependence in DSM-IV to refer to food and eating.[10] Because of the changes made to the diagnostic criteria for substance use disorder in DSM-5, a revised version (YFAS 2.0) has been developed that aims to assess 11 symptoms of "food addiction."[11] Two items assess a clinically significant impairment or distress because of one's eating behavior. These questions are crucial for calculation of a diagnostic score of "food addiction": individuals are only classified as "food addicted" when they endorse at least 2 of the 11 symptoms *and* meet the impairment/distress criterion.

"FOOD ADDICTION" AND OBESITY

"Food addiction" as measured with the YFAS relates to higher body mass index (BMI). In nonobese adults, prevalence rates of "food addiction" range between 5% and 15%. Two studies that used a child version of the YFAS in children and adolescents reported prevalence rates between 3% and 7%.[12,13] In obese adults, prevalence rates range between 15% and 20% but reach up to 30%–50% in treatment-seeking adults with extreme obesity.[14,15] Similarly, 38% of obese adolescents recruited at the beginning of an in-patient weight-loss program were classified as "food addicted."[16] Therefore, although a relationship between "food addiction" and body weight exists, neither can obesity be equated with "food addiction" nor is "food addiction" restricted to individuals with obesity.

"FOOD ADDICTION" AND EATING DISORDERS

Prevalence rates of "food addiction" in adults with binge eating disorder range between 40% and 50% and are even more than 80% in adults with bulimia nervosa.[17,18] There is also a moderate overlap between YFAS scores and night eating severity.[19] Surprisingly, a substantial number of adolescents and adults with restrictive anorexia nervosa also meet the YFAS criteria,[20,21] which may be due to the fact that these individuals interpret items differently and, thus, the scale may be not valid in this population. In conclusion, although there is a relatively weak—but positive—association between "food addiction" as measured with the YFAS and BMI, it appears that there is a much larger overlap between "food addiction" and eating disorders.

IMPLICATIONS AND CONTROVERSIES

Adopting an addiction perspective on eating disorders and obesity has practical implications that include nosology, prevention, and therapy of these disorders. For example, some advocates of the concept argue that "food addiction" is a condition that is distinct from established eating disorders and, thus, should be included as an addictive disorder in diagnostic classification systems. Obesity prevention approaches may be inspired by tobacco control policies.[22] Similar to groups such as Overeaters Anonymous that incorporate an addiction framework,[23] cognitive-behavioral treatments for obesity,[24] or eating disorders such as bulimia nervosa[25,26] may be adjusted accordingly. Finally, pharmacological approaches inspired by addiction treatments have also been proposed.[27]

TABLE 16.1
Approaches to Measure "Food Addiction" or "Eating Addiction" in Humans

Types	Descriptions	References
INTERVIEWS		
Semistructured interview	Themes (e.g., the 11 diagnostic criteria for substance use disorder in DSM-5) mentioned in semistructured interviews on how participants experienced their over- or binge eating were analyzed	Curtis and Davis[37]
Structured interview	The substance dependence module of the Structured Clinical Interview for DSM-IV Axis I Disorders was modified with the term *substance* referring to *binge eating*	Cassin and von Ranson[38]
QUESTIONNAIRES		
Addiction-like Eating Behaviour Scale	15-item questionnaire that conceptualizes addiction-like eating behavior as a behavioral (i.e., not substance-related) addiction	Ruddock et al.[39]
Eating Addiction Questionnaire	22-item questionnaire that conceptualizes addiction-like eating behavior as a behavioral (i.e., not substance-related) addiction	von Ranson[40]
Eating Behaviors Questionnaire	20-item questionnaire that conceptualizes addiction-like eating behavior as a substance-related addiction based on the seven diagnostic criteria for substance dependence in DSM-IV; a child and an adult version are available	Merlo et al.[41]
Yale Food Addiction Scale	25-item questionnaire that conceptualizes addiction-like eating behavior as a substance-related addiction based on the seven diagnostic criteria for substance dependence in DSM-IV; a 9-item short version and a 25-item child version are also available	Gearhardt et al.[10] Gearhardt et al.[12] Flint et al.[42]
Yale Food Addiction Scale 2.0	35-item questionnaire that conceptualizes addiction-like eating behavior as a substance-related addiction based on the 11 diagnostic criteria for substance use disorder in DSM-5; a 13-item short version is also available	Gearhardt et al.[11] Schulte and Gearhardt[43]
SELF-IDENTIFICATION		
Single question	For example, "Are you a chocolate addict?", "Do you agree with the following statement: 'I believe to be a food addict'?", or "Do you feel that you are addicted to some foods?"	Hetherington and Macdiarmid[44] Ruddock et al.[45] Meadows et al.[46]

DSM, Diagnostic and Statistical Manual of Mental Disorders.

Adversaries of the "food addiction" concept, however, have criticized these suggestions. While some of the critiques refer to potential adverse effects of creating a "new" disorder, others refer to the lack of validity of the concept as a whole or that it is simply not necessary.

Table 16.2 presents some of the controversies that are discussed in the "food addiction" field. As a detailed discussion of arguments raised by both sides is beyond the scope of this chapter, readers are referred to the extensive literature on this topic.[9,28–36]

TABLE 16.2
Some Controversies in the "Food Addiction" Field

Issue	Proponents' View	Opponents' View
Definition	"Food addiction" can be defined and assessed by "translating" existing diagnostic criteria for substance use disorder to refer to food and eating.	The category of (processed, high-calorie) foods is too broad, and there is disagreement over the exact "translation" of symptoms or whether this procedure is valid in the first place.
	"Food addiction" refers to processed, high-caloric foods, and thus, these foods can be avoided in exchange for healthy, low-caloric foods.	Eating food is necessary for survival, and thus, abstinence is not possible.
	People usually crave and overconsume palatable, high-fat, and/or high-sugar foods (and not low-caloric, bland foods), and thus, "food addiction" is substance-related and not merely behavioral.	As the addiction potential of each drug of abuse can be traced back to a specific, single substance (e.g., ethanol, nicotine, tetrahydrocannabinol), "food addiction" cannot be a substance-related disorder (but maybe a behavioral addiction).
	There is a large overlap between "food addiction" and problematic eating behaviors such as binge eating, which supports convergent validity of the "food addiction" concept.	There is a large overlap between "food addiction" and problematic eating behaviors such as binge eating, which shows that the "food addiction" concept is not sufficiently different from existing conditions and, thus, does not warrant classification as a distinctive disease phenotype.
Animal models	Animal models support an addictive response to sugar.	The methods applied in animal models create an artificial eating schedule that is not representative of human eating behavior.
Neurobiology	Reward-related brain mechanisms in response to substance use and food consumption are very similar, which supports the "food addiction" model.	Reward-related brain mechanisms in response to substance use and food consumption are overlapping, but a close examination also reveals substantial differences.
	Effects of different drugs of abuse are not uniform (e.g., there is no intoxication syndrome described for tobacco in DSM-5), which means that certain foods can be addictive although they are not intoxicating.	Foods are not intoxicating, which means they cannot be addictive.
Implications	"Food addiction" should be included as an addictive disorder in diagnostic classification systems.	Changes in the diagnostic criteria for eating disorders in DSM-5 reduced the number of EDNOS diagnoses, and most individuals that are classified as "food addicted" are already covered by the diagnostic criteria for full or low-frequency bulimia nervosa and binge eating disorder.
	Obese individuals find the "food addiction" concept helpful, and the focus on addictive foods decreases self-blame and the stigma of personal failure.	The "food addiction" concept distracts attention away from the significant role of exercise for weight loss and maintenance and may create a new stigma.
	The "food addiction" model implies adopting an addiction perspective on eating disorder and obesity treatment, which includes that potentially addictive foods should be abandoned from one's diet.	Success rates of cognitive–behavioral therapy for bulimia nervosa and binge eating disorder are high, and its goal is to achieve a flexible, balanced, and moderate food consumption with no forbidden foods. As only a subset of obese individuals show an addiction-like eating behavior, an addiction framework would be inappropriate for the majority of obese individuals.
	When certain foods can have an addiction potential, public policy actions need to be taken, which may be inspired by tobacco control regulations.	The "food addiction" concept is not necessary to justify such efforts, and the food industry may present "food addiction" as a rare disorder that does not warrant policy changes to influence the general public's eating.

DSM, Diagnostic and Statistical Manual of Mental Disorders; *EDNOS*, Eating Disorder Not Otherwise Specified.

CONCLUSIONS

In contrast to popular beliefs, "food addiction" is not a new idea that was invented in recent years to explain rising prevalence rates of obesity. Instead, an addiction perspective on eating disorders and obesity has been controversially discussed for many decades. Only a subset of obese individuals show an addiction-like eating behavior, and thus, the obesity pandemic cannot be explained by addiction-like eating or addictive foods. On the contrary, many individuals with binge eating meet the proposed "food addiction" criteria, and thus, addiction-like eating appears to be primarily related to eating pathology and only secondarily related to body weight. Although progress in this field has been made by developing measures in an effort to standardize and guide further investigations, researchers are nowhere near to find a consensus about a proper definition of or even about a name for addiction-like eating (e.g., "food addiction," "eating addiction," "food use disorder"), the validity of the concept, or its usefulness and practical implications. Whether or not researchers will someday agree on a unified definition of addiction-like eating, and if "food addiction is real," providing an addiction framework in the prevention and treatment of eating disorders and obesity will likely be helpful in some instances but will be unnecessary or even counterproductive in others. Hopefully, future studies will reveal for which aspects or for whom this is the case.

REFERENCES

1. Hardman CA, Rogers PJ, Dallas R, Scott J, Ruddock HK, Robinson E. "Food addiction is real". The effects of exposure to this message on self-diagnosed food addiction and eating behaviour. *Appetite*. 2015;91:179–184.
2. Ruddock HK, Christiansen P, Jones A, Robinson E, Field M, Hardman CA. Believing in food addiction: helpful or counterproductive for eating behavior? *Obesity*. 2016;24:1238–1243.
3. Ruddock HK, Dickson JM, Field M, Hardman CA. Eating to live or living to eat? Exploring the causal attributions of self-perceived food addiction. *Appetite*. 2015;95:262–268.
4. Meule A. Back by popular demand: a narrative review on the history of food addiction research. *Yale J Biol Med*. 2015;88:295–302.
5. Hormes JM, Rozin P. Does "craving" carve nature at the joints? Absence of a synonym for craving in many languages. *Addict Behav*. 2010;35:459–463.
6. Kavanagh DJ, Andrade J, May J. Imaginary relish and exquisite torture: the elaborated intrusion theory of desire. *Psychol Rev*. 2005;112:446–467.
7. May J, Kavanagh DJ, Andrade J. The Elaborated Intrusion Theory of desire: a 10-year retrospective and implications for addiction treatments. *Addict Behav*. 2015;44:29–34.
8. American Psychiatric Association. *Diagnostic and Statistical Manual of Mental Disorders*. 5th ed. Washington, DC: American Psychiatric Association; 2013.
9. Hebebrand J, Albayrak O, Adan R, et al. "Eating addiction", rather than "food addiction", better captures addictive-like eating behavior. *Neurosci Biobehav Rev*. 2014;47:295–306.
10. Gearhardt AN, Corbin WR, Brownell KD. Preliminary validation of the Yale Food Addiction Scale. *Appetite*. 2009;52:430–436.
11. Gearhardt AN, Corbin WR, Brownell KD. Development of the Yale Food Addiction Scale Version 2.0. *Psychol Addict Behav*. 2016;30:113–121.
12. Gearhardt AN, Roberto CA, Seamans MJ, Corbin WR, Brownell KD. Preliminary validation of the Yale Food Addiction Scale for children. *Eat Behav*. 2013;14:508–512.
13. Mies GW, Treur JL, Larsen JK, Halberstadt J, Pasman JA, Vink JM. The prevalence of food addiction in a large sample of adolescents and its association with addictive substances. *Appetite*. 2017;118:97–105.
14. Hauck C, Weiß A, Schulte EM, Meule A, Ellrott T. Prevalence of 'food addiction' as measured with the Yale Food Addiction Scale 2.0 in a representative German sample and its association with sex, age and weight categories. *Obes Facts*. 2017;10:12–24.
15. Meule A, Müller A, Gearhardt AN, Blechert J. German version of the Yale Food Addiction Scale 2.0: prevalence and correlates of 'food addiction' in students and obese individuals. *Appetite*. 2017;115:54–61.
16. Meule A, Hermann T, Kübler A. Food addiction in overweight and obese adolescents seeking weight-loss treatment. *Eur Eat Disord Rev*. 2015;23:193–198.
17. Gearhardt AN, Boswell RG, White MA. The association of "food addiction" with disordered eating and body mass index. *Eat Behav*. 2014;15:427–433.
18. de Vries S-K, Meule A. Food addiction and bulimia nervosa: new data based on the Yale Food Addiction Scale 2.0. *Eur Eat Disord Rev*. 2016;24:518–522.
19. Nolan LJ, Geliebter A. "Food addiction" is associated with night eating severity. *Appetite*. 2016;98:89–94.
20. Albayrak Ö, Föcker M, Kliewer J, et al. Eating-related psychopathology and food addiction in adolescent psychiatric inpatients. *Eur Eat Disord Rev*. 2017;25:214–220.
21. Granero R, Hilker I, Aguera Z, et al. Food addiction in a Spanish sample of eating disorders: DSM-5 diagnostic subtype differentiation and validation data. *Eur Eat Disord Rev*. 2014;22:389–396.
22. Gearhardt AN, Bragg MA, Pearl RL, Schvey NA, Roberto CA, Brownell KD. Obesity and public policy. *Annu Rev Clin Psychol*. 2012;8:405–430.
23. Russel-Mayhew S, von Ranson KM, Masson PC. How does Overeaters Anonymous help its members? A qualitative analysis. *Eur Eat Disord Rev*. 2010;18:33–42.
24. Davis C, Carter JC. If certain foods are addictive, how might this change the treatment of compulsive overeating and obesity? *Curr Addict Rep*. 2014;1:89–95.

25. Slive A, Young F. Bulimia as substance abuse: a metaphor for strategic treatment. *J Strat Syst Ther.* 1986;5:71–84.

26. Cosci F. Bulimia Nervosa treated with an adapted version of Carroll's cognitive-behavioral approach for treatment of cocaine addiction. *J Neuropsychiat Clin Neurosci.* 2014;26:28–29.

27. Avena NM, Murray S, Gold MS. The next generation of obesity treatments: beyond suppressing appetite. *Front Psychol.* 2013;4(721):1–3.

28. Davis C. A commentary on the associations among 'food addiction', binge eating disorder, and obesity: overlapping conditions with idiosyncratic clinical features. *Appetite.* 2017;115:3–8.

29. Nolan LJ. Is it time to consider the "food use disorder?". *Appetite.* 2017;115:16–18.

30. Schulte EM, Potenza MN, Gearhardt AN. A commentary on the "eating addiction" versus "food addiction" perspectives on addictive-like food consumption. *Appetite.* 2017;115:9–15.

31. Long CG, Blundell JE, Finlayson G. A systematic review of the application and correlates of YFAS-diagnosed 'food addiction' in humans: are eating-related 'addictions' a cause for concern or empty concepts? *Obes Facts.* 2015;8:386–401.

32. Wilson GT. Eating disorders, obesity and addiction. *Eur Eat Disord Rev.* 2010;18:341–351.

33. Ziauddeen H, Fletcher PC. Is food addiction a valid and useful concept? *Obes Rev.* 2013;14:19–28.

34. Finlayson G. Food addiction and obesity: unnecessary medicalization of hedonic overeating. *Nat Rev Endocrinol.* 2017;13:493–498.

35. Rogers PJ, Smit HJ. Food craving and food "addiction": a critical review of the evidence from a biopsychosocial perspective. *Pharmacol Biochem Behav.* 2000;66:3–14.

36. Lee NM, Carter A, Owen N, Hall WD. The neurobiology of overeating. *EMBO Rep.* 2012;13:785–790.

37. Curtis C, Davis C. A qualitative study of binge eating and obesity from an addiction perspective. *Eat Disord.* 2014;22:19–32.

38. Cassin SE, von Ranson KM. Is binge eating experienced as an addiction? *Appetite.* 2007;49:687–690.

39. Ruddock HK, Christiansen P, Halford JC, Hardman CA. The development and validation of the Addiction-like Eating Behaviour Scale. *Int J Obes.* 2017;41:1710–1717.

40. von Ranson KM. Development of the Eating Addiction Questionnaire: evaluation of factor structure among university students. *Poster Presented at the 23rd Annual Meeting of the Eating Disorders Research Society, Leipzig, Germany.* 2017.

41. Merlo LJ, Klingman C, Malasanos TH, Silverstein JH. Exploration of food addiction in pediatric patients: a preliminary investigation. *J Addict Med.* 2009;3:26–32.

42. Flint AJ, Gearhardt AN, Corbin WR, Brownell KD, Field AE, Rimm EB. Food addiction scale measurement in 2 cohorts of middle-aged and older women. *Am J Clin Nutr.* 2014;99:578–586.

43. Schulte EM, Gearhardt AN. Development of the modified Yale Food Addiction Scale Version 2.0. *Eur Eat Disord Rev.* 2017;25:302–308.

44. Hetherington MM, Macdiarmid JI. "Chocolate addiction": a preliminary study of its description and its relationship to problem eating. *Appetite.* 1993;21:233–246.

45. Ruddock HK, Field M, Hardman CA. Exploring food reward and calorie intake in self-perceived food addicts. *Appetite.* 2017;115:36–44.

46. Meadows A, Nolan LJ, Higgs S. Self-perceived food addiction: prevalence, predictors, and prognosis. *Appetite.* 2017;114:282–298.

Stigmatization Associated With Obesity in Children and Adolescents

ANJA HILBERT, PHD • HANS-CHRISTIAN PULS, MSC

INTRODUCTION

Children and adolescents with obesity face weight-related stigmatization across multiple life domains and developmental stages.[1] This enacted weight stigma is defined as "the inclination to form unreasonable judgements based on a person's weight"[2(p. 1)] and includes weight-related stereotypes (i.e., characterizations of people with obesity as lazy, unmotivated, incompetent, noncompliant, sloppy, or lacking in self-discipline and willpower), prejudice (i.e., negative feelings of avoidance or anger toward people with obesity), and discrimination (i.e., actual disadvantages in educational settings, interpersonal relationships, the media, and healthcare). Weight stigma was found to be based on internal controllability attributions regarding body weight,[3] irrespective of the complex causes of obesity.[4]

Children and adolescents with obesity, who report repeated enacted stigma, tend to internalize weight stigma,[5] making them highly vulnerable for a range of adverse health outcomes.[1] Specifically, enacted—and even more, internalized—weight stigma were associated with negative physical and psychological health correlates,[1,6,7] which add to the negative psychological consequences of obesity in children and adolescents.[8,9] Although weight-related stigmatization has been considered to help individuals with obesity to lose weight via shame induction,[2] experiences of weight stigma are actually associated with health-impairing behaviors that might reinforce obesity (i.e., maladaptive eating behavior, decreased physical activity[1]).

The purpose of this chapter is to describe the prevalence of weight stigma in children and adolescents across relevant life domains, to summarize its negative physical and psychological correlates, and to present an overview of interventions aiming at weight stigma reduction in youths.

PREVALENCE OF WEIGHT STIGMA

The prevalence of weight-related discrimination has risen across age groups over the past decades and is now comparable with the prevalence of discrimination due to race or age.[10,11] Thus, weight-related discrimination is common, socially accepted, and widely unquestioned in Western societies.[3] For example, children and adolescents with obesity are at high risk for experiencing weight-related discrimination,[12] which might appear as explicit bullying (e.g., verbal teasing, physical violence, cyberbullying) or implicit relational victimization (e.g., social exclusion, avoidance[1]). Weight-related discrimination and stereotypes occur in many life domains of children and adolescents with obesity, as elaborated below.

Education

Children and adolescents with obesity experience weight stigma across different educational settings, emanating from both peers and educators.[1] For example, they were found to be less socially accepted in school, had less social relationships, and reported more teasing than their normal-weight peers.[13,14] In a recent population-based survey with 5128 middle school students across all weight classes, about one-third of the sample reported experiences of weight-related stigmatization,[15] which is consistent with previous research.[1,16] Regarding educators, cross-sectional studies revealed weight-related stereotypes in teachers (e.g., lower expectations for students with obesity regarding social, reasoning, physical, and cooperation skills than for students with normal weight) both at the implicit[17] and at the explicit level.[18] In addition, weight-related teasing in school children mediated the relationship between higher body mass index (BMI, kg/m^2) and poor school performance.[13] Thus, weight stigma might limit the educational chances for students with obesity.[1,19]

Eating Disorders and Obesity in Children and Adolescents. https://doi.org/10.1016/B978-0-323-54852-6.00017-3

Interpersonal Relationships

Children and adolescents encounter weight-related stigmatization in their interpersonal relationships.[1] A recent study examined self-reported experiences of weight stigma in 60 children aged 9–12 years.[20] Children rated siblings as the most frequent sources of negative weight-related talk, followed by parents. In addition, a retrospective qualitative analysis showed that weight-related stigmatization from family members during youth was described by adults with obesity as most prevalent and pervasive compared with other sources.[21]

Media

Weight-related stereotypes, prejudice, and discrimination are present in and disseminated by entertainment, informational, and social media.[22–24] Within entertainment media, characters with obesity are more likely than normal-weight characters to be depicted in minor roles, to display negative traits (e.g., to be aggressive), and to engage in stereotypical behaviors (e.g., eating large amounts of unhealthy food[1]). Such findings were also demonstrated for entertainment media aimed at children and adolescents.[25,26] In the news media, people with obesity are commonly displayed as headless, with a focus on the lower body parts (i.e., trunk and extremities), and engaging in unhealthy behavior.[24] Further, weight stigma in forms of derogatory posts or comments was documented in the social media landscape.[23] Given the vast impact of media consumption on negative body- and weight-related cognitions, especially in adolescents,[27] identifying and reducing weight-related stereotypes in the media remain central issues in the context of weight stigma reduction.[1]

Healthcare

Because the prevalence of obesity among children and adolescents has risen throughout the past decades,[28] an increasing number of younger patients with obesity seek weight loss treatment. In addition, children and adolescents with obesity are at risk for a range of adverse medical conditions,[8] thus seeking medical advice in fields other than weight loss. These children and adolescents may face weight-related discrimination in multiple healthcare settings, including primary care[1] and specialist weight loss treatment.[11] Indeed, weight-related stereotypes have been reported by physicians,[29] nurses,[30] and dietitians.[31] Weight-related stereotypes toward children with obesity as well as controllability beliefs regarding body weight have been documented in pediatric nurses and clinical support staff.[32] Weight-related discrimination emanates from weight-related stereotypes and has been reported in healthcare settings for adults, reducing the quality of care for patients with obesity.[29]

CORRELATES OF WEIGHT STIGMA IN CHILDREN AND ADOLESCENTS

A growing body of research provides evidence on the associations between experiencing weight stigma and a range of adverse outcomes.[1] Particularly for healthcare professionals, it is essential to be aware of health correlates of weight stigma, most notably behaviors that might reinforce obesity.[1]

Physical Health Correlates

A range of adverse physical health outcomes have been reported for adults who experienced weight stigma, including increased stress levels, increased BMI, and, based on longitudinal evidence, even increased likelihood of developing obesity.[1,6] Aside from indirect effects of weight stigma on children's physical health (e.g., by disordered eating behaviors, chronic dieting, or avoiding gym classes; see the next section Psychological Correlates), less research investigates direct health impairments in youths due to weight stigma. For example, in a sample of 20,277 children and adolescents, experiencing weight stigma was associated with increased psychosomatic symptoms, whereas the BMI did not moderate this association.[33] Longitudinal research on 644 adolescents showed that experiences of weight-related discrimination directly predicted overall self-rated health 2 years later and were indirectly associated with increased systolic blood pressure, diastolic blood pressure, and BMI, mediated by greater emotional symptoms.[34]

Psychological Correlates

Weight stigma is associated with maladaptive health behaviors, which are indirectly impairing the health status of children and adolescents with obesity.[1] For example, in a sample of 1830 adolescents, experiences of weight stigma were longitudinally associated with more disordered eating behaviors 15 years later (e.g., binge eating, unhealthy weight control, eating to cope, and negative body image[35]). In addition, in a sample of 1047 children aged 7–11 years, experiences of weight stigma mediated the association of weight status and psychosocial problems (e.g., restrained eating, emotional problems, and conduct problems) 2 years later.[36] In cross-sectional studies, adolescents with obesity who reported experiencing weight-related discrimination showed reduced physical activity,[37] increased risk for substance use,[38] as well as more symptoms of psychopathology (e.g., depression, anxiety), higher body dissatisfaction, lower self-esteem, and impaired quality of life.[1]

Regarding internalized weight stigma, longitudinal evidence showed its mediating role on the association of weight status and psychosocial problems.[36] In treatment-seeking adolescents with obesity, internalized weight stigma was positively associated with depression, anxiety, social and behavioral problems, and eating, shape, and weight concerns,[5] as well as negatively associated with self-esteem, self-efficacy, and health-related quality of life.[39] Finally, research in adults showed that, especially for healthcare settings, experiences of weight stigma are associated with decreased healthcare utilization[40] and decreased treatment success.[29]

IMPLICATIONS

Given the pervasiveness and social acceptability of weight-related stigmatization in Western societies, evidence-based strategies for stigma reduction are needed.[41] Particularly, there is a lack of interventional studies focusing on weight stigma reduction in children and adolescents.[42] Because weight stigma often occurs in the context of individual controllability beliefs, weight stigma reduction strategies usually aim at modifying such beliefs,[42] for instance, via informing children and adolescents about the multiple causes of obesity via educational videos (e.g., 43) or verbal presentations (e.g., 44). However, especially for children and adolescents, stigma reduction strategies that target individual beliefs about obesity failed to modify the emotional and behavioral reactions toward peers with obesity,[45] and the efficacy of these isolated and short-term interventions has not been sufficiently established.[46] In contrast, more extensive multicomponent interventions (e.g., including information on causes and correlates of weight stigma) seem promising for the long-term reduction of weight stigma.[42,47] Research should provide further evidence on the long-term efficacy of interventions in large community samples across the weight spectrum,[41] ultimately aiming to reduce the weight-related stigmatization on a societal level,[48] thereby decreasing the overall health burden in children and adolescents with obesity.

REFERENCES

1. Puhl RM, King KM. Weight discrimination and bullying. *Best Pract Res Clin Endocrinol Metabol.* 2013;27(2):117–127.

2. Washington RL. Childhood Obesity: Issues of Weight Bias. http://www.cdc.gov/pcd/issues/2011/sep/10_0281.htm/.

3. Puhl RM, Latner JD, O'Brien K, Luedicke J, Danielsdottir S, Forhan M. A multinational examination of weight bias: predictors of anti-fat attitudes across four countries. *Int J Obes.* 2015;39(7):1166–1173.

4. Wright SM, Aronne LJ. Causes of obesity. *Abdom Imag.* 2012;37(5):730–732.

5. Roberto CA, Sysko R, Bush J, et al. Clinical correlates of the weight bias internalization scale in a sample of obese adolescents seeking bariatric surgery. *Obesity.* 2012;20(3):533–539.

6. Papadopoulos S, Brennan L. Correlates of weight stigma in adults with overweight and obesity: a systematic literature review. *Obesity.* 2015;23(9):1743–1760.

7. Hilbert A, Braehler E, Haeuser W, Zenger M. Weight bias internalization, core self-evaluation, and health in overweight and obese persons. *Obesity.* 2014;22(1):79–85.

8. Güngör NK. Overweight and obesity in children and adolescents. *J Clin Res Pediatric Endocrinol.* 2014;6(3):129–143.

9. Rankin J, Matthews L, Cobley S, et al. Psychological consequences of childhood obesity: psychiatric comorbidity and prevention. *Adolesc Health Med Therapeut.* 2016;7:125–146.

10. Andreyeva T, Puhl RM, Brownell KD. Changes in perceived weight discrimination among Americans, 1995–1996 through 2004–2006. *Obesity.* 2008;16(5):1129–1134.

11. Tomiyama AJ, Finch LE, Belsky ACI, et al. Weight bias in 2001 versus 2013: contradictory attitudes among obesity researchers and health professionals. *Obesity.* 2015;23(1):46–53.

12. Haines J, Neumark-Sztainer D. Psychosocial consequences of obesity and weight bias: implications for interventions. In: Heinberg LJ, Thompson JK, eds. *Obesity in Youth: Causes, Consequences, and Cures.* Washington: American Psychological Association; 2009:79–98.

13. Krukowski RA, West DS, Philyaw Perez A, Bursac Z, Phillips MM, Raczynski JM. Overweight children, weight-based teasing and academic performance. *Int J Pediatric Obes.* 2009;4(4):274–280.

14. Lumeng JC, Forrest P, Appugliese DP, Kaciroti N, Corwyn RF, Bradley RH. Weight status as a predictor of being bullied in third through sixth grades. *Pediatrics.* 2010;125(6):e1301–e1307.

15. Juvonen J, Lessard LM, Schacter HL, Suchilt L. Emotional implications of weight stigma across middle school: the role of weight-based peer discrimination. *J Clin Child and Adolesc Psychol.* 2017;46(1):150–158.

16. Puhl RM, Luedicke J. Weight-based victimization among adolescents in the school setting: emotional reactions and coping behaviors. *J Youth Adolesc.* 2012;41(1):27–40.

17. Lynagh M, Cliff K, Morgan PJ. Attitudes and beliefs of nonspecialist and specialist trainee health and physical education teachers toward obese children: evidence for "anti-fat" bias. *J Sch Health.* 2015;85(9):595–603.

18. Peterson JL, Puhl RM, Luedicke J. An experimental assessment of physical educators' expectations and attitudes: the importance of student weight and gender. *J Sch Health*. 2012;82(9):432–440.

19. MacCann C, Roberts RD. Just as smart but not as successful: obese students obtain lower school grades but equivalent test scores to nonobese students. *Int J Obes*. 2013;37(1):40–46.

20. Berge JM, Hanson-Bradley C, Tate A, Neumark-Sztainer D. Do parents or siblings engage in more negative weight-based talk with children and what does it sound like? a mixed-methods study. *Body Image*. 2016;18:27–33.

21. Rand K, Vallis M, Aston M, et al. "It is not the diet; it is the mental part we need help with." a multilevel analysis of psychological, emotional, and social well-being in obesity. *Int J Qual Stud Health Well Being*. 2017;12(1):1306421.

22. Ata RN, Thompson JK. Weight bias in the media: a review of recent research. *Obes Facts*. 2010;3(1):41–46.

23. Chou W-YS, Prestin A, Kunath S. Obesity in social media: a mixed methods analysis. *Transl Behav Med*. 2014;4(3):314–323.

24. Puhl RM, Peterson JL, DePierre JA, Luedicke J. Headless, hungry, and unhealthy: a video content analysis of obese persons portrayed in online news. *J Health Commun*. 2013;18(6):686–702.

25. Eisenberg ME, Carlson-McGuire A, Gollust SE, Neumark-Sztainer D. A content analysis of weight stigmatization in popular television programming for adolescents. *Int J Eat Disord*. 2015;48(6):759–766.

26. Robinson T, Callister M, Jankoski T. Portrayal of body weight on children's television sitcoms: a content analysis. *Body Image*. 2008;5(2):141–151.

27. Voelker DK, Reel JJ, Greenleaf C. Weight status and body image perceptions in adolescents: current perspectives. *Adolesc Health Med Therapeut*. 2015;6:149–158.

28. Ogden CL, Carroll MD, Lawman HG, et al. Trends in obesity prevalence among children and adolescents in the United States, 1988-1994 through 2013-2014. *J Am Med Assoc*. 2016;315(21):2292–2299.

29. Phelan SM, Burgess DJ, Yeazel MW, Hellerstedt WL, Griffin JM, van Ryn M. Impact of weight bias and stigma on quality of care and outcomes for patients with obesity. *Obes Rev*. 2015;16(4):319–326.

30. Ward-Smith P, Peterson JA. Development of an instrument to assess nurse practitioner attitudes and beliefs about obesity. *J Am Assoc Nurse Pract*. 2016;28(3):125–129.

31. Jung FUCE, Luck-Sikorski C, Wiemers N, Riedel-Heller SG. Dietitians and nutritionists: stigma in the context of obesity. a systematic review. *PLoS One*. 2015;10(10):e0140276.

32. Garcia JT, Amankwah EK, Hernandez RG. Assessment of weight bias among pediatric nurses and clinical support staff toward obese patients and their caregivers. *J Pediatric Nurs*. 2016;31(4):e244–e251.

33. Warkentin T, Borghese MM, Janssen I. Associations between weight-related teasing and psychosomatic symptoms by weight status among school-aged youth. *Obes Sci Pract*. 2017;3(1):44–50.

34. Rosenthal L, Earnshaw VA, Carroll-Scott A, et al. Weight- and race-based bullying: health associations among urban adolescents. *J Health Psychol*. 2015;20(4):401–412.

35. Puhl RM, Wall MM, Chen C, Bryn Austin S, Eisenberg ME, Neumark-Sztainer D. Experiences of weight teasing in adolescence and weight-related outcomes in adulthood: a 15-year longitudinal study. *Prev Med*. 2017;100:173–179.

36. Zuba A, Warschburger P. The role of weight teasing and weight bias internalization in psychological functioning: a prospective study among school-aged children. *Eur Child Adolesc Psychiatry*. 2017;26(10):1245–1255.

37. Gray WN, Janicke DM, Ingerski LM, Silverstein JH. The impact of peer victimization, parent distress and child depression on barrier formation and physical activity in overweight youth. *J Dev Behav Pediatrics*. 2008;29(1):26–33.

38. Bucchianeri MM, Eisenberg ME, Wall MM, Piran N, Neumark-Sztainer D. Multiple types of harassment: associations with emotional well-being and unhealthy behaviors in adolescents. *J Adolesc Health*. 2014;54(6):724–729.

39. Ciuputu-Plath C, Wiegand S, Babitsch B. The weight bias internalization scale for youth: validation of a specific tool for assessing internalized weight bias among treatment-seeking German adolescents with overweight. *J Pediatric Psychol*. 2018;43(1):40–51.

40. Hernandez-Boussard T, Ahmed SM, Morton JM. Obesity disparities in preventive care: findings from the National Ambulatory Medical Care Survey, 2005-2007. *Obesity*. 2012;20(8):1639–1644.

41. Puhl RM, Himmelstein MS, Gorin AA, Suh YJ. Missing the target: including perspectives of women with overweight and obesity to inform stigma-reduction strategies. *Obes Sci Pract*. 2017;3(1):25–35.

42. Daníelsdóttir S, O'Brien KS, Ciao A. Anti-fat prejudice reduction: a review of published studies. *Obes Facts*. 2010;3(1):47–58.

43. Hennings A, Hilbert A, Thomas J, Siegfried W, Rief W. Reduktion der Stigmatisierung Übergewichtiger bei Schülern: Auswirkungen eines Informationsfilms. *Psychotherapie, Psychosomatik, Medizinische Psychologie*. 2007;57(9–10):359–363.

44. Anesbury T, Tiggemann M. An attempt to reduce negative stereotyping of obesity in children by changing controllability beliefs. *Health Educ Res*. 2000;15(2):145–152.

45. Barnett MA, Wadian TW, Sonnentag TL, Nichols MB. Role of various fault attributions and other factors in children's anticipated response to hypothetical peers with undesirable characteristics. *Soc Dev*. 2015;24(1):113–127.

46. Lee M, Ata RN, Brannick MT. Malleability of weight-biased attitudes and beliefs: a meta-analysis of weight bias reduction interventions. *Body Image*. 2014;11(3):251–259.

47. Hilbert A. Weight stigma reduction and genetic determinism. *PLoS One*. 2016;11(9):e0162993.

48. Alberga AS, Russell-Mayhew S, von Ranson KM, McLaren L. Weight bias: a call to action. *J Eat Disord*. 2016;4:34.

CHAPTER 18

Cognitive-Behavioral Therapy in Adolescent Eating Disorders

RICCARDO DALLE GRAVE, MD

INTRODUCTION

Eating disorders (EDs) have a profound impact on the psychosocial and physical health of adolescents. It is therefore crucial that they are treated early and effectively to avoid long-lasting negative effects. The leading evidence-based treatment for adolescents with anorexia nervosa is currently family-based treatment (FBT), a specific form of family therapy,[1] which also has some support in young people with bulimia nervosa and its variants.[2] However, FBT is not accepted by all families and patients, it is labor-intensive and therefore costly, and fewer than half of its patients exhibit a full response,[3] suggesting that alternative treatments may be more suitable for many young patients. In this regard, enhanced cognitive-behavioral therapy (CBT-E) for adolescents is considered the most valid alternative to FBT and has been recommended for children or young people with anorexia nervosa or bulimia nervosa when FBT is unacceptable, contraindicated, or ineffective by the recent National Institute for Health and Clinical Excellence (NICE) guidelines.[2]

RATIONALE BEHIND CBT-E FOR ADOLESCENTS

CBT-E is an evidence-based treatment for adults with eating disorders that has been specifically adapted for adolescents.[4] CBT-E was initially developed by the Centre for Research on Eating Disorders at Oxford (CREDO) to address the psychopathology of ED, rather than a specific diagnosis as classified in the *Diagnostic and Statistical Manual of Mental Disorders* (*DSM-5*).[5] The treatment, originally designed for adult outpatients with a body mass index (BMI) between 15.0 and 39.9,[6] has been evaluated in numerous controlled and cohort clinical trials and is now recommended for all clinical forms of adult eating disorders.[2]

In collaboration with the CREDO, the Department of Eating and Weight Disorders of Villa Garda Hospital, Italy, has adapted CBT-E for adolescents of at least 13 years of age.[7] Indeed, CBT-E has a number of features that make it well suited to younger patients with eating disorders.[4] Firstly, CBT-E adopts a flexible and personalized approach, which is easily adaptable to the needs of adolescents' cognitive development. Moreover, CBT-E is both comprehensible and easy to receive and promotes the pursuit of control, autonomy, and independence; these are issues of major relevance to younger patients, who therefore respond favorably to a collaborative treatment such as CBT-E. Last but not least, CBT-E includes several strategies for engaging patients in the treatment, a feature that is vital for the management of adolescents who, by nature, are usually ambivalent about their treatment.

Standard CBT-E has been adapted for adolescents taking into account two distinctive characteristics, namely, physical health and parental involvement.[4] Indeed, some medical complications associated with eating disorders (e.g., osteopenia and osteoporosis) are particularly severe in this age range, and periodical medical assessments and a lower threshold for hospital admission are therefore integral parts of CBT-E for adolescents. In addition, parents need to be involved in the treatment in the great majority of cases.

TREATMENT GOALS

CBT-E for adolescents has four general goals:
1. To engage patients in the treatment and involve them actively in the process of change
2. To remove the eating disorder psychopathology, i.e., the dietary restraint and restriction (and low weight if present), extreme weight control behaviors, and preoccupation with shape, weight, and eating

Eating Disorders and Obesity in Children and Adolescents. https://doi.org/10.1016/B978-0-323-54852-6.00018-5

3. To correct the mechanisms maintaining the eating disorder psychopathology
4. To ensure lasting change

GENERAL STRATEGIES OF THE TREATMENT

CBT-E is a time-limited, personalized psychologic treatment designed to treat all diagnostic categories of eating disorders (transdiagnostic approach) by addressing the behavioral and cognitive processes maintaining the patient's individual psychopathology.[6] Unlike FBT—which postulates that the problem or symptoms belongs to the entire family, separates the illness from the patient (externalization), and promotes parents' "taking control" of their child's eating[1]—CBT-E maintains that the problem belongs to the individual. As such, it treats the illness as part of the patient and encourages the patient, rather than the parents, to take control.

To promote a feeling of self-control, CBT-E treatment procedures are designed to involve patients actively in all phases of treatment, from the decision to start treatment, to the choice of problems to be addressed, and the procedures used to address them. Patients are told that overcoming the eating problem will be difficult, but worth it, and treatment should therefore be considered a priority. Another essential feature of CBT-E is that the therapist always ensures that the patients understand what is happening and encourages them to become active participants in the process of change. In short, CBT-E is a collaborative means of overcoming eating problems (collaborative empiricism).

Hence CBT-E for adolescents never adopts "coercive" or "prescriptive" procedures; patients are never asked to do things that they do not agree to, as this may increase their resistance to change.[4] The key strategy is to collaboratively create a personal formulation of the main processes maintaining the patient's individual psychopathology, as these will become the targets of treatment (see Fig. 18.1). The formulation helps create a tailor-made treatment to address the evolving individual psychopathology of each patient and can be modified midcourse to address any emerging processes. To promote self-empowerment, patients are educated about the processes in their personal formulation and actively involved in the decision to address them. If they do not reach the conclusion that they have a problem to address, the treatment cannot start or must be suspended, but this is a very rare occurrence.

Once the patient is engaged in the process of change, their personal eating disorder psychopathology is addressed via a flexible set of sequential cognitive and behavioral strategies and procedures, integrated with progressive patient education. In common with other forms of CBT, self-monitoring and success in completing strategically planned homework tasks are of paramount importance. Because in some cases these can create anxiety, the therapist needs to be not only empathetic but also aware of when to keep the patient firmly on track.[6]

To achieve cognitive change, patients are encouraged to observe, using real-time self-monitoring, how the processes in their personal formulation operate in real life. They are asked to make gradual behavioral changes and analyze their effects and implications on their way of thinking. In the later stages of CBT-E, when the main maintenance processes have been interrupted and the patient reports having periods free from shape, weight, and eating concerns, the treatment focuses on helping them recognize the early warning signs of eating disorder mind-set reactivation, and to decenter from it quickly, thereby avoiding relapse.[6]

TREATMENT STRUCTURE AND MAIN PROCEDURES

CBT-E for adolescents involves two preparatory/assessment sessions followed by three main steps (see Fig. 18.2). Treatment is delivered by a single therapist in 30–40 50-min sessions in patients with a BMI between the 3rd and 25th centile, and in 20 sessions in those with a BMI > the 25th centile. Like CBT-E for adults,[6,8] it can be delivered in two forms: (1) a "focused" form, which exclusively addresses the specific psychopathology of eating disorders or (2) a "broad" form, which features specific modules to address one or more of the adjunctive mechanisms maintaining the eating disorder (i.e., clinical perfectionism, core low self-esteem, and interpersonal difficulties). The focused form is indicated for most patients, whereas the broad form should be reserved only for patients in whom the adjunctive mechanisms maintaining the eating disorder psychopathology hinder treatment. The decision to use the broad form is taken in a review session held after 4 weeks in nonunderweight patients or in one of the review sessions in Step 2 in underweight patients.

Preparing Adolescent Patients for Treatment

Assessment of the eating problem in young patients is similar to that for adults. The adult version of the Eating Disorder Examination (EDE) is suitable for patients aged 16 or above,[9] but a modified version is also available for younger patients.[10]

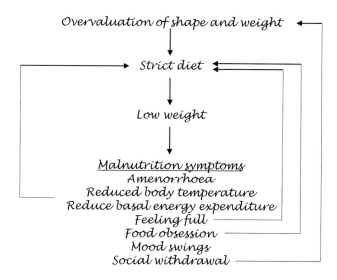

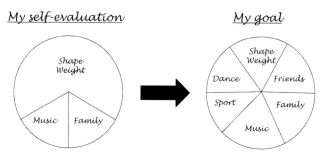

FIG. 18.1 An example of personal formulation of a young underweight patient with eating disorder (the slice in the pie chart represent the domain of self-evaluation).

The initial interview has two aims: (1) to establish the nature of the eating problem (assessment) and (2) to begin to engage the patient by fostering a positive therapeutic relationship (preparation). Although adolescent patients are often not fully aware that they have a problem, the majority can be adequately engaged via appropriately delivered CBT-E procedures. Specifically, parents are asked for their consent to the CBT-E practitioner initially seeing adolescent alone, as a one-to-one approach will not only facilitate exploration of the adolescent's perspective on the consultation and the nature of their problems but also lay the foundations for a sound therapeutic relationship. Other key features of engaging adolescents in CBT-E are to emphasize that the therapist will be operating entirely on their behalf, rather than as agents of their parents, and to dedicate time to listening to their views on their eating problem and treatment. Indeed, one major obstacle to engaging younger patients is that they often ignore or underestimate the negative effects of their eating problem, perceiving only positive effects. In these cases, engagement can be facilitated by a joint exploration of whether their control over eating, shape, and weight is a choice, or whether it has become a burden.

If CBT-E is indicated, the therapist should describe the treatment in detail to the patients and ask them to do the following homework assignments for the second assessment session: (1) considering the pros and cons of starting the treatment and (2) creating a list of questions about the treatment. In the second preparatory session, generally fixed 1 week after the first, the therapist reviews this homework with the patient, reinforces their interest in change, and addresses any questions.

Step 1—Starting Well

The first CBT-E step also has the aim of engaging patients and helping them to decide to address their overvaluation of shape and weight and weight regain if indicated. It is generally delivered over 4 weeks of twice-weekly sessions, but in underweight patients may be reduced to 2–3 weeks, if after few sessions they manifest the desire to address weight regain. During Step 1, patients are introduced to the following procedures (described in detail in the main CBT-E guide)[8]: real-time self-monitoring, collaborative in-session weighing, personal formulation creation (including underweight symptoms if applicable), and regular eating patterns (see Fig. 18.2).

There is also a collaborative decision whether to pass in Step 2; if underweight patients do not reach the conclusion that they need to address their low weight after 4 weeks, CBT-E should be discontinued, and they should be referred to other forms of treatment that do not require their active involvement in the process of change.

Step 2—Addressing the Change

The goals of Step 2 are to remove the patient's eating disorder psychopathology (including low weight if applicable) and correct the mechanisms maintaining it using one or more of the modules shown in Fig. 18.2 (described in detail the main CBT-E guide).[8] In not-underweight patients, Step 2 is delivered in once-weekly sessions over 10 weeks, whereas in those who are underweight its duration can vary from 20 to 30 weeks, depending on the difficulties encountered by the patients in addressing weight regain; in these patients, two sessions a week are advised until the rate of weight regain is stable. Additionally, every 4 weeks a session should be partially devoted to reviewing progress, identifying any emerging barriers to change, modifying the formulation as necessary, and planning the next 4 weeks (in not-underweight patients, a review is conducted solely at the end of Step 1).

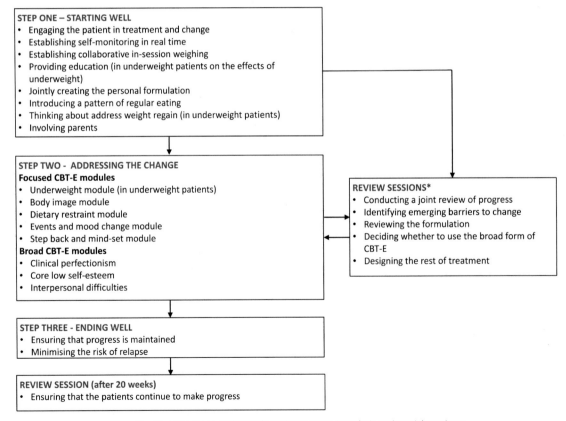

FIG. 18.2 The steps and the main procedures of CBT-E for adolescents.

*One after Step One in non-underweight patients; every 4 weeks in underweight patients

Step 3—Ending Well

Step 3 is the final stage and involves three sessions every 2 weeks. Its focus is to help patients become accomplished at weight maintenance and consolidate the other changes they have made. This includes developing personalized strategies for minimizing the risk of relapse and rapidly reversing any setbacks, ensuring that progress is maintained until a review session held at 20 weeks.

PARENTAL INVOLVEMENT

A joint interview with the patients and their parents (or other relevant family members) is held after the first preparatory session with the patient alone. The therapist should inform parents about both the nature of the adolescent's eating problem and the general features of CBT-E, focusing in particular on their role in the treatment; because parents can influence a patient's decision to start treatment, they should be encouraged to help their child evaluate the pros and cons, taking care to stress that they approach this in an inquisitive, rather than authoritative, manner and that the final decision will belong to the patient alone. In a second joint interview (after the patient's second preparatory session), parents are informed as to the young person's decisions regarding the treatment.

Parents are then asked to participate alone in an interview of about 90 min during the first week of Step 1. This has the aim of identifying and addressing any family-related factors that might hinder the patient's attempts to change. Subsequently, the patient and parents are seen together in 4–6 (in patients who are not underweight) or 8–10 (in patients who are underweight) 15–20 min sessions held immediately after the patient's individual session. These joint sessions should inform parents about what is happening and the patient's progress; they should also be used to discuss, with the patient's prior agreement, how they might help the patient make changes. Additional sessions with parents may take place in the event of family crises, extreme difficulties at mealtimes, or parental hostility toward the young patient.

ADAPTATION FOR INTENSIVE LEVELS OF CARE

Two forms of intensive CBT-E for adolescents have been developed and have been described in detail elsewhere[11,12]: inpatient CBT-E (which also includes a day-hospital component) and intensive outpatient CBT-E. Aside from the increased intensiveness, the main

difference between these forms and outpatient CBT-E is that treatment is delivered by a multidisciplinary team (rather than a single therapist) comprising physicians, psychologists, dieticians, and nurses, all fully trained in CBT-E. Moreover, the treatment also includes some group sessions and assistance with eating in the first weeks of treatment to help patients get over their difficulties in real time. These versions of CBT-E provide patients who are not responding to standard outpatient CBT-E with a more intensive form, without creating discontinuity in the treatment itself. To the same end, intensive CBT-E is followed by a stepped-down CBT-E-based treatment delivered in an outpatient setting.

EFFECTIVENESS OF CBT-E FOR ADOLESCENTS

CBT-E for adolescents has been evaluated in four cohort studies on patients aged between 13 and 19 years—three on patients with severe anorexia nervosa and one not-underweight adolescents with other eating disorders. The first evaluated the effect of CBT-E in 46 of 49 adolescents with anorexia nervosa.[13] The two-thirds who completed the 40 treatment sessions displayed a significant increase in BMI centile, from 3.36 (SD = 3.73) to 30.3 (SD = 16.7), associated with a marked improvement in eating disorder psychopathology and general psychiatric features. There was little change in these positive outcomes over the 60-week post-treatment follow-up period, despite minimal subsequent treatment.

The second study compared the effect of CBT-E in 46 adolescents and 49 adults with anorexia nervosa.[14] Significantly, more adolescents than adults reached normal weight (65.3% vs. 36.5%; $P = .003$). Moreover, the mean time required by adolescents to restore body weight was about 15 weeks less than that required by adults [14.8 (SE = 1.7) weeks versus 28.3 (SE = 2.0) weeks, log-rank = 21.5, $P < .001$], suggesting that a shorter CBT-E may be effective in adolescent patients.

The third study assessed the effect of inpatient CBT-E in 27 adolescents with severe anorexia nervosa.[15] All but one patient completed treatment. From baseline to discharge, the mean BMI centile increased from 2.7 (SD 4.3) to 34.2 (SD 15.7), and there was marked reduction in eating disorder and general psychopathologies. These outcomes were maintained at 12-month follow-up, when the mean BMI centile was 29.9 (SD 20.1) and 81.5% of patients retained normal weight.

The fourth study evaluated the effects of CBT-E on 68 nonunderweight adolescents with an eating disorder.[16] Three-quarters completed the full 20 sessions. At intent-to-treat analysis, 68% of patients had minimal residual eating disorder psychopathology by the end of treatment, and 50% of those with binge eating or purging episodes at baseline reported no longer having them.

CONCLUSIONS

CBT-E is a promising treatment for adolescents with eating disorder. It is well accepted by adolescents, probably due to its collaborative approach, which grants ambivalent young patients a feeling of being in control, and has several other advantages. In particular, the transdiagnostic nature of CBT-E makes it suitable for treating all the main eating disorders that afflict adolescent patients. Associated with the promising results obtained in cohort studies, this suggests that CBT-E for adolescents is a potentially good alternative to FBT, the other leading approach for adolescent eating disorders. Future studies should compare CBT-E with FBT across the full range of eating disorder presentations to provide useful information regarding treatment in adolescents and to identify moderators and mediators of the twos.

REFERENCES

1. Lock J, Le Grange D. *Treatment Manual for Anorexia Nervosa: A Family-based Approach*. 2nd ed. New York: Guilford Press; 2013.
2. NICE. *Eating Disorders: Recognition and Treatment (NG69)*. London: National Institute for Clinical Excellence; 2017.
3. Lock J, Le Grange D, Agras WS, Moye A, Bryson SW, Jo B. Randomized clinical trial comparing family-based treatment with adolescent-focused individual therapy for adolescents with anorexia nervosa. *Arch Gen Psychiatry*. 2010;67(10):1025–1032.
4. Dalle Grave R, Cooper Z. Enhanced cognitive behavior treatment adapted for younger patients. In: Wade T, ed. *Encyclopedia of Feeding and Eating Disorders*. Singapore: Springer Singapore; 2016:1–8.
5. American Psychiatric Association. *Diagnostic and Statistical Manual of Mental Disorders, Fifth Edition (DSM-5)*. Washington, DC: American Psychiatric Association; 2013.
6. Fairburn CG, Cooper Z, Shafran R. Cognitive behaviour therapy for eating disorders: a "transdiagnostic" theory and treatment. *Behav Res Ther*. 2003;41(5):509–528.
7. Cooper Z, Dalle Grave R. Chapter 14-Eating disorders: transdiagnostic theory and treatment. In: Asmundson SG, Gordon JG, eds. *The Science of Cognitive Behavioral Therapy*. San Diego: Academic Press; 2017:337–357.
8. Fairburn CG. *Cognitive Behavior Therapy and Eating Disorders*. New York: Guilford Press; 2008.
9. Fairburn CG, Cooper Z, O'Connor M. Eating disorder examination (Edition 16.0D). In: Fairburn CG, ed. *Cognitive Behavior Therapy and Eating Disorders*. New York: Guilford Press; 2008:265–308.
10. Carter JC, Stewart DA, Fairburn CG. Eating disorder examination questionnaire: norms for young adolescent girls. *Behav Res Ther*. 2001;39(5):625–632.
11. Dalle Grave R. *Multistep Cognitive Behavioral Therapy for Eating Disorders: Theory, Practice, and Clinical Cases*. New York: Jason Aronson; 2013.
12. Dalle Grave R. *Intensive Cognitive Behavior Therapy for Eating Disorders*. Hauppauge, NY: Nova; 2012.
13. Dalle Grave R, Calugi S, Doll HA, Fairburn CG. Enhanced cognitive behaviour therapy for adolescents with anorexia nervosa: an alternative to family therapy? *Behav Res Ther*. 2013;51(1):R9–R12.
14. Calugi S, Dalle Grave R, Sartirana M, Fairburn CG. Time to restore body weight in adults and adolescents receiving cognitive behaviour therapy for anorexia nervosa. *J Eat Disord*. 2015;3:21.
15. Dalle Grave R, Calugi S, El Ghoch M, Conti M, Fairburn CG. Inpatient cognitive behavior therapy for adolescents with anorexia nervosa: immediate and longer-term effects. *Front Psychiatry*. 2014;5:14.
16. Dalle Grave R, Calugi S, Sartirana M, Fairburn CG. Transdiagnostic cognitive behaviour therapy for adolescents with an eating disorder who are not underweight. *Behav Res Ther*. 2015;73:79–82.

CHAPTER 19

Family-Based Treatment for Adolescent Eating Disorders

ABIGAIL R. COOPER, BA • ASHLEY F. JENNINGS, BS •
KATHARINE L. LOEB, PHD • DANIEL LE GRANGE, PHD

Family-based treatment (FBT) is considered a first-line treatment for adolescents with anorexia nervosa (AN) who are medically stable for outpatient care.[1,2] Since its first randomized controlled trial (RCT),[4] FBT has continued to develop as an intervention, as well as garner increasing empirical evidence for its utility with a range of eating disorder (ED) populations, generally with superiority over comparison interventions in speed or degree of symptom reduction, as well as need for hospitalization.[5–8] Four studies to date have also shown that positive outcomes persist 4–5 years after a course of FBT.[9–12] In light of its research support, the FBT model is expanding to include a wider range of diagnoses, age ranges, delivery methods, and care settings.[8,13–15]

In FBT, "family" is not operationally defined, meaning that although it is most often comprised of those who live in the same household as the patient, the family ultimately defines its composition and participation.[2] The entire family system—siblings, parents, and others who are consistently present for meal times with the patient—is involved. However, it is the *parents'* engagement that is integral in weight restoration and to the overall success of treatment.

FBT is a short-term treatment comprised of three distinct, necessarily sequential phases. By subverting the maintaining factors of the ED, FBT for adolescent AN aims for full-weight restoration (i.e., a return to the premorbid, healthy place on the patient's growth curve) and guides the adolescent back to an age-appropriate developmental trajectory. Phase I involves weekly sessions to rapidly restore the adolescent's physical health as managed by the parents. Specifically, the parents are in charge of monitoring and orchestrating the adolescent's food intake and minimizing his/her physical activity as they, their FBT clinician, and the collaborating physician deem appropriate. Siblings and other in-household family members play a more indirect role in treatment, i.e., one of support rather

than symptom management.[16] Phase I continues until the adolescent no longer resists renourishment by the parents, has steadily gained the minimal weight required, and has begun to experience a reduction in the ego-syntonic nature of ED thoughts and behaviors. At this point, the therapist assists the parents in titrating down the parent's involvement in treatment as the AN recedes. This transition signals the start of the second phase of FBT, which typically lasts 2–3 months, with sessions occurring biweekly. Issues around adolescent ED behaviors (e.g., food rituals) that may have been deferred so that initial weight restoration could more smoothly progress are addressed during this phase. Phase III of FBT, with sessions occurring every 1–2 months, begins once the adolescent has achieved a healthy and stable weight and no longer engages in self-starvation or excessive exercise. This phase focuses on the general challenges of adolescent development and restoration of a parent-adolescent relationship that is not centered around the ED and also addresses termination of treatment.

CORE PRINCIPLES AND TECHNIQUES

There are several core principles of FBT for the treatment of adolescent AN. As FBT is atheoretical in its foundation, it is derived from various interventions to pragmatically alleviate and correct maladaptive family-level behaviors that have developed in response to the ED and that may inadvertently maintain it. A fundamental assumption of FBT is that the illness is complex and stemming from a myriad of factors—none of which implicates the parents or child in blame for the ED—that converge for the ED to emerge.[2] However, rather than focusing on the past to uncover these factors, FBT focuses on the present and future, helping parents identify the steps that need to be taken to ensure recovery.

Eating Disorders and Obesity in Children and Adolescents. https://doi.org/10.1016/B978-0-323-54852-6.00019-7

A second assumption of the FBT approach is that parents' ability to feed their child appropriately has not been lost, and indeed, has always been present. FBT empowers parents to decide what will be most effective in treatment. Because they are the main resource for recovery and change in FBT—rather than the therapist as in most treatments—parents are given countless opportunities to build their confidence.

Lastly, there is a focus on externalization of the illness from the adolescent. Because of the ego-syntonic nature of an ED, it is imperative for recovery that the parents and adolescent be able to differentiate the "voice" of the ED from the self. The ED "commandeers" the adolescent's beliefs, affect, and behavior regarding food, shape, weight, and eating-related instances. Given the pivotal role that parents play in this therapy, and to facilitate parental empathy while reducing blame and criticism, FBT emphasizes that the parents must understand that the adolescent is powerless over the disorder.

The techniques of FBT are derived from these principles and are the purported therapeutic mechanisms by which the end goal of full recovery is attained.[9,17] One technique of FBT involves a unique therapeutic style that is nondirective yet offers ED expertise that complements the parents' expertise regarding their child and family, when necessary. Another technique that supports the symptom focus is to meet alone with the adolescent at the start of each session to obtain weight, help manage response to the weight, and inquire about treatment-specific issues the adolescent may want support with during the session with the rest of the family present. A third core treatment strategy is an in vivo family meal during the second session, in which parents practice prevailing over AN resistance by helping their child consume at least "one more bite" than he/she is willing, as a symbolic representation of how they will facilitate the many such bites that will take place at home between sessions. The family is responsible for bringing and eating a meal they would normally have at home, which provides a window through which the therapist can begin to identify any challenging aspects of family coalitions, dynamics, and authority structure (e.g., an overly permissive parenting style around eating, siblings in a parental role, adult relationship discord, etc.). However, parent-focused treatment (PFT) and separated family therapy, two empirically supported variants of traditional FBT, exclude the family meal without degradation of results and indeed can yield superior outcomes.[18,19] Despite its face-valid appeal, no research to date has indicated that the family meal is a core mechanism of change in FBT models.[18]

There have been questions raised in the FBT field regarding whether implementing a manualized treatment diminishes the ability to treat families as individual cases, thus compromising their autonomy.[20] Flexibility requires competence, and flexibility in the delivery of therapeutic techniques is necessary to target each family system, which is undoubtedly different from the next. Research has explored the benefits of FBT clinicians adhering to manualized techniques rather than deviating by case.[21] Likewise, clinical studies have been conducted to modify the techniques or the delivery system to fit individual cases while adhering to the principles of FBT.[6,22,23]

APPLICATIONS OF FBT

The efficacy of FBT as an intervention for adolescents with AN has catalyzed more recent research on expanding the applications of FBT.

Dose of Treatment

FBT generally involves a total of ~20 outpatient sessions, although previous research has shown that a shorter course is at times more cost-effective and just as beneficial.[11,24] Conversely, some families may benefit from an augmented FBT relative to the standard intervention. Research demonstrates that patients who fail to reach an established, early weight gain criterion predictive of a good prognosis[25,26] can "catch up" to their successful early weight gain counterparts with a targeted additive protocol. A pilot study randomly assigned individuals who failed to meet the early weight gain marker to either continue FBT as usual or receive an augmentation package of FBT.[3,27] The augmented package involved identifying early obstacles that were interfering with treatment, framing the failure to meet weight gain as a crisis, and increasing the direct in vivo meal coaching sessions with parents. Results showed that initial nonresponders in the augmented treatment condition eventually met the same level of outcome as those who had naturally reached the early prognostic cutoff, suggesting that a good outcome can be induced through intensified FBT.[27]

Target Population

The application of FBT has also been modified to fit various target populations. Using the core approach as the foundation, changes in techniques are made to accommodate the unique clinical needs of each population. For example, the bulimia nervosa (BN) FBT protocol[28] has an earlier focus on fostering a collaborative parent-child relationship to promote behavioral change while acknowledging that BN is more ego-dystonic than AN.[29] FBT for BN was found to reduce bulimic symptoms more than a control treatment[28] and to be superior to cognitive-behavioral therapy at end of treatment and at 6-month follow-up.[30] Another study compared FBT for BN with separated family therapy and found both to be effective in improving psychologic functioning; however, FBT had more success with bulimic symptom reduction in the younger age group of the sample.[31] FBT has also been shown to be an effective intervention for medically stable adolescents with atypical anorexia,[22] through less emphasis on weight restoration and more focus on decreasing ED cognitions and behaviors.

Additional research has tested FBT modifications with older adolescents/emerging adults (i.e., transition age youth, or TAY).[6,13,14,23,32] One developmental consideration with TAY is that they may present for treatment independent of their parents, indicating at least a minimal degree of motivation.[23] FBT for TAY has a similar format to the original FBT protocol; however, to accommodate and appropriately strengthen developmental autonomy, clients meet with therapists individually for a longer period rather than having longer family sessions.[14] Additionally, a modification of FBT for young adults (FBT-Y) was developed and tested and contains adaptations to fit their development by allowing them to choose their support adult (i.e., a parent, sibling, or close friend). Nonetheless, research has found that typically, young adults continue to pick their parent as their primary support.[13,14,23]

Implementation

Format. The expansion of FBT into new levels of care and target populations has propelled research to consider new ways to implement FBT. For instance, FBT has expanded to include multiple family therapy (MFT).[33,34] MFT is a combination of family and group therapy in which several families attend who are confronted with similar pathology.[34] In ED pathology, this method is an intensive form of intervention that involves an initial consecutive 4-day program followed by six 1-day meetings at 4- to 8-week intervals for 9 months.[33] In the first randomized controlled trial comparing MFT and single family therapy (FT) in adolescent AN population, better treatment outcomes were found at the end of a 12-month postbaseline in MFT-AN compared with FT-AN. At the 18-month follow-up, MFT-AN produced a higher weight restoration compared with FT-AN.[34] Research regarding the application of MFT is limited, although results in the few studies

conducted have suggested promising results in regard to cost-effectiveness and a possible alternative to FT.[35] MFT has also been applied successfully to adolescents with BN[36] as well as adults with AN.[13] Both MFT and FT were found to be equivalent in effectiveness for adults with AN; thus further consideration of discrepant clinical advantages of each treatment may be useful in determining the choice of treatment.[13]

Another recent adaptation of FBT involves PFT intervention in which the parents are the primary participants in therapy. Unlike the standard FBT protocol, this intervention removes the family meal and the adolescent is monitored medically and psychiatrically, and does not participate in therapy sessions. A recent RCT found PFT to be a more efficacious alternative to FBT in terms of weight restoration as well as improvement in psychologic functioning.[29] Internet-based applications of ED interventions, such as the implementation of FBT via telehealth platforms,[38] have also been a recent undertaking in attempt to broaden treatment dissemination and increase accessibility.[37] In a small sample study, the use of telehealth communication was reportedly better able to recruit and retain patients and was more advantageous for parents.[38]

Levels of care. It is imperative to maintain FBT's core principles as the system of delivery changes to accommodate diverse settings, patients, and their families. This challenge is particularly salient as clinicians begin to apply the intervention to higher levels of care, specifically, partial hospitalization programming (PHP), intensive outpatient programming (IOP), and inpatient programing.[39,40] Girz et al.[15] found 6 months in PHP with FBT integration to be an adequate duration in which to improve psychologic functioning of the adolescent, increase parents' knowledge and confidence of specific treatment strategies, and decrease caregiver burden with dysregulated behavior. Day programming has also been found to have the potential for faster weight gain, which is a strong predictive factor for successful outcomes with FBT.[26] Overall, research demonstrates that family involvement in day programming appears to be more beneficial than programs without parental involvement,[15] which further emphasizes the need for a family-oriented treatment intervention within this more intensive setting.

Although the introduction of FBT in an inpatient setting reduces length of hospitalization,[41] this level of care is critical for patients in need of intensive medical stabilization and monitoring. The removal of the adolescent from the home environment is a natural challenge to FBT implementation, but recent research[39,42] has started to explore how the core FBT principles can begin to be activated within this level of care, without introducing "competition" between the concepts of AN-as-crisis and parents-as-agents-of-change. A naturalistic outcome report of FBT in a hospital-based treatment center in Norway demonstrated that over half of the participants achieved normal body weight and over a third were classified as recovered.[43] Murray[44] emphasizes the distinction between medical stabilization and weight restoration in hospital settings, making the argument that once medical stabilization is achieved, a less intensive treatment setting with increased parent-driven symptom reduction may be a more effective way to apply FBT to severe cases.

CONCLUSION

FBT has made an overarching impact on the field of EDs. Beyond its demonstrated efficacy,[7] the agnostic perspective of FBT shifts blame away from sufferers and their parents and allows therapists to correct maladaptive ED behaviors by integrating multiple interventions. The clearly delineated core principles of FBT (e.g., parental empowerment) and utilization of techniques maintaining these principles (e.g., nondirective therapeutic style) enable a delivery system that is moldable to different levels of care as well as other target populations. New forms of implementation show promise for utilization of FBT in hard-to-reach populations with disordered eating.

Although superior to other interventions,[7] FBT is not a "cure-all" for adolescent EDs. There are some individuals for whom FBT is not an effective treatment and fail to meet weight gain criteria throughout treatment.[27] There is a need for continual development of alternative interventions as well as improvements of FBT within clinical research. Future research needs to continue to consider the factors of the intervention that can be amplified or combined with other treatments to improve response and outcomes.

REFERENCES

1. Couturier J, Kimber M, Szatmari P. Efficacy of family-based treatment for adolescents with eating disorders: a systematic review and meta-analysis. *Int J Eat Disord.* 2013;46(1):3–11. https://doi.org/10.1002/eat.22042.
2. Lock J, Le Grange D. *Treatment Manual for Anorexia Nervosa: A Family-Based Approach.* New York, NY: Guilford Press; 2013.
3. Rienecke R. Family-based treatment of eating disorders in adolescents: current insights. *Adolesc Health Med Ther.* 2017;8:69–79. https://doi.org/10.2147/AHMT.S115775.
4. Russell GF, Szmukler GI, Dare C, Eisler I. An evaluation of family therapy in anorexia nervosa and bulimia nervosa. *Arch Gen Psychiatry.* 1987;44(12):1047–1056. http://www.ncbi.nlm.nih.gov/pubmed/3318754.
5. Agras WS, Lock J, Brandt H, et al. Comparison of 2 family therapies for adolescent anorexia nervosa. *JAMA Psychiatry.* 2014;71(11):1279. https://doi.org/10.1001/jamapsychiatry.2014.1025.
6. Chen EY, Weissman JA, Zeffiro TA, et al. Family-based therapy for young adults with anorexia nervosa restores weight. *Int J Eat Disord.* 2016;49(7):701–707. https://doi.org/10.1002/eat.22513.
7. Lock J, Le Grange D, Agras WS, Moye A, Bryson SW, Jo B. Randomized clinical trial comparing family-based treatment with adolescent-focused individual therapy for adolescents with anorexia nervosa. *Arch Gen Psychiatry.* 2010;67(10):1025. https://doi.org/10.1001/archgenpsychiatry.2010.128.
8. Loeb KL, Le Grange D, Lock J, James D. *Family Therapy for Adolescent Eating and Weight Disorders: New Applications.* New York, NY: Routledge; 2015.
9. Eisler I, Dare C, Russell GF, Szmukler G, le Grange D, Dodge E. Family and individual therapy in anorexia nervosa. A 5-year follow-up. *Arch Gen Psychiatry.* 1997;54(11):1025–1030. http://www.ncbi.nlm.nih.gov/pubmed/9366659.
10. Eisler I, Simic M, Russell GFM, Dare C. A randomised controlled treatment trial of two forms of family therapy in adolescent anorexia nervosa: a five-year follow-up. *J Child Psychol Psychiatry.* 2007;48(6):552–560. https://doi.org/10.1111/j.1469-7610.2007.01726.x.
11. Lock J, Couturier J, Agras WS. Comparison of long-term outcomes in adolescents with anorexia nervosa treated with family therapy. *J Am Acad Child Adolesc Psychiatry.* 2006;45(6):666–672. https://doi.org/10.1097/01.chi.0000215152.61400.ca.
12. Le Grange D, Lock J, Accurso EC, et al. Relapse from remission at two- to four-year follow-up in two treatments for adolescent anorexia nervosa. *J Am Acad Child Adolesc Psychiatry.* 2014;53(11):1162–1167. https://doi.org/10.1016/j.jaac.2014.07.014.
13. Dimitropoulos G, Farquhar JC, Freeman VE, Colton PA, Olmsted MP. Pilot study comparing multi-family therapy to single family therapy for adults with anorexia nervosa in an intensive eating disorder program. *Eur Eat Disord Rev.* 2015;23(4):294–303. https://doi.org/10.1002/erv.2359.
14. Dimitropoulos G, Landers AL, Freeman VF, et al. Open trial of family-based treatment of anorexia nervosa for transition age youth. *J Can Acad Child Adolesc Psychiatry.* 2018;27:50–61.
15. Girz L, Lafrance Robinson A, Foroughe M, Jasper K, Boachie A. Adapting family-based therapy to a day hospital programme for adolescents with eating disorders: preliminary outcomes and trajectories of change. *J Fam Ther.* 2013;35(suppl 1):102–120.

16. Van Langenberg T, Sawyer SM, Le Grange D, Hughes EK. Psychosocial well-being of siblings of adolescents with anorexia nervosa. *Eur Eat Disord Rev.* 2016;24(6):438–445. https://doi.org/10.1002/erv.2469.

17. Eisler I, Wallis A, Dodge E. What's new is old and what's old is new: the origins and evolution of eating disorders family therapy. In: Loeb K, Le Grange D, eds. *Family Therapy for Adolescent Eating and Weight Disorders: New Applications.* New York, NY: Routledge; 2015:6–42.

18. Hughes E, Le Grange D, Yeo M, et al. Parent-focused treatment for adolescent anorexia nervosa: a study protocol of a randomised controlled trial. *BMC Psychiatry.* 2014;14(1):105.

19. Eisler I, Dare C, Hodes M, Russell G, Dodge E, Le Grange D. Family therapy for adolescent anorexia nervosa: the results of a controlled comparison of two family interventions. *J Child Psychol Psychiatry.* 2011;41(6):727–736.

20. Fitzpatrick KK, Accurso EC, Aspen V, Forsberg SE, Le Grange D, Lock J. Conceptualizing fidelity in FBT as the field moves forward: how do we know when we're doing it right?. In: Loeb K, Le Grange D, eds. *Family Therapy for Adolescent Eating and Weight Disorders: New Applications.* New York, NY: Routledge; 2015:418–439.

21. Kosmerly S, Waller G, Robinson AL. Clinician adherence to guidelines in the delivery of family-based therapy for eating disorders. *Int J Eat Disord.* 2015:223–230. https://doi.org/10.1002/eat.22276.

22. Hughes EK, Le Grange D, Court A, Sawyer SM. A case series of family-based treatment for adolescents with atypical anorexia nervosa. *Int J Eat Disord.* 2017;50(4):424–432. https://doi.org/10.1002/eat.22662.

23. Pisetsky EM, Utzinger LM, Peterson CB. Incorporating social support in the treatment of anorexia nervosa: special considerations for older adolescents and young adults. *Cogn Behav Pract.* 2017;23(3):316–328. https://doi.org/10.1016/j.cbpra.2015.09.002.

24. Knatz S, Walter KH, Marzola E, Boutelle KN. A brief intensive application of family-based treatment for eating disorders. In: Loeb K, Le Grange D, eds. *Family Therapy for Adolescent Eating and Weight Disorders: New Applications.* New York, NY: Routledge; 2015:72–91.

25. Le Grange D, Accurso EC, Lock J, Agras S, Bryson SW. Early weight gain predicts outcome in two treatments for adolescent anorexia nervosa. *Int J Eat Disord.* 2014;47(2):124–129. https://doi.org/10.1002/eat.22221.

26. Swenne I, Parling T, Salonen Ros H. Family-based intervention in adolescent restrictive eating disorders: early treatment response and low weight suppression is associated with favourable one-year outcome. *BMC Psychiatry.* 2017;17(1):1–10. https://doi.org/10.1186/s12888-017-1486-9.

27. Lock JD, Le Grange D, Agras WS, et al. Can adaptive treatment improve outcomes in family-based therapy for adolescents with anorexia nervosa? Feasibility and treatment effects of a multi-site treatment study. *Behav Res Ther.* 2015;28(10):1304–1314.

28. Le Grange D, Lock J. *Treating Bulimia in Adolescents: A Family-Based Approach.* New York: Guilford; 2007.

29. Le Grange D, Hughes EK, Court A, Yeo M, Crosby RD, Sawyer SM. Randomized clinical trial of parent-focused treatment and family-based treatment for adolescent anorexia nervosa. *J Am Acad Child Adolesc Psychiatry.* 2016;55(8):683–692. https://doi.org/10.1016/j.jaac.2016.05.007.

30. Le Grange D, Lock J, Agras WS, Bryson SW, Jo B. Randomized clinical trial of family-based treatment and cognitive-behavioral therapy for adolescent bulimia nervosa. *J Am Acad Child Adolesc Psychiatry.* 2015;54(11):886–894.e2. https://doi.org/10.1016/j.jaac.2015.08.008.

31. Ciao A, Accurso EC, Fitzsimmons-Craft EE, Le Grange D. Predictors and moderators of psychological changes during treatment of adolescent bulimia nervosa. *Behav Res Ther.* 2015;69:48–53. https://doi.org/10.1016/j.brat.2015.04.002.

32. Dimitropoulous G, Lock J, Le Grange D, Anderson K. Family therapy for transition youth. In: Loeb K, Le Grange D, eds. *Family Therapy for Adolescent Eating and Weight Disorders: New Applications.* New York, NY: Routledge; 2015:230–255.

33. Dare C, Eisler I. A multi-family group day treatment programme for adolescent eating disorder. *Eur Eat Disord Rev.* 2000;8(1):4–18. https://doi.org/10.1002/(SICI)1099-0968(200002)8:1<4::AID-ERV330>3.0.CO;2-P.

34. Eisler I, Simic M, Hodsoll J, et al. A pragmatic randomised multi-centre trial of multifamily and single family therapy for adolescent anorexia nervosa. *BMC Psychiatry.* 2016;16(1):1–14. https://doi.org/10.1186/s12888-016-1129-6.

35. Gelin Z, Cook-Darzens S, Hendrick S. The evidence base for Multiple Family Therapy in psychiatric disorders: a review (part 1). *J Fam Ther.* 2017:1–24. https://doi.org/10.1111/1467-6427.12178.

36. Stewart C, Voulgari S, Eisler I, Hunt K, Simic M. Multifamily therapy for bulimia nervosa in adolescence. *Eat Disord.* 2015;23(4):345–355. https://doi.org/10.1080/10640266.2015.1044348.

37. Aardoom JJ, Dingemans AE, Van Furth EF. E-health interventions for eating disorders: emerging findings, issues, and opportunities. *Curr Psychiatry Rep.* 2016;18(4):42. https://doi.org/10.1007/s11920-016-0673-6.

38. Anderson KE, Byrne CE, Crosby RD, Le Grange D. Utilizing Telehealth to deliver family-based treatment for adolescent anorexia nervosa. *Int J Eat Disord.* 2017;50(10):1235–1238. https://doi.org/10.1002/eat.22759.

39. Anderson LK, Reilly EE, Berner L, et al. Treating eating disorders at higher levels of care: overview and challenges. *Curr Psychiatry Rep.* 2017;19(8):48. https://doi.org/10.1007/s11920-017-0796-4.

40. Hoste RR. Incorporating family-based therapy principles into a partial hospitalization programme for adolescents with anorexia nervosa: challenges and considerations. *J Fam Ther.* 2015;37(1):41–60.

41. Wallis A, Rhodes P, Kohn M, Madden S. Five-years of family-based treatment for anorexia nervosa: the Maudsley model at the children's hospital at westmead. *Int J Adolesc Med Health*. 2007;19:277–283.

42. Peebles R, Lesser A, Park CC, et al. Outcomes of an inpatient medical nutritional rehabilitation protocol in children and adolescents with eating disorders. *J Eat Disord*. 2017;5(1):7. https://doi.org/10.1186/s40337-017-0134-6.

43. Halvorsen I, Reas DL, Nilsen J-V, Rø Ø. Naturalistic outcome of family-based inpatient treatment for adolescents with anorexia nervosa. *Eur Eat Disord Rev*. December 2017. https://doi.org/10.1002/erv.2572.

44. Murray SB, Anderson LK, Rockwell R, Griffiths S, Le Grange D, Kaye WH. Adapting family-based treatment for adolescent anorexia nervosa across higher levels of patient care. *Eat Disord*. 2015;23(4):302–314. https://doi.org/10.1080/10640266.2015.1042317.

Inpatient and Day Patient Treatment of Adolescents With Eating Disorders

BEATE HERPERTZ-DAHLMANN, MD

INTRODUCTION

Eating disorders (ED) are serious mental disorders with a high prevalence of medical and psychiatric comorbidity. The mortality risk of anorexia nervosa (AN) with a standardized mortality ratio (SMR) of 11.5 by 1 year after discharge among individuals aged 15–24 years is higher than that for other serious diseases in adolescence such as asthma, type 1 diabetes, and any other psychiatric disorders. Bulimia nervosa (BN) also has an increased risk with an SMR of approximately 4 in adolescents and young adults, whereas eating disorders not otherwise specified (EDNOS according to DSM-IV), including binge eating disorder (BED), have a mortality rate of 1.4 in this age group.[1]

Severely affected patients with EDs require clinical settings that are able to provide intensive treatment modalities to cope with medical and psychologic complications. Moreover, children and adolescents might require inpatient (IP) treatment because starvation-induced underweight has a considerable effect on physical growth and brain development. In Germany (www.gbe-bund.de) and the United Kingdom,[2] admission rates for children and adolescents with AN rose substantially in the past several years, although the reasons are not quite clear. However, young patients with AN often do not want to be hospitalized and experience hospitalization as more coercive than adult patients.[3] Consequently, dropout rates in adolescents from an IP treatment program amount to approximately 25%.[4]

There is a broad consensus that patients with BN or BED should be treated on an outpatient basis; however, serious depression, suicidality, and substance abuse in both disorders or severe electrolyte disturbances in BN might also lead to emergency treatment.

TREATMENT SETTINGS

Inpatient Treatment

Although there are different admission policies to IP treatment depending on the healthcare system of each country, there has been a consensus on medical/psychiatric/psychosocial indications that would make admission to hospitals mandatory (for more details, see Ref. 5) (Table 20.1).

Most clinical guidelines recommend a child and adolescent (CAP) or pediatric unit experienced in the treatment of EDs with a team aware of developmental changes and sensitive to the patients' needs.[6] Moreover, the unit should provide educational and other age-appropriate activities to facilitate reintegration into everyday life.[7] IP treatment should take a multimodal approach with an interdisciplinary team of child and adolescent psychiatrists and/or pediatricians, psychotherapists, nurses familiar with the problems of ED patients, dieticians, physiotherapists, and additional professions such as occupational therapists. This also applies to any other treatment setting for EDs, e.g., day patient (DP) treatment or residential care. There is some evidence that the treatment outcome in a general medical or psychiatric setting is poorer than in a specialized ED unit.[8] Moreover, the duration of IP treatment should be as short as possible because children and adolescents are potentially at risk of becoming institutionalized. In an Australian randomized controlled trial (RCT), two different lengths of hospitals stays were compared: a short stay for medical stabilization and a more prolonged stay for weight restoration. In the shorter intervention, all patients received additional family-based therapy (FBT) on an outpatient basis. At the 12-month follow-up, there was no difference in outcome; however, there were some methodological problems with this study.[9]

Table 20.2 demonstrates the most important goals of a multidisciplinary treatment program.

Eating Disorders and Obesity in Children and Adolescents. https://doi.org/10.1016/B978-0-323-54852-6.00020-3

TABLE 20.1
Medical and Psychosocial Indications for Hospital Admission for Adolescent AN

- Body weight (BMI) below the third age-adapted percentile or complete food refusal during the last days or marked weight loss in a short space of time
- Metabolic risk (e.g., hypoglycemia, pancreas or liver affection, electrolyte disturbances)
- Cardiologic risk (e.g., abnormally slow heart rate [<40 beats/min] or hypotension, pericardial effusion, ECG changes [e.g., prolonged QT interval])
- Low body temperature
- Dehydration, especially in children
- Suicidality or another severe psychologic comorbidity
- Severe problems with caregivers
- Insufficient weight gain despite appropriate outpatient treatment

Summary Clinical Guidelines[6,7,10] (for a review, see Ref. 11).

TABLE 20.2
IP Multidisciplinary Treatment Program for Adolescents With AN[5]

- Treatment of medical complications and nutritional restoration (physician, nurses, dietician)
- Nutritional counseling (individual and/or group psychoeducation) to regain healthy eating behavior (dietician, nurses)
- Psychotherapy (individual and group psychotherapy) (psychotherapist, child and adolescent psychiatrist)
- Joint or separate family-based approaches (psychotherapist or psychiatrist)
- Psychoeducation for carers and close friends

Nutritional Rehabilitation

One of the major goals of IP treatment is weight restoration and resumption of menses. Nevertheless, there is no generally determined target weight, although BMI at discharge is one of the most important prognostic indicators.[12]

Previous investigations in adolescent AN indicate the 25th age-adapted BMI percentile as the threshold for the reoccurrence of menses, which thus might serve as a recommendation for target weight.[13] In the United States, target weight is mostly defined as % of expected body weight (EBW) (EBW corresponds to the median age-adjusted BMI [50th BMI percentile]; %EBW is the observed BMI/EBW × 100). A recent study examined resumption of menses in relation to %EBW and found that two-thirds of the adolescent patients resumed menses at weights of approximately 95% EBW.[14] However, there is no clinical consensus on how to define EBW. In a very recent survey, less than half of the clinicians in the United States, when asked for their definition of EBW, used growth curve data.[15]

Several recent studies point to the fact that nutritional rehabilitation is probably practiced too slowly for mildly and moderately starved patients because clinicians are afraid of the so-called refeeding syndrome[16,17] (for a review, see Ref. 11). The refeeding syndrome is induced by hypophosphatemia caused by realimentation and may result in cardiac and renal failure as well as in neurological complications such as epileptic seizures. However, there was no higher prevalence of a refeeding syndrome when comparing high- versus low-caloric nutritional restoration.[11] Rather, refeeding syndrome occurred in very-low-weight adolescent patients and those with a reduced white blood cell count, which is mostly a symptom of a protracted course of AN.

To support weight gain and a normal eating behavior, a meal plan consisting of three main meals and three snacks should be established. In patients with very severe weight loss and food refusal, nasogastric tube feeding or liquid high-energy meals may be recommended.

Psychotherapy

Besides family-oriented approaches, individual or group psychotherapy are among a number of essential therapeutic strategies during IP, DP, or outpatient treatment. Recently, cognitive-behavioral therapy (CBT) has been modified for adolescents (see Chapter 18). Another individual psychologic approach is adolescent-focused therapy (AFT) mainly performed in the United States. AFT is a manualized treatment approach that is based on the concept that EDs represent dysfunctional behavior patterns for coping with the developmental demands of adolescence, such as identity formation or delineation from parents.[18] In a longer-term follow-up study, the outcome in AFT was not worse than in FBT, although remission by FBT was achieved in a shorter period of time.[19]

Family-based approaches such as FBT are an essential part of ED treatment and have proven to be effective (see Chapter 19).[20] However, there are far too few investigations that compared FBT with other psychologic approaches (for more detailed comments, see Ref. 11).

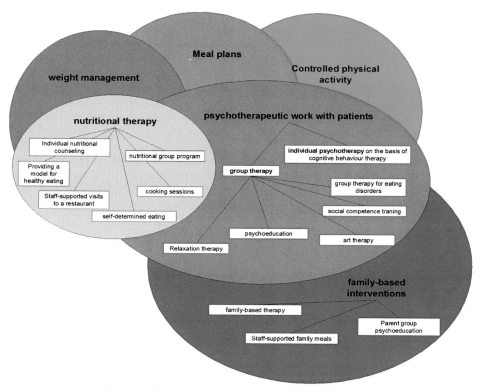

FIG. 20.1 Multimodal treatment program in adolescent AN.

Group psychotherapy is also seen as an important therapeutic tool for adolescent patients with AN, although there is still not sufficient scientific evidence. Many adolescents find it helpful to discuss their problems with other affected peers as well as everyday problems that emerge when they return to school and everyday life.

Other Therapeutic Approaches

Additional interventions such as body image therapy, physiotherapy, and sports therapy may support the patient's motivation to regain health and overcome ED-associated rituals and habits (Fig. 20.1).

Medication

Currently, no medication has been approved by the FDA or the European Medicines Agency for the treatment of adolescent AN (for a more detailed review, see Chapter 22). However, in very agitated and anxious patients, the application of neuroleptics, specifically olanzapine, may prove beneficial. Very recently, the effect of the D2-dopamine receptor agonist aripiprazole has been evaluated in adolescent patients.[21] In a retrospective chart analysis, patients medicated with aripiprazole experienced a significantly higher weight gain than those without the medication.

Relapse and Rehospitalization

Although there is high variability in the definition of relapse, most authors use body weight or BMI thresholds and/or recurrence of psychologic ED symptoms or both as criteria for relapse. The majority of studies with different durations of follow-up report relapse rates higher than 25%, with the highest probability of relapse occurring during the first year after treatment (for a review, see Ref. 22). With a longer duration of observation time, relapse rates decline (for a review, see Chapter 26).

In a European 6-year follow-up study in individuals with adolescent AN, 50% of the sample required a second hospitalization, and 40% required three or more hospitalizations.[23] In our 2.5-year follow-up study of DP (see above[24]), readmission rates during this period were approximately 30%.

Because of these high rehospitalization rates, especially in the first year after discharge, the recommendation is to create a contract with the patient and his/her parents about the necessity of readmission if the patient's weight falls below a defined threshold or if he/she suffers from severely disturbed eating disorder behavior. Furthermore, the rate of weight gain parallel to development of growth should be determined. This contract should be enforced as long as the patient has an adequate body weight; severe weight loss often diminishes insight into the illness and makes readmission difficult. If the patient is at a critical medical level, parents should be advised about the legal issues, and all therapists working with ED patients should be informed about the procedures involved in obtaining allowance for compulsory treatment.

Day Patient Treatment

Depending on the health status of the patient, DP treatment or partial hospitalization may be initiated as a first-line treatment or may follow IP treatment in a stepped care approach. However, there is great variety in the intensity and duration of DP treatment. Whereas some patients attend DP programs only after school in the afternoon, others visit DP treatment 4–7 whole days/week; in addition, the duration of DP treatment varies between several weeks to several months.

In addition to the financial advantages associated with DP, the skills patients obtain while in DP treatment may be more easily transferred to the home setting and thus are more generalizable to everyday life. Moreover, DP may be more likely to increase patients' autonomy and self-confidence than IP. In DP, the family is more involved in managing refeeding, which is a strategy that has been shown to be effective in the treatment of adolescent AN. In addition, during DP, adolescents are able to maintain contact with their peers and take part in school activities and other social networking, thus supporting social competence. This is of considerable importance because patients with AN are known to have a range of social difficulties. It may be hypothesized that in DP, the patient is confronted more with the "real world" than in IP, which makes the transition to the home environment at the end of treatment smoother and could thus lower the risk for rapid relapses.

Evidence for Different Treatment Settings

In a systematic review of five studies, with three also including adolescents, different settings in AN were compared: two evaluated IP in comparison with outpatient treatment, one compared IP with DP treatment, another evaluated different lengths of treatment, and one compared DP with outpatient treatment. BMI and ED symptoms were defined as outcome variables. There was no substantial difference between all three settings, with IP being by far the most expensive.[9,25]

One of these studies comparing IP with DP treatment was conducted by us. A total of 172 adolescents with a first onset of AN and an average age of 15 years from six specialized treatment centers were included. After a short hospital stay for medical stabilization, the patients were treated on a DP basis until the late afternoon. During the weekend, patients stayed at home; otherwise, the treatment program was identical. After 1 year, DP treatment after a short IP care was not inferior to continued IP treatment for restoration and maintenance of body weight.[24] Patients in the DP group had a significantly better psychosexual outcome and a better mental state than those who remained in IP treatment. The number of adverse events was low and comparable in both treatment arms.

In a narrative trial, 22 studies on DP/partial hospitalization in ED treatment were evaluated. Most of the investigations were open trials that reported weight gain and a reduction of ED symptoms at discharge. Those which reported follow-up data at some time interval after discharge also described a significant improvement but included a large number of noncompleters or dropouts.[26]

Bulimia Nervosa

Very few adolescent patients with BN or BED need IP. Sometimes, admission to the hospital is helpful for interrupting a vicious cycle of fasting and binge attacks and/or binge attacks and vomiting. Several binge attacks per day, frequent vomiting, or regular laxative abuse might be indicators for admission to IP. In addition, medical complications of BN may lead to hospitalization (see Table 20.1); in BN, ECG changes are often related to hypokalemia caused by frequent vomiting. Moreover, gastroesophageal complications may occur, such as esophagitis and erosions (for more detailed information, see Chapter 7). Finally, comorbid psychiatric disorders, e.g., borderline personality disorder associated with severe self-harm, suicidal behavior, depression, or substance abuse, might also make more intensive treatment necessary. In BN, the primary need is for regular meals and snacks to prevent fasting-associated binge attacks. In addition, nutritional counseling is necessary to become accustomed to normal eating and abstain from low calorie food; moreover, patients should learn to include so-called "forbidden foods" in their diet to stop cravings for sweets or other high-calorie products.

In an RCT comparing IP with DP in patients with BN, the latter was not inferior to IP in terms of remission rates or general psychopathology.[27,28] However, this study only included adult patients.

CONCLUSION

Several clinicians and researchers argue that long hospital stays contribute to the severe social impairment of patients with AN and other EDs and add to delayed adolescent development of these patients.[29] According to the WHO report (2005), "children and adolescents should be treated in the least restrictive and stigmatizing environment." There is emerging evidence that less intensive treatment settings, such as DP or a higher frequency outpatient treatment, achieve similar or even better outcomes as IP treatment in medically stable adolescents.[11] In addition, IP treatment is costly and significantly more expensive than DP.[24] Nevertheless, the relapse rate remains very high independent of the treatment setting. The patient status at the end of the intervention does not predict recovery in the medium or long-term follow-up. In the 4-year follow-up report of outpatient FBT in AN, only 30% of the former patients remained weight restored.[19] Thus, there is an ongoing, urgent need for research for more effective and affordable treatment strategies that help the adolescent overcome his/her ED and return to an age-appropriate quality of life.

REFERENCES

1. Hoang U, Goldacre M, James A. Mortality following hospital discharge with a diagnosis of eating disorder: national record linkage study, England, 2001-2009: mortality following a diagnosis of eating disorder. *Int J Eat Disord.* 2014;47:507–515.
2. Holland J, Hall N, Yeates DG, Goldacre M. Trends in hospital admission rates for anorexia nervosa in Oxford (1968-2011) and England (1990-2011): database studies. *J R Soc Med.* 2016;109(2):59–66.
3. Guarda AS, Pinto AM, Coughlin JW, et al. Perceived coercion and change in perceived need for admission in patients hospitalized for eating disorders. *Am J Psychiatry.* 2007;164(1):108–114.
4. Godart NT, Rein Z, Perdereau F, et al. Predictors of premature termination of anorexia nervosa treatment. *Am J Psychiatry.* 2005;162(12):2398–2399.
5. Herpertz-Dahlmann B. *Intensive Treatments. Encyclopedia of Feeding and Eating Disorders;* 2017. Meteor.Springer.com.
6. Lock J, La Via MC. American Academy of Child and Adolescent Psychiatry (AACAP) committee on quality issues (CQI). Practice parameter for the assessment and treatment of children and adolescents with eating disorders. *J Am Acad Child Adolesc Psychiatry.* 2015;54:412–425.
7. NICE 2017. *National Institute for Health and Care Excellence. Eating Disorders: Recognition and Treatment. National Institute for Health and Clinical Excellence Guideline (NG69);* May 2017. Website http://www.nice.org.uk. Published.
8. House J, Schmidt U, Craig M, et al. Comparison of specialist and non-specialist care pathways for adolescents with anorexia nervosa and related eating disorders. *Int J Eat Disord.* 2012;45(8):949–956.
9. Madden S, Miskovic-Wheatley J, Wallis A, et al. A randomized controlled trial of in-patient treatment for anorexia nervosa in medically unstable adolescents. *Psychol Med.* 2015;45:415–427.
10. Hay P, Chinn D, Forbes D, et al. Royal Australian and New Zealand College of Psychiatrists: Clinical practice guidelines for the treatment of eating disorders. *Aust N Z J Psychiatry.* 2014;48:977–1008.
11. Herpertz-Dahlmann B. Treatment of eating disorders in child and adolescent psychiatry. *Curr Opin Psychiatry.* 2017;30:438–445.
12. Kaplan AS, Walsh BT, Olmsted M, et al. The slippery slope: prediction of successful weight maintenance in anorexia nervosa. *Psychol Med.* 2009:1037–1045.
13. Dempfle A, Herpertz-Dahlmann B, Timmesfeld N, et al. Predictors of the resumption of menses in adolescent anorexia nervosa. *BMC Psychiatry.* 2013;39.
14. Faust JP, Goldschmidt AB, Anderson KE, et al. Resumption of menses in anorexia nervosa during a course of family-based treatment. *J Eat Disord.* 2013;1:12.
15. Lebow J, Sim LA, Accurso EC. Is there clinical consensus in defining weight restoration for adolescents with anorexia nervosa? *Eat Disord.* 2018;26:270–277.
16. Garber AK, Sawyer SM, Golden NH, et al. A systematic review of approaches to refeeding in patients with anorexia nervosa. *Int J Eat Disord.* 2016;49:293–310.
17. O'Connor G, Nicholls D, Hudson L, Singhal A. Refeeding low weight hospitalized adolescents with anorexia nervosa: a multicenter randomized controlled trial. *Nutr Clin Pract.* 2016;31:681–689.
18. Moye A, Fitzpatrick K, Hoste RR. Adolescent-focused psychotherapy for anorexia nervosa. In: *Eating Disorders in Children and Adolescents.* New York, London: The Guildford Press; 2011.
19. Le Grange D, Lock J, Accurso EC, et al. Relapse from remission at two- to four-year follow-up in two treatments for adolescent anorexia nervosa. *J Am Acad Child Adolesc Psychiatry.* 2014;53:1162–1167.
20. Le Grange DI, Eisler I. Family interventions in adolescent anorexia nervosa. *Child Adolesc Psychiatr Clin N Am.* 2009;18(1):159–173.
21. Frank GKW, Shott ME, Hagman JO, et al. The partial dopamine D2 receptor agonist aripiprazole is associated with weight gain in adolescent anorexia nervos. *Int J Eat Disord.* 2017;50(4):447–450.
22. Khalsa SS, Portnoff LC, McCurdy-McKinnon D, Feusner JD. What happens after treatment? A systematic review of relapse, remission, and recovery in anorexia nervosa. *J Eat Disord.* 2017;5:20.
23. Steinhausen H-C. Outcome of eating disorders. *Child Adolesc Psychiatr Clin N Am.* 2009;18:225–242.
24. Herpertz-Dahlmann B, Schwarte R, Krei M, et al. Day-patient treatment after short inpatient care versus

continued inpatient treatment in adolescents with anorexia nervosa (ANDI): a multicentre, randomised, open-label, non-inferiority trial. *Lancet.* 2014;383:1222–1229.

25. Madden S. Systematic review of evidence for different treatment settings in anorexia nervosa. *World J Psychiatry.* 2015;5:147.

26. Friedman K, Ramirez AL, Murray SB, et al. A narrative review of outcome studies for residential and partial hospital-based treatment of eating disorders. *Eur Eat Disord Rev.* 2016;24:263–276.

27. Zeeck A, Weber S, Sandholz A, et al. Inpatient versus day treatment for bulimia nervosa: results of a one-year follow-up. *Psychother Psychosom.* 2009;78:317–319.

28. Zeeck A, Weber S, Sandholz A, Joos A, Hartmann A. Stability of long-term outcome in bulimia nervosa: a 3-year follow-up. *J Clin Psychol.* 2011;67:318–327.

29. Treasure J, Claudino AM, Zucker N. Eating disorders. *Lancet.* 2010;375:583–593.

Early Intervention for Eating Disorders in Young People

MICHAELA FLYNN, BPSY (HONS) • ULRIKE SCHMIDT, MD, PHD, FRCPSYCH

INTRODUCTION

The principle of early diagnosis and treatment to optimize disease outcomes is intuitively appealing and widely accepted in medicine. Accumulating evidence from epidemiological, neurobiological, and clinical studies has provided a compelling case for early intervention in eating disorders (EDs). As such, the development and investigation of early intervention in EDs is a clinical and research priority. This chapter defines key concepts, provides an overview of the current knowledge on early intervention in EDs, and highlights areas for future research.

What Is Early Intervention?

Early intervention in psychiatric disorders is critically dependent on the early detection of illness and the prompt initiation of effective treatment. The rationale is that detection and treatment of symptoms in the early stages of illness may prevent the development of full-syndrome disorder, facilitate recovery or improve outcomes, and prevent development of long-term secondary disabilities. Early intervention is distinct from, but on a spectrum with, preventative interventions, which target modifiable risk factors. A detailed review of the literature relating to the prevention of EDs is presented elsewhere in this edition.

Why Is Early Intervention Important in Eating Disorders?

There are several reasons to prioritize early intervention in EDs. Firstly, it is widely accepted that response to treatment is greatest in the early stages of the illness and diminishes the longer the disorder persists.[1] Similarly, longer illness duration is associated with poorer long-term outcomes. This is proposed to arise from "neuroprogression," i.e., neurobiological changes that unfavorably alter the trajectory of a mental illness (e.g., Passos et al.[2]). Growing neuroimaging data and cognitive neuroscience models support the idea of neuroprogression in EDs. For example, increasing illness duration in anorexia nervosa (AN) appears to be associated with pathological thoughts and behaviors becoming more rewarding, habitual, and neurobiologically "entrenched."[3,4] Similar processes are thought to be involved in bulimic eating disorders.[5] Secondly, the peak time for ED onset is adolescence/emerging adulthood, a critical period during which the brain is undergoing significant development, particularly in the prefrontal regions.[6] During this developmental period the brain is likely to be particularly susceptible to the effects of poor nutrition and stress. Thirdly, the onset of EDs during adolescence derails social and emotional development and compromises successful transition into adulthood. Early intervention may minimize disruption to development by favorably altering the illness trajectory, increasing rates of full recovery, and reducing the need for more intensive forms of treatment. Finally, given the high physical, psychosocial, and financial burden of EDs, treating symptoms early is valuable from both an ethical and economical standpoint.

Laying the Foundations: Learning From Early Intervention in Psychosis

In psychiatry, the principles of early intervention have been most widely and effectively implemented in psychosis, with the key strategy being the reduction of the duration of untreated psychosis (DUP), i.e., the period from the first emergence of clinical symptoms to the start of treatment.[7] This is based on the idea that untreated psychosis has a "toxic" or neuroprogressive effect on the brain, potentially compromising recovery. Accordingly, studies have shown that a shorter DUP is associated with better long-term outcomes in relation to symptoms, social and psychological functioning, and relapse rates. This has led to vigorous attempts to reduce DUP through education campaigns, the development

Eating Disorders and Obesity in Children and Adolescents. https://doi.org/10.1016/B978-0-323-54852-6.00021-5

of early intervention services for first-episode and pro-dromal cases, and the streamlining of care pathways. In bipolar disorder, growing evidence again suggests that treatment in early-stage illness results in better outcomes, further strengthening the rationale.[8] Early intervention has been a clinical and research focus in psychotic disorders for more than 20 years, and there is much that the ED field can learn from these endeavors in terms of the development and investigation of early intervention models.

Key Concepts and Issues in Early Intervention in Eating Disorders

Early intervention across medical and psychiatric disor-ders (e.g., psychosis) is typically based on a stage model of illness, with the idea that clearly defined illness stages have prognostic and treatment implications. Such a stage of illness model for EDs has recently been proposed. In this model, early-stage illness has been defined as an illness duration of ≤3 years, based on evidence available from clinical studies in AN which suggest that thereafter response to treatment becomes more muted. However, equivalent evidence is lacking for bulimia nervosa (BN) and binge eating disorder (BED).[1]

As in psychosis, early intervention models for EDs might fruitfully focus on reducing the duration of untreated ED (DUED). To date, two systematic reviews and several individual studies have examined this unique period between clinical onset and first treat-ment (i.e., DUED) in different EDs.

In anorexia nervosa, an early systematic review of six studies from different countries found an average duration of untreated illness of 21.6 months.[9] More recently, three related studies on first-episode AN were conducted by a German research network. In the first of these, Neubauer et al.[10] examined the way in which age of onset influenced care pathways for first-episode AN. This study reported that DUED exceeded 2 years for all patients (M = 25.1 months) and was longest (38.4 months) for individuals with an early age of onset (onset ≤14 years of age). Two further studies by Weigel et al.[11] and Gumz et al.[12] investigated the average DUED for AN patients across the life span receiving specialist treatment for their first episode of AN and found mean DUEDs of 31.8 and 36.5 months, respectively.

In bulimia nervosa, one systematic review attempted to assess DUED and the relationship between illness duration and treatment outcome.[13] However, four out of five identified studies also included patients with previous treatment (i.e., who did not have a first-episode illness). The fifth study had no information about previous treatment.

Two further studies assessed DUED across ED diagnoses. A large patient survey by the UK charity Beat (including 1478 patients treated between 2007 and 2017) found a mean DUED of 44 months (or 176 weeks).[14] These 176 weeks were divided further as follows: on average, it took 91 weeks for the person to realize they had an ED, and a further 58 weeks to seek help. Following this they wait 11 weeks between the first visit to their general practitioner and referral, and 8 weeks each between referral to and assessment by specialist services, and specialist assessment and start of treatment. In children and adolescents, DUED was 130 weeks compared with 256 weeks in adults.

Finally, in a catchment area–based sample of emerg-ing adults with short-duration EDs (<3 years), we found a mean DUED of 19.1 months.[15]

These data clearly reflect that across studies, indi-viduals with EDs are unwell for significant periods of time before accessing treatment. The lack of consistency between studies most likely reflects methodological dif-ferences between studies (e.g., definition and assessment of DUED, study samples). The Beat survey, although limited by a self-selected sample, the self-report nature of the data, and the inclusion of people who had their first treatment 10 years before the survey, nonetheless highlights that, in terms of their sheer length, the main barriers to early intervention seem to be lack of ED rec-ognition by those affected, and delays in help-seeking. However, service level delays also have an important role to play and different approaches might be needed to shorten each of the different components of DUED.

Key Features of Early Intervention in Eating Disorders

Efforts to reduce DUED, and to provide optimally coor-dinated evidence-based early care, are essential aspects of early intervention for EDs. Reduction of key components of DUED might usefully include awareness raising and information/education campaigns for young people, parents, schools, university staff, sports coaches, and other stakeholders to facilitate early detection, help-seek-ing, and referral. Similarly, DUED might be improved by reducing service-related delays. This may involve training of general practitioners in early detection and manage-ment of EDs, and establishing clear access and waiting time standards for specialist ED services.

In addition to reducing DUED, there is also a need to adapt/tailor interventions to both the developmen-tal and illness stage of the young person, as treatment content or intensity may be more or less effective/rel-evant at different developmental/illness stages. Service/ care pathway–related factors concerning how, when, and where services are offered may also help or hinder a young people presenting for treatment. Thus, an argument can be made for specially designed early intervention services for EDs for young people, akin to those set up in psychosis.[16] Below, we have outlined how a model early intervention service for EDs would differ from a more conventional ED service (see Table 21.1).

MAJOR FINDINGS

Three different, more or less evidence-based, approaches to early intervention for EDs have been described.

A Systemic Public Health Intervention for Early Intervention in Anorexia Nervosa Across the Life Span

A very ambitious attempt to comprehensively address the different components of DUED through a systemic public health intervention was made by a German research group.[12,17] The multicomponent intervention was designed to increase awareness, reduce stigma, and promote timely help-seeking. It involved (1) a health literacy campaign with presentation of informative short films about EDs in cinemas and corresponding posters, (2) the introduction of a school-based

TABLE 21.1
What Might a Model Early Intervention Service for EDs Look Like?

	Early Intervention	Conventional ED Service
Prioritization	Applies an illness model that emphasizes "biological malleability"[26] during early illness stages and prioritizes early-stage cases.	Prioritization based on diagnosis and/or illness severity.
Access	Easy to access, ideally via self-referral, or alternatively early referral from primary care.	Systemic and service barriers delay access to service. Early referral from primary care discouraged.
Aims	To deliver a person-centered and evidence-based service to young people that reduces DUED and promotes early full recovery.	To deliver best possible care to all patients seen.
Approach	Person-centered care informed by stage of illness.	Service-centred, "one size fits all" care package determined by age, diagnosis, and/or illness severity.
Engagement	Active outreach using multiple modes of contact (e.g., emails, SMS). Clinician as initial contact. Increased flexibility (e.g., appointments). Informative psychoeducation tailored to young people's needs and interests (e.g., guidance social media use).	Limited outreach using traditional modes of contact (e.g., letters). Administrator as initial contact. Limited flexibility. Generic psychoeducation resources using a "one size fits all" approach.
Assessment	Biopsychosocial and person-centered approach. Strong emphasis on family involvement. Strategic use of psychoeducation emphasizing "biological malleability" to increase patient motivation for early change.	Standard assessment focusing on diagnosis and illness severity. Variable family involvement. Limited psychoeducation.
Treatment	Evidence-based treatments tailored to developmental and illness stage. Focus on early nutritional change for all ED diagnoses. Emphasis on family education, skills training, and support. Use of technology (e.g., online interventions, apps). Focus on transition management (e.g., university starter groups)	Standardized treatment determined by age, diagnosis, and/or illness severity. Variable focus on nutritional change. Variable emphasis on family involvement. Variable use of technology. Few supported transitions.

prevention program, (3) the development of an online treatment guide for EDs, (4) the establishment of a network of healthcare professionals within the field of EDs, and (5) the establishment of a specialist outpatient clinic for AN. In a pre-post evaluation of the intervention, mean DUED was reported as 36.5 months before the implementation of the intervention and remained unchanged thereafter (40.1 months). Further, mean duration of untreated illness at first contact with health services (usually with a general practitioner) was 25.0 months before introduction of the intervention and 32.8 months thereafter. Thus, the intervention did not have an impact on either DUED or time to first contact with health services. The authors themselves reflected on possible reasons for why the intervention was not successful, e.g., the sample size was small and the intervention period was short. However, it is also possible that the intervention simply was not effective and/or that public health interventions may not be an appropriate tool for reaching patients with AN in the early stages of illness. Nonetheless, the study highlights very lengthy delays (>1 year) from first contact with the healthcare system to start of specialist treatment for patients with AN.

A Government-Led, Country-Wide Approach to Early Intervention for Adolescents With EDs

In England, the National Health Service (NHS) has recently introduced access and waiting-time standards for child and adolescent ED services (CAEDS)[18] in an attempt to reduce delays, deterioration, and distress. This has been coupled with a sizeable investment in the establishment and training of CAEDS teams throughout the country to facilitate timely evidence-based care. This welcome change to service provision was influenced by concern about rising admission rates in young people with EDs.[19] In addition, there was the recognition that specialist outpatient services have better treatment engagement and outcomes and fewer hospital admissions. As such, specialist services are more cost-effective than nonspecialist services.[20-23] Although data reflecting the impact of these profound changes to service provision for children and young people are presently lacking, it is anticipated that reducing wait-times and increasing access to specialist care will markedly improve treatment outcomes for young people and reduce costs. This is a significant achievement; however, this initiative only covers those presenting with a first episode of an ED below age 18 years and does not extend to emerging adults.

A Service-Led Model of Early Intervention for Emerging Adults With EDs

We developed a service model for early intervention,[16] based on ideas from the psychosis field and the key principles of youth mental healthcare described by McGorry et al.[24] The model aims to significantly reduce DUED by offering rapid access to high-quality evidence-based interventions that are carefully tailored to both developmental and illness stage, i.e., a service model that is very similar to that described in Table 21.1. The "First Episode Rapid Early Intervention for Eating Disorders (FREED) service" is a novel early intervention service, developed specifically for adolescents and young adults (16–25 years) in the early stages of an ED (<3 years illness duration).[15,25] FREED is a "service within a service" that was initially piloted at a large ED service in South East England with a catchment area population of 2 million people.

Preliminary data from this pilot suggest that the FREED model is feasible and associated with better outcomes from treatment than conventional ED care.[15,25] Patients who received treatment via the FREED care pathway (N = 60) were compared with those from a comparison group (N = 86) of patients previously seen in our service who were of similar age and illness duration. FREED reduced DUED from previously 19 months to just over 13 months in patients from areas where there was minimal NHS gatekeeping. FREED also significantly reduced waiting times and improved treatment uptake. Furthermore, FREED patients showed significant improvements in ED and other symptoms over the course of the 12-month study period. Notably, weight-related outcomes for FREED patients with AN were significantly improved; although body mass index (BMI) at assessment was similar to that of the comparison group, by start of treatment, FREED-AN patients had gained some weight, whereas patients from the comparison cohort had deteriorated, most likely because they had waited much longer to start treatment. This BMI difference continued throughout treatment, and at 12 months, nearly 60% FREED-AN patients had returned to a BMI of 18.5 kg/m^2 or greater, whereas only 16.6% of participants in the comparison group achieved weight restoration during this period. This pilot study demonstrated that FREED has promise as a service model for emerging adults and has provided a platform for further evaluation of the model. We are currently scaling FREED to three other large ED services in England, with integrated qualitative and quantitative assessments of clinical effectiveness.

CONCLUSION

Although there is a strong rationale for early intervention in EDs, research shows that across different Western countries, the period from first onset of symptoms to the start of treatment (DUED) is typically at least 2 years and can be considerably longer. Different components of DUED may differ between countries in their length. Different models of early intervention for EDs have been proposed, either disorder-specific or transdiagnostic, and either covering children and adolescents, young adults or going across the age divide. These models have shown varying degrees of promise, but robust evaluations are so far lacking.

OUTLOOK

Future studies would benefit from a standardized definition of DUED and an observer-rated tool for assessing this. Such a tool would enable the exploration of symptom trajectories and the investigation of the relationships between components of DUED, i.e., ED awareness, help-seeking efforts, and service-related delays. This would allow a more nuanced and complete knowledge of facilitators/barriers to accessing care and the development of more targeted early intervention, fit for different healthcare systems. To date, no high-quality (i.e., randomized controlled) evaluations of early intervention service models for EDs exist. These are difficult but not impossible to design, as our colleagues working with psychosis have amply shown,[7] and will be an important component of future research.

REFERENCES

1. Treasure J, Stein D, Maguire S. Has the time come for a staging model to map the course of eating disorders from high risk to severe enduring illness? An examination of the evidence. *Early Interv Psychiatry*. 2015;9(3):173–184.
2. Passos IC, Mwangi B, Vieta E, Berk M, Kapczinski F. Areas of controversy in neuroprogression in bipolar disorder. *Acta Psychiatr Scand*. 2016;134(2):91–103.
3. O'Hara C, Campbell I, Schmidt U. A reward-centred model of anorexia nervosa: a focussed narrative review of the neurological and psychophysiological literature. *Neurosci Biobehav Rev*. 2015;52:131–152.
4. Steinglass JE, Walsh BT. Neurobiological model of the persistence of anorexia nervosa. *J Eat Disord*. 2016;4(1):19.
5. Berner L, Marsh R. Frontostriatal circuits and the development of bulimia nervosa. *Front Behav Neurosci*. 2014;8:395.
6. Dahl RE, Allen NB, Wilbrecht L, Suleiman AB. Importance of investing in adolescence from a developmental science perspective. *Nature*. 2018;554(7693):441.
7. Oliver D, Davies C, Crossland G, et al. Can we reduce the duration of untreated psychosis? A systematic review and meta-analysis of controlled interventional studies. *Schizophr Bull*. 2018;sbx166.
8. Joyce K, Thompson A, Marwaha S. Is treatment for bipolar disorder more effective earlier in illness course? A comprehensive literature review. *Int J Bipolar Disord*. 2016;4(1):19.
9. Schoemaker C. Does early intervention improve the prognosis in anorexia nervosa? A systematic review of the treatment-outcome literature. *Int J Eat Disord*. 1997;21(1):1–15.
10. Neubauer K, Weigel A, Daubmann A, et al. Paths to first treatment and duration of untreated illness in anorexia nervosa: are there differences according to age of onset? *Eur Eat Disord Rev*. 2014;22(4):292–298.
11. Weigel A, Rossi M, Wendt H, et al. Duration of untreated illness and predictors of late treatment initiation in anorexia nervosa. *J Publ Health*. 2014;22(6):519–527.
12. Gumz A, Uhlenbusch N, Weigel A, Wegscheider K, Romer G, Löwe B. Decreasing the duration of untreated illness for individuals with anorexia nervosa: study protocol of the evaluation of a systemic public health intervention at community level. *BMC Psychiatry*. 2014;14(1):300.
13. Reas D, Schoemaker C, Zipfel S, Williamson D. Prognostic value of duration of illness and early intervention in bulimia nervosa: a systematic review of the outcome literature. *Int J Eat Disord*. 2001;30(1):1–10.
14. BEAT. Delayed for years, denied for months: the health, emotional and financial impact on sufferers. In: *Families and the NHS of Delaying Treatment for Eating Disorders in England*. 2017. Available from: https://www.beateatingdisorders.org.uk/uploads/documents/2017/11/delaying-for-years-denied-for-months.pdf.
15. Brown A, McClelland J, Boysen E, Mountford V, Glennon D, Schmidt U. The FREED Project (first episode and rapid early intervention in eating disorders): service model, feasibility and acceptability. *Early Interv Psychiatry*. 2016;12(2):250–257.
16. Schmidt U, Brown A, McClelland J, Glennon D, Mountford V. Will a comprehensive, person-centered, team-based early intervention approach to first episode illness improve outcomes in eating disorders? *Int J Eat Disord*. 2016;49(4):374–377.
17. Gumz A, Weigel A, Wegscheider K, Romer G, Löwe B. The psychenet public health intervention for anorexia nervosa: a pre–post-evaluation study in a female patient sample. *Prim Health Care Res Dev*. 2018;19(1):42–52.
18. NHS E. *Access and Waiting Time Standard for Children and Young People with an Eating Disorder*; 2015. Available from: https://www.england.nhs.uk/wp-content/uploads/2015/07/cyp-eating-disorders-access-waiting-time-standard-comm-guid.pdf.
19. Holland J, Hall N, Yeates D, Goldacre M. Trends in hospital admission rates for anorexia nervosa in Oxford (1968–2011) and England (1990–2011): database studies. *J R Soc Med*. 2016;109(2):59–66.

20. House J, Schmidt U, Craig M, et al. Comparison of specialist and nonspecialist care pathways for adolescents with anorexia nervosa and related eating disorders. *Int J Eat Disord.* 2012;45(8):949–956.

21. Byford S, Barrett B, Roberts C, et al. Economic evaluation of a randomised controlled trial for anorexia nervosa in adolescents. *Br J Psychiatry.* 2007;191(5): 436–440.

22. Schmidt U, Sharpe H, Bartholdy S, et al. Treatment of anorexia nervosa: translating experimental neuroscience into clinical practice. *NIHR J Libr.* 2017. [Chapter 10].

23. Gowers SG, Clark AF, Roberts C, et al. A randomised controlled multicentre trial of treatments for adolescent anorexia nervosa including assessment of cost-effectiveness and patient acceptability-the TOuCAN trial. *Health Technol Assess.* 2010;14(15):1–98.

24. McGorry P, Goldstone S, Parker A, Rickwood D, Hickie I. Cultures for mental health care of young people: an Australian blueprint for reform. *Lancet Psychiatry.* 2014;1(7):559–568.

25. McClelland J, Hodsoll J, Brown A, et al. A pilot evaluation of a novel first episode and rapid early intervention service for eating disorders (FREED). *Eur Eat Disord Rev.* 2018;26(2):129–140.

26. Farrell N, Lee A, Deacon B. Biological or psychological? Effects of eating disorder psychoeducation on self-blame and recovery expectations among symptomatic individuals. *Behav Res Ther.* 2015;74:32–37.

CHAPTER 22

Pharmacotherapy of Eating Disorders in Children and Adolescents

EVELYN ATTIA, MD • PAULA TABARES, MD

PHARMACOTHERAPY OF EATING DISORDERS IN CHILDREN AND ADOLESCENTS

Eating disorders are serious psychiatric illnesses associated with significant morbidity and mortality. Pharmacologic strategies are frequently considered in the treatment of eating disorders, yet information is limited regarding the safety and utility of medications in child and adolescent patients. In this chapter, we will review the available literature on the use of medications for eating disorders, including anorexia nervosa, bulimia nervosa, and binge eating disorder. We will describe only briefly the treatments of avoidant-restrictive food intake disorder (ARFID), pica, and rumination disorder as there is no established evidence base for their treatment with medications. Across all of the feeding and eating disorders, very few clinical trials have included adolescent participants; therefore, in this chapter, we will describe findings from adult samples and their possible application to younger patients.

Pharmacotherapy of Anorexia Nervosa

Treatment for anorexia nervosa emphasizes restoration of both normal weight and normal eating behaviors. Because of the symptom overlap between anorexia nervosa and several other psychiatric illnesses (e.g., mood disorders, anxiety disorders, psychotic disorders), many medications that are useful in the treatments of other conditions have been considered for anorexia nervosa but consistently have been found to be of little or no benefit. Consensus guidelines therefore do not recommend medication treatments as part of first-line interventions for children and adolescents with anorexia nervosa.[1,2] Not infrequently, however, they are considered for refractory cases or for management of comorbid conditions.[2] Below is a summary of relevant studies.

Antidepressant medications for the treatment of anorexia nervosa

Patients with anorexia nervosa often present with symptoms of depression, anxiety, and obsessive-compulsive disorder. Several selective serotonin reuptake inhibitors (SSRIs) have been approved for the treatment of these disorders in children and adolescents and thus have been considered for use in anorexia nervosa. However, in a retrospective study of 35 hospitalized adolescents with anorexia nervosa, evaluations during their hospital stay, as well as 3 and 6 months following discharge, illustrated no differences in BMI ($P = .84$), symptoms of core eating disorder ($P = .79$), depression ($P = .75$), or obsessive-compulsive symptoms ($P = .40$) between the 19 patients treated with SSRIs and the 16 patients who did not receive SSRIs.[3]

Although there have been several randomized clinical trials examining SSRIs versus placebo in adults with anorexia nervosa,[4–6] there have not been similar trials in younger populations, likely due to the challenges of recruiting younger patients, as well as the sizeable evidence base for behavioral (i.e., nonmedication) treatments for adolescents with anorexia nervosa, including family-based therapy (FBT).[7]

In adults, Attia et al.[4] compared fluoxetine 60 mg with placebo in 31 hospitalized underweight women with anorexia nervosa. All participants received behaviorally focused treatment in addition to study medication during hospital stay, and at 7 weeks, no significant differences in body weight ($F = 0.23$; df = 1.28; p = n.s.), or measures of psychologic state or eating behavior, were detected between study groups. Participants with binge-purge subtype responded no differently than did those with restricting subtype.[4] Similarly, an open randomized trial with citalopram, which was conducted by Fassino et al.,[5] included 26 patients with anorexia nervosa restricting subtype. Researchers found no differences in BMI between the patients who received the medication and a control group who did not take medication.[5] Hypothesizing that weight-restored patients might respond to SSRIs differently than underweight individuals, Walsh et al.[6] conducted a multisite randomized controlled trial in which 93 weight-restored women with anorexia nervosa received cognitive-behavioral therapy, aimed at relapse prevention, and were randomly assigned to fluoxetine 60 mg or placebo. The investigators found no significant difference between fluoxetine and placebo in time-to-relapse (hazard ratio, 1.12; 95% CI, 0.65–2.01; $P = .64$).[6] Randomized, placebo-controlled trials with other classes of antidepressant medications including tricyclics (TCAs) have been completed in adults with anorexia nervosa without any findings to support their utility.[8]

Antipsychotic medications for the treatment of anorexia nervosa

The typical cognitions associated with anorexia nervosa, including overvalued beliefs concerning body shape and weight, and near fixed ideation about fear of fat, and likelihood of weight gain, have led to interest in the possible utility of antipsychotic medications for anorexia nervosa. The greater tolerability of second-generation (also known as atypical) antipsychotic medications coupled with their collateral weight gain effect has made their use compelling in the treatment of anorexia nervosa. However, in spite of several open trials suggesting the benefit of antipsychotics in the treatment of anorexia nervosa in children and adolescents, three small, randomized controlled trials that included adolescents with anorexia nervosa demonstrated no difference between medication and placebo in weight restoration.[9–11]

Kafantaris and colleagues[9] studied 20 underweight adolescents with anorexia nervosa–restrictive subtype in a 10-week, double-blind, placebo-controlled pilot trial using olanzapine. Medication dose was titrated up from 2.5 mg to a target dose of 10 mg daily. Completion rates were similar for medication (n = 7) and placebo (n = 8) groups, as were rates of increase in mean body weight (t = −2.68, $P < .01$) and improvements in eating attitudes and behaviors. The olanzapine group, however, demonstrated a trend of increasing fasting glucose and insulin levels at week 10 of treatment.[9] Hagman et al.[10] conducted a randomized double-blind, placebo-controlled trial with risperidone in 41 adolescents with a primary diagnosis of anorexia nervosa, in weight restoration phase. Participants received risperidone (n = 18) or placebo (n = 22). Mean dose of risperidone was 2.5 mg/day. After 9 weeks, there were no significant

differences between the groups for increase in body weight ($P < .76$). As expected, prolactin levels increased in the group receiving risperidone ($P < 0.001$). No other differences in laboratory parameters or extrapyramidal symptoms were present between groups. Sixteen of the study patients also received antidepressant medications for treatment of comorbidities, including depression, anxiety, and obsessive-compulsive disorder.[10] Court et al.[11] conducted an open label, 12-week randomized controlled trial with quetiapine (100–400 mg/day) versus treatment as usual, in 33 patients with anorexia nervosa. The mean age of those who completed the study was 23.8 years (range 15–42) for the quetiapine group and 21.0 years (range 16–27) for the control group. Both groups showed modest weight gain over the 12-week trial period. The quetiapine group demonstrated no significant difference on the Center for Epidemiological Studies Depression Scale (CES-D), compared with the treatment as usual group at the end of treatment ($F = 0.01$, $P < .93$). However, the study did not control for comorbidity and for the concomitant use of antidepressant and benzodiazepine medications.[11] Norris et al.[12] conducted a retrospective matched-group comparison study of 43 adolescents, aged 10–17 years, with mainly restrictive eating disorder (anorexia nervosa and eating disorder not otherwise specified—EDNOS) treated with olanzapine up to a maximum of 5 mg/day, and matched controls. The investigators found no significant differences in weight and psychologic measures between groups.[12] Frank et al.[13] recently published a retrospective chart review, including 106 adolescents with anorexia nervosa who received treatment in a specialized eating disorders treatment program. There were 22 patients treated with aripiprazole (mean dose of 3.59 mg/day) and 84 patients included in the control group who did not receive the medication. The aripiprazole group showed greater increase in BMI and BMI percentile than the control group.[13]

In adults, however, olanzapine has shown some effect on weight gain. In 2008, Bissada et al. compared olanzapine 10 mg (mean dose for completers = 6.6 mg/day) with placebo, in 34 patients with anorexia nervosa participating in a partial hospital treatment program. The olanzapine group demonstrated a higher rate of weight gain, earlier achievement of target weight, and a reduction of obsessive symptoms on the Yale Brown Obsessive Compulsive Scale (Y-BOCS) compared with the placebo group.[14] Attia et al.[15] conducted a double-blind randomized controlled trial in 23 patients with anorexia nervosa, in an outpatient setting. The increase in BMI was significantly greater in the group receiving olanzapine [$F(1,20) = 6.64$, $P = .018$] at the end of

8 weeks of treatment, with initial BMI as a covariate. There were no differences in psychologic symptoms between the groups, and no adverse metabolic effects, with sedation being the only frequent side effect.[15] Attia et al. conducted a more definitive multisite study that included 152 adults with anorexia nervosa, who were randomly assigned to olanzapine or placebo. The authors found a statistically significant treatment by time interaction, $(F_{[1,1435]} = 4.98; P = .026)$ indicating that the increase in BMI over time was greater in the olanzapine group $(0.259 \pm 0.051$ SE kg/m^2 per month vs. 0.095 ± 0.053 kg/m^2 per month) (Attia E, MD. Unpublished data, 2018). Powers et al.[16] conducted a small placebo-controlled study with quetiapine in which 15 patients with anorexia nervosa were randomized. Only 10 patients completed the study, and researchers found no difference in weight gain or core symptoms between the medication and placebo group.[16] A metaanalysis conducted by Dold et al.[17] examining seven randomized controlled trials using second-generation antipsychotics in the treatment of anorexia nervosa concluded that there was lack of evidence for the efficacy of this group of medications for increasing BMI compared with placebo. However, looking at the studies of olanzapine only, these investigators described a weight effect that did not achieve statistical significance.[17]

Other medications used in the treatment of anorexia nervosa

Premeal anxiety has been associated with reduced caloric intake in patients with anorexia nervosa, suggesting that eating-related anxiety may be a useful target for treatment. Steinglass et al.[18] conducted a randomized, double-blind, placebo-controlled, crossover study in 17 weight-restored patients with anorexia nervosa, who received alprazolam or placebo before a laboratory meal in an inpatient setting. There was no difference between the medication and the placebo group in levels of anxiety or in caloric intake.[18]

Andries et al.[19] conducted a randomized controlled trial with 24 adult anorexia nervosa patients with dronabinol, a synthetic cannabinoid agonist used in other clinical populations for the treatment of appetite suppression, nausea, and vomiting. The authors found a significant increase of weight in the group receiving dronabinol compared with placebo.[19]

Intranasal oxytocin was studied in a randomized controlled trial by Russell et al. (2017) in 41 patients with anorexia nervosa. After 4–6 weeks of treatment, the investigators found no differences in BMI between the placebo and the oxytocin group. However, measures of eating concern and cognitive rigidity were significantly lower in the oxytocin group. There were no adverse effects reported with the medication.[20]

D-Cycloserine (DCS) has been used as an adjunct to exposure therapy for the treatment of specific phobias, and because anorexia nervosa is characterized by fear of foods, Steinglass[21] hypothesized that DCS may be useful to individuals with anorexia nervosa receiving exposure therapy. Steinglass and colleagues conducted a pilot randomized controlled trial comparing DCS with placebo in 11 inpatients receiving exposure therapy and found no benefits associated with medication.[21] However, Levinson et al. studied a somewhat larger group of 36 patients in a randomized placebo-controlled trial and found an increase of weight associated with DCS compared with placebo.[22]

In summary, psychotropic medications are consistently of little or no benefit to patients with anorexia nervosa, with the possible exception of olanzapine, which appears to be associated with modest weight gain.

Medications used in the treatment of osteopenia in anorexia nervosa

Reduction in bone mineral density (BMD) in patients with anorexia nervosa can be irreversible in some cases, predisposing patients to fractures for years following presentation of illness. Misra and colleagues demonstrated promising effects associated with transdermal estrogen replacement with cyclic progesterone. They found increased bone accrual rates in 110 adolescents with anorexia nervosa compared with placebo.[23] Golden et al.[24] also conducted a double-blinded randomized trial comparing alendronate and placebo in 32 adolescents with anorexia nervosa. After 1 year of treatment, they found significantly increased BMD in the medication group compared with placebo $(P < .05).$[24] Recent data from a randomized controlled trial with teriparatide, an injected form of parathyroid hormone, showed that spine BMD increased significantly after 6 months of the treatment compared with placebo $(P < .01)$ in 21 women with anorexia nervosa.[25]

Pharmacotherapy of Bulimia Nervosa

In contrast to the lack of clear benefit for medications in anorexia nervosa treatment, several medications have demonstrated significant effects in the treatment of adults with bulimia nervosa, although the underlying mechanisms for their effectiveness remain unclear. There has only been one study conducted in adolescents with bulimia nervosa, which showed fluoxetine to be effective and well tolerated.[26]

Antidepressant medication for the treatment of bulimia nervosa

Most classes of antidepressant medications, including tricyclic antidepressants,[27] monoamine oxidase inhibitors (MAOIs),[28] and SSRIs,[29,30] have been examined for utility in bulimia nervosa using randomized placebo-controlled trials and consistently conclude that medication is superior to placebo in decreasing binge eating and purging episodes. Studies have been conducted almost exclusively in adults, but there is a small amount of evidence that these medications may be safe and effective in younger patients.[26.]

The most widely examined medication for bulimia nervosa treatment is fluoxetine. The Fluoxetine Bulimia Nervosa Collaborative Study Group[29] conducted a multicenter randomized controlled trial, which included 387 adults with bulimia nervosa who were treated with fluoxetine 60 mg/day versus matched placebo. The investigators found significant decreases in binge eating and purging episodes in the medication group compared with placebo, without group differences in side effects experienced.[29] This study along with others[30] led to the US Food and Drug Administration (FDA) approval for the use of fluoxetine 60 mg/day in adults with bulimia nervosa, the only medication commonly used for bulimia nervosa that has this formal status. Notably, the antidepressant fluoxetine is similarly effective in treating bulimia nervosa, whether or not depression is present.[31] Also, fluoxetine is effective even among individuals with bulimia nervosa who have failed psychotherapy.[32]

In an open trial using fluoxetine 60 mg/day in 10 adolescents with bulimia nervosa, Kotler and colleagues[26] demonstrated similar clinical response to that seen in adult patients, with adequate acceptability and tolerability of medication, suggesting that this medication may be used effectively and safely in younger patients.[26] The fact that fluoxetine has received FDA approval for the treatment of depression in children and adolescents 8–18 years old strengthens its choice for safe use in younger patients with eating disorder symptoms.[33] Other SSRI medications, including fluvoxamine,[34] sertraline,[35] and citalopram[36] have been examined for utility in adults with bulimia nervosa using randomized placebo-controlled studies. Study findings generally support that these other medications may also be effective strategies for treating bulimia nervosa.

Bupropion was studied in a randomized controlled trial by Horne et al.[37] in 81 adult patients with bulimia nervosa and was found to be more effective than placebo for treating binge eating and purging behaviors.

However, 4 of the 55 patients who received the medication had seizures, contributing to a current FDA "black box" warning against using this medication for individuals with eating disorders.[37]

Antiepileptics and mood stabilizers for the treatment of bulimia nervosa

No studies examining the efficacy of antiepileptics and mood stabilizers for the treatment of bulimia nervosa have been conducted in children or adolescents. However, in adults, phenytoin, carbamazepine, oxcarbazepine, and topiramate have been well studied for the treatment of bulimia nervosa, but only topiramate has been shown to be effective.[38–40] Topiramate is FDA approved for treatment of tonic-clonic seizures in children and is therefore likely safe for use in younger patients.[41] Although effective at decreasing binge eating episodes in adults with bulimia nervosa, topiramate is associated with nuisance side effects, including nonspecific cognitive symptoms and paresthesias that interfere with medication treatment adherence, making it an unlikely first-choice medication for youth. In addition, topiramate may induce weight loss and has been described in association with relapse of anorexia nervosa, both of which renders its use in eating disordered patients potentially problematic.

Among mood stabilizers, lithium versus placebo was studied by Hsu et al.[42] in 91 adult patients with bulimia nervosa and medication was found to be no better than placebo.[42]

Other medications used for the treatment of bulimia nervosa

The antinausea and antivomiting medication ondansetron was examined for potential utility in bulimia nervosa by Faris et al.,[43] who conducted a randomized controlled trial comparing 4 mg/day of active medication with placebo in 26 adults with bulimia nervosa. Investigators found that the medication was associated with decreased binge eating and purging and normalized eating behaviors compared with placebo at 4 weeks of treatment. However, this medication is not recommended for routine use for treatment of bulimia nervosa due to its side effect profile.[43]

Given the longstanding question about whether binge eating resembles addictive behavior, there have been studies of opiate antagonists to treat conditions that include binge eating such as bulimia nervosa. There are several placebo-controlled trials that have been conducted with naltrexone in bulimic patients, but they have shown conflicting results.[44–46]

Pharmacotherapy for Binge Eating Disorder

Binge eating disorder became a formally recognized diagnosis in the most recent edition of the *Diagnostic and Statistical Manual*, Fifth Edition (*DSM-5*)[47] but has been studied extensively as a research construct before it is joining the formal diagnostic list. Medications that appear to have the greatest utility for decreasing binge eating behaviors include antidepressant medications as well as medications known to suppress appetite such as stimulant medications, and others that include appetite lessening as a side effect. As with other eating disorders, medication studies for binge eating disorder have traditionally excluded children and adolescents.

Antidepressant medications for the treatment of binge eating disorder

Overall, across several randomized clinical trials, SSRI medications are modestly more helpful than placebo in decreasing frequency of binge eating episodes. Specifically, fluoxetine,[48,49] sertraline,[50,51] citalopram,[52] and escitalopram[53] have been considered modestly helpful. In contrast to bulimia nervosa, binge eating disorder treatment studies commonly report high placebo response rates, estimated in one metaanalysis as approximately 33%,[54] suggesting that several nonspecific factors likely contribute to symptom reduction in binge eating disorder treatment. Notably, the symptom reductions described in antidepressant treatments for binge eating disorder include decreased frequency of binge episodes but do not include weight reduction, frustrating some treatment-seeking patients, and sometimes contributing to their pursuing other adjunctive treatment strategies.

Other Medication treatments for binge eating disorder

Because of its appetite and weight-reducing side effects, topiramate has been studied and found to be helpful in both decreasing binge frequency and reducing weight,[55,56] although medication side effects were associated with significant study dropout rates. As mentioned in the discussion of bulimia nervosa, this medication is not considered first-line treatment for children and adolescents with loss of control eating despite FDA approval for use in children with seizure disorders.

Stimulants have been used in the treatment of binge eating disorder following a large industry-sponsored multisite placebo-controlled study that demonstrated symptom reduction associated with lisdexamfetamine (LDX), which became the first medication to receive FDA approval for treatment of binge eating disorder in adults. Medication at 50 mg/day and 70 mg/day doses ($P = .08$ and $P < .001$, respectively) was superior to placebo at reducing binge episodes after 11 weeks of treatment.[57] Notably, this medication has FDA approval for use in children and adolescents with attention-deficit/hyperactivity disorder, so its safety profile for short and intermediate use is considered good for younger patients. Clinical experience regarding this medication in binge eating disorder treatments is relatively sparse, however, and it should not be considered as a first-line treatment for adolescents with binge eating disorder. Also, because young patients with eating disorders may be prone to a range of eating behavior disturbances, stimulants should be used with caution for anyone at risk of significant food restriction, such as patients with a history of anorexia nervosa or associated disorders.

Pharmacotherapy for Avoidant-Restrictive Food Intake Disorder

Currently, there are no evidence-based treatments for ARFID; however, therapies that target comorbid anxieties have been empirically used. D-Cycloserine (DCS) as an adjunct of behavioral therapy has been recently studied, in a placebo-controlled trial, for the treatment of ARFID by Sharp and colleagues.[58] They found significant improvement in median number of bites swallowed in each meal ($P < .001$) and decrease in mealtime disruptions ($P < .005$); additionally the medication was well tolerated.[58]

Pharmacotherapy for Rumination Disorder

Pharmacologic agents for rumination disorder are of limited utility and when used, target illness complications or cooccurring disorders. Proton-pump inhibitors, gastric motility–enhancing agents, antidepressant, and anxiolytic medications have been considered for symptom relief in this population.[59]

Pharmacotherapy for Pica

Pharmacotherapy is indicated for treating comorbidities in individuals with pica, but medications are not generally used to target the core symptoms of this disorder.[60]

CONCLUSION

Medications for the treatment of eating disorders are most useful for bulimia nervosa and binge eating disorder, and most medication studies have included only adult participants. Behavioral treatments are generally considered first line for children and adolescents with any of the feeding and eating disorders described in DSM-5, because many younger patients with eating disorders respond to behavioral strategies, and because many of them have conditions such as anorexia nervosa and ARFID that are not as responsive to pharmacotherapy.

Children and adolescents who do not respond to behavioral treatments, or who present with significant comorbidities, may be appropriate for medication treatments as adjunctive strategies. Examples include olanzapine for anorexia nervosa and fluoxetine for bulimia nervosa.

REFERENCES

1. National Guideline Alliance (UK). *Eating Disorders: Recognition and Treatment.* London: National Institute for Health and Care Excellence (UK); 2017.
2. Lock J, La Via MC. American Academy of Child and Adolescent Psychiatry (AACAP) Committee on Quality Issues (CQI). Practice parameter for the assessment and treatment of children and adolescents with eating disorders. *J Am Acad Child Adolesc Psychiatry.* 2015;54(5):412–425. https://doi.org/10.1016/j.jaac.2015.01.018.
3. Holtkamp K, Konrad K, Kaiser N. A retrospective study of SSRI treatment in adolescent anorexia nervosa: insufficient evidence for efficacy. *J Psychiatr Res.* 2005;39(3): 303–310.
4. Attia E, Haiman C, Walsh BT, Flater SR. Does fluoxetine augment the inpatient treatment of anorexia nervosa? *Am J Psychiatry.* 1998;155(4):548–551.
5. Fassino S, Leombruni P, Daga G. Efficacy of citalopram in anorexia nervosa: a pilot study. *Eur Neuropsychopharmacol.* 2002;12(5):453–459.
6. Walsh BT, Kaplan AS, Attia E. Fluoxetine after weight restoration in anorexia nervosa: a randomized controlled trial. *J Am Med Assoc.* 2006;295(22):2605–2612. [Erratum in: JAMA. 2006;296(8):934. JAMA. 2007;298(17):2008].
7. Lock J, Le Grange D, Agras WS, Moye A, Bryson SW, Jo B. Randomized clinical trial comparing family-based treatment with adolescent-focused individual therapy for adolescents with anorexia nervosa. *Arch Gen Psychiatry.* 2010;67(10):1025–1032. https://doi.org/10.1001/archgenpsychiatry.2010.128.
8. Halmi KA, Eckert E, LaDu TJ, Cohen J. Anorexia nervosa. Treatment efficacy of cyproheptadine and amitriptyline. *Arch Gen Psychiatry.* 1986;43(2):177–181.
9. Kafantaris V, Leigh E, Hertz S. A placebo-controlled pilot study of adjunctive olanzapine for adolescents with anorexia nervosa. *J Child Adolesc Psychopharmacol.* 2011;21(3):207–212. https://doi.org/10.1089/cap.2010.0139.
10. Hagman J, Gralla J, Sigel E. A double-blind, placebo-controlled study of risperidone for the treatment of adolescents and young adults with anorexia nervosa: a pilot study. *J Am Acad Child Adolesc Psychiatry.* 2011;50(9):915–924. https://doi.org/10.1016/j.jaac.2011.06.009. [Epub 2011 Aug 5].
11. Court A, Mulder C, Kerr M. Investigating the effectiveness, safety and tolerability of quetiapine in the treatment of anorexia nervosa in young people: a pilot study. *J Psychiatr Res.* 2010;44(15):1027–1034. https://doi.org/10.1016/j.jpsychires.2010.03.011. [Epub 2010 May 5].
12. Norris ML, Spettigue W, Buchholz A. Olanzapine use for the adjunctive treatment of adolescents with anorexia nervosa. *J Child Adolesc Psychopharmacol.* 2011;21(3):213–220. https://doi.org/10.1089/cap.2010.0131. [Epub 2011 Apr 21].
13. Frank GK, Shott ME, Hagman JO, Schiel MA, DeGuzman MC, Rossi B. The partial dopamine D2 receptor agonist aripiprazole is associated with weight gain in adolescent anorexia nervosa. *Int J Eat Disord.* 2017;50(4):447–450. https://doi.org/10.1002/eat.22704. [Epub 2017 Mar 23].
14. Bissada H, Tasca GA, Barber AM, Bradwejn J. Olanzapine in the treatment of low body weight and obsessive thinking in women with anorexia nervosa: a randomized, double-blind, placebo-controlled trial. *Am J Psychiatry.* 2008;165(10):1281–1288. https://doi.org/10.1176/appi.ajp.2008.07121900. [Epub 2008 Jun 16].
15. Attia E, Kaplan AS, Walsh BT. Olanzapine versus placebo for out-patients with anorexia nervosa. *Psychol Med.* 2011;41(10):2177–2182. https://doi.org/10.1017/S0033291711000390. [Epub 2011 Mar 22].
16. Powers PS, Klabunde M, Kaye W. Double-blind placebo-controlled trial of quetiapine in anorexia nervosa. *Eur Eat Disord Rev.* 2012;20(4):331–334. https://doi.org/10.1002/erv.2169. [Epub 2012 Apr 26].
17. Dold M, Aigner M, Klabunde M, Treasure J, Kasper S. Second-generation antipsychotic drugs in anorexia nervosa: a meta-analysis of randomized controlled trials. *Psychother Psychosom.* 2015;84(2):110–116.
18. Steinglass JE, Kaplan SC, Liu Y, Wang Y, Walsh BT. The (lack of) effect of alprazolam on eating behavior in anorexia nervosa: a preliminary report. *Int J Eat Disord.* 2014;47(8):901–904. https://doi.org/10.1002/eat.22343. [Epub 2014 Aug 19].
19. Andries A, Frystyk J, Flyvbjerg A, Støving RK. Dronabinol in severe, enduring anorexia nervosa: a randomized controlled trial. *Int J Eat Disord.* 2014;47(1):18–23. https://doi.org/10.1002/eat.22173. [Epub 2013 Sep 14].
20. Russell J, Maguire S, Hunt GE. Intranasal oxytocin in the treatment of anorexia nervosa: randomized controlled trial during re-feeding. *Psychoneuroendocrinology.* 2018;87:83–92. https://doi.org/10.1016/j.psyneuen.2017.10.014. [Epub 2017 Oct 14].
21. Steinglass J, Sysko R, Schebendach J, Broft A, Strober M, Walsh BT. The application of exposure therapy and D-cycloserine to the treatment of anorexia nervosa: a preliminary trial. *J Psychiatr Pract.* 2007;13(4):238–245.
22. Levinson CA, Rodebaugh TL, Fewell L. D-Cycloserine facilitation of exposure therapy improves weight regain in patients with anorexia nervosa: a pilot randomized controlled trial. *J Clin Psychiatry.* 2015;76(6):e787–e793. https://doi.org/10.4088/JCP.14m09299.

23. Misra M, Katzman D, Miller KK. Physiologic estrogen replacement increases bone density in adolescent girls with anorexia nervosa. *J Bone Miner Res.* 2011;26(10):2430–2438. https://doi.org/10.1002/jbmr.447.

24. Golden NH, Iglesias EA, Jacobson MS. Alendronate for the treatment of osteopenia in anorexia nervosa: a randomized, double-blind, placebo-controlled trial. *J Clin Endocrinol Metab.* 2005;90(6):3179–3185. [Epub 2005 Mar 22].

25. Fazeli PK, Wang IS, Miller KK. Teriparatide increases bone formation and bone mineral density in adult women with anorexia nervosa. *J Clin Endocrinol Metab.* 2014;99(4):1322–1329. https://doi.org/10.1210/jc.2013-4105. [Epub 2014 Jan 23].

26. Kotler LA, Devlin MJ, Davies M, Walsh BT. An open trial of fluoxetine for adolescents with bulimia nervosa. *J Child Adolesc Psychopharmacol.* 2003;13(3):329–335.

27. Hughes PL, Wells LA, Cunningham CJ, Ilstrup DM. Treating bulimia with desipramine. A double-blind, placebo-controlled study. *Arch Gen Psychiatry.* 1986;43(2):182–186.

28. Walsh BT, Gladis M, Roose SP, Stewart JW, Stetner F, Glassman AH. Phenelzine vs placebo in 50 patients with bulimia. *Arch Gen Psychiatry.* 1988;45(5):471–475.

29. Fluoxetine Bulimia Nervosa Collaborative Study Group. Fluoxetine in the treatment of bulimia nervosa. A multicenter, placebo-controlled, double-blind trial. *Arch Gen Psychiatry.* 1992;49(2):139–147.

30. Goldstein DJ, Wilson MG, Thompson VL, Potvin JH, Rampey Jr AH. Long-term fluoxetine treatment of bulimia nervosa. Fluoxetine bulimia nervosa research group. *Br J Psychiatry.* 1995;166(5):660–666.

31. Goldstein DJ, Wilson MG, Ascroft RC, al-Banna M. Effectiveness of fluoxetine therapy in bulimia nervosa regardless of comorbid depression. *Int J Eat Disord.* 1999;25(1):19–27.

32. Walsh BT, Agras WS, Devlin MJ. Fluoxetine for bulimia nervosa following poor response to psychotherapy. *Am J Psychiatry.* 2000;157(8):1332–1334.

33. Bridge JA, Iyengar S, Salary CB. Clinical response and risk for reported suicidal ideation and suicide attempts in pediatric antidepressant treatment: a meta-analysis of randomized controlled trials. *J Am Med Assoc.* 2007;297(15):1683–1696.

34. Fichter MM, Krüger R, Rief W, Holland R, Döhne J. Fluvoxamine in prevention of relapse in bulimia nervosa: effects on eating-specific psychopathology. *J Clin Psychopharmacol.* 1996;16(1):9–18.

35. Milano W, Petrella C, Sabatino C, Capasso A. Treatment of bulimia nervosa with sertraline: a randomized controlled trial. *Adv Ther.* 2004;21(4):232–237.

36. Leombruni P, Amianto F, Delsedime N. Citalopram versus fluoxetine for the treatment of patients with bulimia nervosa: a single-blind randomized controlled trial. *Adv Ther.* 2006;23(3):481–494.

37. Horne RL, Ferguson JM, Pope Jr HG. Treatment of bulimia with bupropion: a multicenter controlled trial. *J Clin Psychiatry.* 1988;49(7):262–266.

38. Hoopes SP, Reimherr FW, Hedges DW. Treatment of bulimia nervosa with topiramate in a randomized, double-blind, placebo-controlled trial, part 1: improvement in binge and purge measures. *J Clin Psychiatry.* 2003;64(11):1335.

39. Hedges DW, Reimherr FW, Hoopes SP. Treatment of bulimia nervosa with topiramate in a randomized, double-blind, placebo-controlled trial, part 2: improvement in psychiatric measures. *J Clin Psychiatry.* 2003;64(12):1449–1454.

40. Nickel C, Tritt K, Muehlbacher M. Topiramate treatment in bulimia nervosa patients: a randomized, double-blind, placebo-controlled trial. *Int J Eat Disord.* 2005;38(4):295–300.

41. Faught E. Topiramate in the treatment of partial and generalized epilepsy. *Neuropsychiatr Dis Treat.* 2007;3(6):811–821.

42. Hsu LK, Clement L, Santhouse R, Ju ES. Treatment of bulimia nervosa with lithium carbonate. A controlled study. *J Nerv Ment Dis.* 1991;179(6):351–355.

43. Faris PL, Kim SW, Meller WH. Effect of decreasing afferent vagal activity with ondansetron on symptoms of bulimia nervosa: a randomised, double-blind trial. *Lancet.* 2000;355(9206):792–797.

44. Marrazzi MA, Bacon JP, Kinzie J, Luby ED. Naltrexone use in the treatment of anorexia nervosa and bulimia nervosa. *Int Clin Psychopharmacol.* 1995;10(3):163–172.

45. Alger SA, Schwalberg MD, Bigaouette JM, Michalek AV, Howard LJ. Effect of a tricyclic antidepressant and opiate antagonist on binge-eating behavior in normoweight bulimic and obese, binge-eating subjects. *Am J Clin Nutr.* 1991;53(4):865–871.

46. Mitchell JE, Christenson G, Jennings J. A placebo-controlled, double-blind crossover study of naltrexone hydrochloride in outpatients with normal weight bulimia. *J Clin Psychopharmacol.* 1989;9(2):94–97.

47. American Psychiatric Association. *American Psychiatric Association. DSM-5 Task Force. Diagnostic and Statistical Manual of Mental Disorders: DSM-5.* American Psychiatric Association; 2013.

48. Marcus MD, Wing RR, Ewing L, Kern E, McDermott M, Gooding W. A double-blind, placebo-controlled trial of fluoxetine plus behavior modification in the treatment of obese binge-eaters and non-binge-eaters. *Am J Psychiatry.* 1990;147(7):876–881.

49. Arnold LM, McElroy SL, Hudson JI, Welge JA, Bennett AJ, Keck PE. A placebo-controlled, randomized trial of fluoxetine in the treatment of binge-eating disorder. *J Clin Psychiatry.* 2002;63(11):1028–1033.

50. McElroy SL, Casuto LS, Nelson EB. Placebo-controlled trial of sertraline in the treatment of binge eating disorder. *Am J Psychiatry.* 2000;157(6):1004–1006.

51. O'Reardon JP, Allison KC, Martino NS, Lundgren JD, Heo M, Stunkard AJ. A randomized, placebo-controlled trial of sertraline in the treatment of night eating syndrome. *Am J Psychiatry.* 2006;163(5):893–898.

52. McElroy SL, Hudson JI, Malhotra S, Welge JA, Nelson EB, Keck Jr PE. Citalopram in the treatment of binge-eating disorder: a placebo-controlled trial. *J Clin Psychiatry*. 2003;64(7):807–813.

53. Guerdjikova AI, McElroy SL, Kotwal R. High-dose escitalopram in the treatment of binge-eating disorder with obesity: a placebo-controlled monotherapy trial. *Hum Psychopharmacol*. 2008;23(1):1–11.

54. Carter WP, Hudson JI, Lalonde JK, Pindyck L, McElroy SL, Pope Jr HG. Pharmacologic treatment of binge eating disorder. *Int J Eat Disord*. 2003;34:S74–S88.

55. McElroy SL, Arnold LM, Shapira NA. *Topiramate in the Treatment of Binge Eating Disorder Associated with Obesity: A Randomized, Placebo-controlled Trial.*

56. McElroy SL, Arnold LM, Shapira NA. Topiramate in the treatment of binge eating disorder associated with obesity: a randomized, placebo-controlled trial. *Am J Psychiatry*. 2003;160(2):255–261. [Erratum in: Am J Psychiatry. 2003;160(3):612].

57. McElroy SL, Hudson J, Ferreira-Cornwell MC, Radewonuk J, Whitaker T, Gasior M. Lisdexamfetamine dimesylate for adults with moderate to severe binge eating disorder: results of two pivotal phase 3 randomized controlled trials. *Neuropsychopharmacology*. 2016;41(5):1251–1260. https://doi.org/10.1038/npp.2015.275. [Epub 2015 Sep. 9].

58. Sharp WG, Allen AG, Stubbs KH. Successful pharmacotherapy for the treatment of severe feeding aversion with mechanistic insights from cross-species neuronal remodeling. *Transl Psychiatry*. 2017;7(6):e1157. https://doi.org/10.1038/tp.2017.126.

59. Freidl E, Attia E. Treatment of other eating problems, including Pica and rumination. In: *Handbook of Assessment and Treatment of Eating Disorders*. 1st ed. Arlington, VA: American Psychiatric Association Publishing; 2006:297–310.

60. Matson JL, Hattier MA, Belva B, Matson ML. Pica in persons with developmental disabilities: approaches to treatment. *Res Dev Disabil*. 2013;34(9):2564–2571. https://doi.org/10.1016/j.ridd.2013.05.018. [Epub 2013 Jun 7].

CHAPTER 23

Conventional Weight Loss Programs

YVONNE MÜHLIG, PHD • MIRIAM REMY, MSC PSYCH •
MARTIN WABITSCH, MD, PHD • JOHANNES HEBEBRAND, MD

OVERWEIGHT AND OBESITY IN CHILDHOOD AND ADOLESCENCE

Over the past decades, overweight and obesity have reached "pandemic proportions" in low-, middle-, and high-income countries all over the world.[1] Worldwide, overweight or obesity affected 41 million children below the age of 5 years and over 340 million children and adolescents aged 5–19 years in 2016.[2] Prevalence rates for overweight or obesity in children and adolescents aged 5–19 years were 18% or 6% in girls and 19% or 8% in boys, respectively.[2] According to internationally accepted standards, overweight or obesity in children and adolescents aged 5–19 years is defined by a body mass index (BMI) for age greater than one or two standard deviations above the WHO Growth Reference median, respectively.[3]

The etiologic basis of childhood and adolescent obesity is regarded as a complex interaction of multiple factors including a polygenic predisposition and an obesogenic environment.[4] Especially the growing availability of energy-dense food and an increasingly sedentary lifestyle are held to account for the global rise of overweight and obesity prevalence.[5] Obesity in childhood and adolescence is associated with a wide range of somatic comorbidities (e.g., sleep apnea, hypertension, early markers of cardiovascular disease, insulin resistance, and type 2 diabetes mellitus) as well as premature death and disability in adulthood.[2] Psychologic problems due to a reduced quality of life, low self-esteem, and stigmatization are also very common.[6] Given the high number of serious long-term consequences of obesity in childhood and adolescence, there is a great demand for effective treatment programs to reduce the extent of overweight and obesity as well as their associated complications.

CONVENTIONAL WEIGHT LOSS PROGRAMS: STATE OF THE ART

In 2016, the World Health Organization published their "Report of the Commission on Ending Childhood Obesity."[7] According to this report, the main treatment aims for children and adolescents must be the reduction in the level of overweight and the improvement in obesity-related comorbidities and in risk factors for excess weight gain. To reach these aims, "family-based multi-component lifestyle weight management" is regarded as the gold standard of treatment.[7] Such treatment programs comprise the elements "nutrition counseling," "physical activity," and "behavior therapy," which are commonly offered by a multiprofessional team and presented in group sessions.[8] The core treatment rational is the promotion of a healthy lifestyle and weight loss resulting from the development of healthy dietary patterns and increased physical activity. Attendance requirements and duration of the available treatment programs vary largely, and the involvement of parents mainly depends on the age of children and adolescents.[9]

Usually, this type of treatment is also called "conventional weight loss treatment" in distinction to pharmacologic or surgical treatments of severe obesity for patients not sufficiently responding to conventional weight loss treatment.[7] Treatment success is most often evaluated in terms of anthropometric measures (e.g., change in weight, BMI, BMI z score, or body composition) and sometimes also in terms of somatic (e.g., blood pressure, insulin sensitivity, lipid profiles) or psychologic (e.g., health-related quality of life, self-esteem) parameters.[9] Considering the natural height and weight gain in the process of growth, the BMI z score (standard deviation score of the BMI) appears as the most exact measure for weight loss in childhood and adolescence[2]; BMI percentiles do not allow an adequate differentiation of subjects with a very high body weight.

CONVENTIONAL WEIGHT LOSS PROGRAMS: EVIDENCE

The WHO recommendation of conventional weight loss programs as the preferred treatment strategy for obesity in childhood and adolescence[7] is based on several systematic reviews and metaanalyses.[10,11] One main conclusion drawn from those metaanalyses was that 6 months after the initiation of treatment, the effect size of conventional weight loss programs was small (–0.06 or –0.14 BMI z score units in children younger than 12 years or adolescents aged 12 years and older, respectively), but statistically significant and clinically relevant.[11] At 12 months after the initiation of treatment, the effect only remained statistically significant in adolescents aged 12 years or older. Dropout rates and the loss-to-follow-up rates were estimated at up to 42% and 43%, respectively.

These findings are in line with our own systematic review and update of the literature based on randomized controlled trials of conventional weight loss programs published in the period from 2008 to 2013.[9] In distinction to the aforementioned metaanalysis in which different conventional weight loss interventions were compared against each other, we focused on the overall amount of weight loss that can be expected from conventional weight loss programs in childhood and adolescence. We included 48 randomized controlled trials with a total of 5025 participants in our systematic review. The included studies had to consist of at least one element of dietary, physical activity-based or behavioral intervention with a follow-up period of at least 6 months after the initiation of treatment and the inclusion of BMI z score and/or BMI as primary outcome measures. Participants had to be younger than 18 years at the time of study enrollment. Based on the eight trials with the highest methodological quality, our systematic review revealed BMI z score reductions in the range from 0.05 to 0.42 units over the period of 12–24 months after the initiation of treatment. We found dropout rates of up to 50% and a loss-to-follow-up rate of up to 71% in the included trials.

Most recently, a further update of the evidence was performed in a metaanalysis of trials assessing behavioral weight loss interventions in children aged 6–11 years.[12] The authors included 70 randomized controlled trials into their systematic review comparing different treatments based on physical activity, diet, and/or behavioral interventions in a total of 8461 children with overweight or obesity. Most of the trials (N = 55) compared a behavioral weight loss intervention group with a "no treatment" or "usual care" control group, and some trials (N = 15) assessed the effectiveness of adding a specific treatment element to a behavioral weight loss intervention. The average age of the children was 10 years, and the median BMI z score was 2.2 units. The total duration of the trials from treatment initiation to the final follow-up ranged from 6 months

to 3 years. Metaanalyses were calculated, each including all final (longest) follow-up data of the trials.

Of the 70 trials, 37 studies in 4019 children reporting BMI z score as a primary outcome measure were included in a metaanalysis,[12] resulting in a mean BMI z score reduction of 0.06 units in the treatment (–0.02 to –0.10 units) compared with the nontreatment control groups at the final follow-up. The authors also summarized the results of 24 trials reporting BMI as a main outcome measure involving 2785 children. BMI was 0.53 kg/m² lower in the treatment (–0.24 to –0.84 kg/m²) compared with the nontreatment control (+2.8 to –0.3 kg/m²) groups at the final follow-up. Seventeen trials reported weight loss in kilogram as a main outcome measure in 1774 children. In the intervention groups (–1.02 to –1.88 kg), weight was 1.45 kg lower than in the control groups (+17.1 to +1.95 kg) at the final follow-up. Data on serious adverse events were reported in 31 trials and occurred in only two of them (4/2105 participants in the intervention vs. 7/1991 participants in the control groups). The authors also discuss that other potentially beneficial effects beyond measures of weight loss (e.g., reduction of comorbidities or improvement of health-related quality of life) could not be assessed in the metaanalysis due to the high heterogeneity and low methodological quality of the trials. Overall, the quality of evidence was judged as low or very low. Finally, the authors concluded that in children aged 6–11 years, multicomponent behavior-changing interventions "may be beneficial in achieving small, short-term reductions in BMI, BMI z score, and weight."[12]

Parallel to this systematic review,[12] a metaanalysis was conducted for preschool children up to the age of 6 years.[13] Similarly, in this review, the effects of behavioral weight loss programs based on physical activity, dietary, and/or behavioral interventions were assessed in seven randomized controlled trials with a total of 923 preschool children with overweight or obesity. The included trials were based on multicomponent or dietary interventions. The total duration of the trials from treatment initiation to the final follow-up ranged from 6 months to 3 years (data at 12–18 months of follow-up were included in the metaanalysis). A metaanalysis including four trials with a total of 202 preschool children was calculated, revealing a lower BMI z score (–0.4 units) and weight (–2.8 kg) in the intervention (multicomponent weight loss programs: –0.2 to –0.6 units and –1.2 to –4.4 kg) compared with the control (usual care/information control/wait-list control: +0.4 to –0.3 units and +5.2 to +3.1 kg) groups 12–18 months after the initiation of treatment. Adverse events were not reported except in one trial stating that no serious adverse events had occurred. No metaanalyses could be performed for any other outcome measures due to the high methodological heterogeneity of the included trials. The authors concluded that "multicomponent interventions appear to be an effective treatment option for overweight and obese preschool children," whereas the overall quality of evidence was judged low or very low.[13]

CONVENTIONAL WEIGHT LOSS PROGRAMS: PROBLEMS AND LIMITATIONS

To draw clinical implications from the cited evidence, the meaning of the results must be put into an individual perspective. Hypothesizing a middle weight loss of −0.3 BMI z score units 12 months after the initiation of a conventional weight loss program, a 15-year-old female with extreme obesity (1.70 m [77th length for age percentile] and 102 kg [>99.5th BMI for age percentile]) would have lost 4.8 kg (1.71 m [77th length for age percentile] and 97.2 kg [>99.5th BMI-for-age-percentile]) 1 year after treatment initiation, assuming a steady height development. In the same example, the respective weight change for an obese 8-year-old male (130 cm [50th length for age percentile] and 40 kg [99th BMI for age percentile]) would be +3.5 kg (136.4 cm [50th length for age percentile] and 43.5 kg [98th BMI for age percentile]) 1 year later, also assuming a steady height development. Based on these values, the adolescent female with extreme obesity would still remain extremely obese 1 year after participating in a conventional weight loss treatment and the prepubertal male with obesity would only experience a small improvement in the degree of obesity.

Apart from the limited effectiveness of conventional weight loss programs on weight status, there are several methodological problems diminishing the quality of evidence of the available systematic reviews and meta-analyses. The most important methodological problems of the cited systematic reviews and metaanalyses include a high heterogeneity with regard to the age of the participants, their initial weight, treatment settings, number and types of comparators, duration of the intervention and follow-up period, socioeconomic factors, and varying outcome measures, thus hampering the generalizability of the results.[9,12] Importantly, the high attrition rates (dropout and loss-to-follow-up) represent a strong potential bias in evaluating the overall effects of conventional weight loss programs on body weight.[9,12] Apart from this methodological problem, the question why so many children and

adolescents discontinue treatment arises. Potentially, patients realize that despite their intensive efforts, they do not substantially lose weight and consequently give up before the end of the treatment program. In this case, it seems possible that patients might experience this as a personal failure with potential harmful consequences for their psychologic well-being.[9] Perhaps the beneficial effects of conventional weight loss programs pertain to an improvement of comorbidities or health-related quality of life rather than a change in weight status. Although a significant improvement of somatic markers associated with comorbidities of obesity[14] or in health-related quality of life[15] was revealed in single trials, these parameters were too rarely assessed to be included into the cited metaanalyses.[11–13]

CLINICAL IMPLICATIONS: SUGGESTION FOR A MULTILEVELED TREATMENT APPROACH

Derived from the consistent evidence of a limited effectiveness of conventional weight loss programs on weight status, the focus of clinical care should be shifted to a multileveled treatment approach with different pathways according to the individual needs of children, adolescents, and their families. There are mainly three therapeutic approaches in the treatment of obesity in childhood and adolescence depending on age, treatment history, comorbidities, and the individual needs of children and adolescents. Our suggestion for a multilevel treatment approach is depicted in Fig. 23.1. Conventional weight loss programs still remain the treatment of first choice for children and adolescents, especially for those younger than 16 years with moderate obesity and no or little experience in conventional weight loss treatments (pathway 1; see Fig. 23.1). Based on the evidence, treatment-seeking families should be informed about the limited effectiveness of conventional weight loss programs on weight status and that children and adolescents with obesity cannot be expected to normalize their body weight within such a treatment program.[9] Instead of weight status, clinicians and therapists should focus on promoting a healthy lifestyle and emphasizing beneficial consequences of physical activity and a healthy diet apart from weight loss (e.g., physical well-being, feelings of strength and fitness). More research is required to assess such potential effects in a systematic manner.

In cases of extreme obesity and/or a history of unsuccessful conventional treatment, the individual needs as well as potential physical and/or psychiatric comorbidities should be evaluated thoroughly. If the adolescents

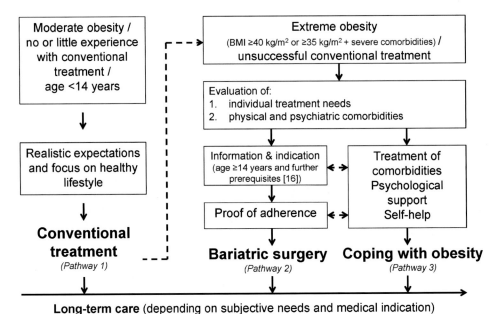

FIG. 23.1 Multilevel treatment approach for obesity in childhood and adolescence.

express interest in surgical treatment of obesity, the individual indication should be assessed and the adolescents and their caregivers should be informed in detail about bariatric surgery, its prerequisites, and risks[16] (pathway 2; see Fig. 23.1). Access to bariatric surgery should be based on the adherence of adolescents. To prevent postsurgical complications, only those adolescents should be classified as eligible for bariatric surgery, who are able to attend medical assessments and treatment sessions regularly.[17] Before bariatric surgery, adolescents and their caregivers should be offered to participate in a structured interdisciplinary information and preparation course on bariatric surgery, and they should be enrolled in a structured multiprofessional program for postsurgical care.[18]

For those adolescents with no interest in bariatric surgery or those who do not (yet) fulfill the prerequisites for bariatric surgery, "coping with obesity" should become the treatment focus (pathway 3; see Fig. 23.1). Adolescents should be offered a nonstigmatizing treatment of their comorbidities, as well as psychologic support to deal with the impairments in daily life and potential psychologic problems (e.g., bullying, low self-esteem) and have access to self-help groups. If adolescents experience acceptance of their obesity and a nonstigmatizing communication from health professionals, they are more likely to stay adherent and make regular use of healthcare services. This in turn is deemed important to treat comorbidities in the long term and to prevent possible deteriorations of health associated with a withdrawal from medical care.

ACKNOWLEDGMENTS

This work was supported by the German Federal Ministry of Education and Research (BMBF; project no. 01GI1120A/B, 01GI1401) and was integrated within the German Competence Network Obesity (Consortium "Youth with Extreme Obesity").

REFERENCES

1. World Obesity Federation. About Obesity. Version 2012, Online resource. http://www.worldobesity.org/aboutobesity/.
2. World Health Organization. *Obesity and Overweight. Fact sheet;* October 2017. Online resource http://www.who.int/mediacentre/factsheets/fs311/en/.
3. World Health Organization. Growth Reference 5-19 Years. BMI-for-Age (5-19 Years), Version 2007. Online resource. http://www.who.int/growthref/who2007_bmi_for_age/en/.
4. Hebebrand J, Hinney A. Environmental and genetic risk factors in obesity. *Child Adolesc Psychiatr Clin N Am.* 2009;18:83–94.
5. Black JR, Macinko J. Neighborhoods and obesity. *Nutr Rev.* 2008;66:2–20.

6. Hebebrand J, Herpertz-Dahlmann B. Psychological and psychiatric aspects of pediatric obesity. *Child Adolesc Psychiatr Clin N Am.* 2009;18:49–65.

7. World Health Organization. *Final report of the Commission on Ending Childhood Obesity;* 2016. Online resource http://apps.who.int/iris/bitstream/10665/204176/1/9789241510066_eng.pdf?ua=.

8. Barlow SE, Dietz WH. Obesity evaluation and treatment: expert committee recommendations. *Pediatrics.* 1998;102:e29.

9. Mühlig Y, Moss A, Wabitsch M, Hebebrand J. Weight loss in children and adolescents – a systematic review and evaluation of conservative, non-pharmacological obesity treatment programs. *Dtsch Arztebl Int.* 2014;111(48):818–824.

10. Summerbell CD, Waters E, Edmunds LD, Kelly SAM, Brown TJ, Campbell KJ. Interventions for preventing obesity in children. *Cochrane Database Syst Rev.* 2005;3:1–70.

11. Oude Luttikhuis H, Baur L, Jansen H, et al. Interventions for treating obesity in children. *Cochrane Database Syst Rev.* 2009:CD001872. https://doi.org/10.1002/14651858.CD001872.pub2.

12. Mead E, Brown T, Rees K, et al. Diet, physical activity and behavioural interventions for the treatment of overweight or obese children from the age of 6 to 11 years (Review). *Cochrane Database Syst Rev.* 2017;(6):CD012651. https://doi.org/10.1002/14651858.CD012651.

13. Colquitt JL, Loveman E, O'Malley C, et al. Diet, physical activity and behavioural interventions for the treatment of overweight or obesity in preschool children up to the age of 6 years (Review). *Cochrane Database Syst Rev.* 2016;(3):CD012105. https://doi.org/10.1002/14651858.CD012105.

14. Ho M, Garnett SP, Baur LA, et al. Impact of dietary and exercise interventions on weight change and metabolic outcomes in obese children and adolescents: a systematic review and meta-analysis of randomized trials. *JAMA Pediatr.* 2013;167:759–768.

15. Walpole B, Dettmer E, Morrongiello BA, McCrindle BW, Hamilton J. Motivational interviewing to enhance self-efficacy and promote weight loss in overweight and obese adolescents: a randomized controlled trial. *J Pediatr Psychol.* 2013;38:944–953.

16. Wabitsch M, Lennerz B. Safety of bariatric surgery in adolescents. In: Preedy VR, Rajendram R, Martin CR, eds. *Metabolism and Pathophysiology of Bariatric Surgery. Nutrition, Procedures, Outcomes, and Adverse Effects.* Academic Press, Elsevier; 2017.

17. Mühlig Y, Scherag A, Bickenbach A, et al. A structured, manual-based low-level intervention vs. treatment as usual evaluated in a randomized controlled trial for adolescents with extreme obesity – the STEREO trial. *Obes Facts.* 2017;10:341–352.

18. Lennerz B, Wabitsch M, Geisler A, et al. Manual-based approach for pre- and post-operative treatment following bariatric surgery in adolescents. *Adipositas.* 2014;8:5–11.

CHAPTER 24

Metabolic and Bariatric Surgery as a Treatment for Adolescent Severe Obesity

JUSTIN R. RYDER, PHD

INTRODUCTION

Pediatric severe obesity [body mass index (BMI) ≥ 1.2 × 95th percentile or >35 kg/m²] affects 9% of adolescents in the United States and is frequently accompanied by prediabetes, type 2 diabetes (T2D), hypertension, nonalcoholic fatty liver disease (NAFLD), and/or dyslipidemia.[1-6] Current treatment options for severe obesity are lifestyle modification, pharmacotherapy, and metabolic and bariatric surgery (MBS). Typically, MBS is reserved for those with significant obesity-associated comorbidities and failed attempts at other modes of treatment before consideration. Current guidelines suggest MBS can be considered for adolescents with a BMI ≥35 kg/m² with serious comorbidities such as type 2 diabetes, nonalcoholic hepatic steatohepatitis (NASH), pseudotumor cerebri, hypertension, gastroesophageal reflux disease, and/or chronic obstructive sleep apnea, or for adolescents with BMI ≥40 kg/m² with less severe comorbidities.[7-9] Early guidelines recommend that adolescent candidates should be close to postpuberty in development (Tanner stage 4 or 5) or have completed at least 95% of expected linear growth to be eligible for surgery; however, the most recent guidelines from 2018 have removed this recommendation because of lack of data to support it.[9] Ages in large prospective studies typically range from 13 to under 20 years. Contraindications for surgery include ongoing substance abuse in the past year, a medical, psychiatric, psychosocial, or cognitive condition that prevents adherence to postoperative dietary and medication regimens, or planned pregnancy within 12–18 months of the procedure. In addition to the clinical inclusion and exclusion criteria, from a psychosocial perspective, candidates should have a strong understanding of the lifestyle changes required after surgery, demonstrate mature decision-making ability, and have evidence of strong social support. An extensive psychologic evaluation should be undertaken before MBS. From a decisional capacity standpoint, both the adolescent and the caregivers should provide assent. However, if the eligible adolescent is unable to do so (due to, for example, a medical and/or genetic condition), only the parents can consent; in such cases, the patient must be able to demonstrate the ability to make lifestyle changes required by MBS with or without the assistance of a dedicated caregiver. Both parents and the multidisciplinary team of providers with consultation of the ethics committee, where appropriate, should agree that MBS is the best course of action for the adolescent. It should be noted that these guidelines are consistently being refined and challenged as the body of evidence surrounding adolescent MBS expands.

Major Findings

Among adolescents, who are eligible for surgery, significant clinical comorbidities and subclinical risk factors often exist. In the Teen-Longitudinal Assessment of Bariatric Surgery (Teen-LABS), cohort comorbidity rates before surgery were highly prevalent: 74% presented with dyslipidemia, 57% with sleep apnea, 46% with back and joint pain, 45% with hypertension, 37% with NAFLD, 18% with microalbuminuria, and 13% met stage 1 of chronic kidney disease.[10] A similar distribution of comorbidities and risk factors has been observed in other bariatric surgery cohorts of adolescents and underscores the serious nature of the disease. Importantly, although other treatment options aimed at weight loss and risk factor reduction in adolescents with severe obesity come with a lower risk than something as invasive as surgery, the outcomes are notoriously poor and not durable in the long term.[3,11,12]

From a weight loss and risk factor modification perspective, MBS is irrefutably the most effective treatment for adolescent severe obesity. The two primary

Eating Disorders and Obesity in Children and Adolescents. https://doi.org/10.1016/B978-0-323-54852-6.00024-0

procedures that have been evaluated are Roux-en-Y gastric bypass (RYGB) and the vertical sleeve gastrectomy (VSG). The adjustable gastric band has fallen out of favor and is seldomly used because of its inferior weight loss efficacy compared with RYGB and VSG and concerns regarding band slippage and other side effects. RYGB has been studied extensively in adults and involves the rearrangement of the alimentary canal and a portion of the proximal jejunum. This allows food, once digested, to bypass the majority of the stomach and the duodenum. This results in a restrictive and malabsorptive mechanism, which is indicated as the primary mechanism for weight loss. VSG has recently overtaken RYGB as the preferred surgery for severe obesity because of its lower risk profile with similar weight loss results. VSG involves separation of the greater curvature from the omentum and splenic attachment, which results in a significant portion (65%–75%) of the stomach being excised. This results in a restrictive procedure but does not appear to be as malabsorptive as RYGB. Both procedures have been evaluated in adolescents but probably because of the lack of statistical power, no difference in weight loss or risk factor modification has been observed between MBS types. Future studies with greater power may be able to better describe differences.

In prospective studies among adolescents with severe obesity, medium-term weight loss (1–3 years) ranges from 30% to 40% BMI reduction and long-term weight loss (5–8 years) shows sustainability of BMI reduction at around 30%.[13–16] The largest study in the United States [Teen-Longitudinal Assessment of Bariatric Surgery (Teen-LABS)][13] and the largest study in Europe [Adolescent Morbid Obesity Surgery (AMOS) study; Sweden][15] intend to continue to study adolescents for 10 years to understand both the long-term risks and benefits of undertaking MBS during this critical development period. When compared with nonsurgical interventions followed over the same period of time, the results of bariatric surgery are unequivocally superior by every metric, except for the greater risk of surgery.[14,15,17] Therefore, although surgery is superior to lifestyle modification and pharmacotherapy, these lower risk options should be attempted before considering this higher risk procedure. To date, all studies have been prospective, observational studies as enrollment into an MBS randomized controlled trial raises ethical concerns and is challenging to justify in a pediatric population. Once pharmacotherapy or other means establish similar weight loss efficacy to surgery, randomized controlled trials might be considered.

Perhaps the most pronounced medical effect of MBS in adolescents is its ability to consistently alter and offer durable change to a number of comorbid conditions and risk factors for chronic disease. Studies have noted an 85%–95% remission in T2D, 64%–73% resolution of dyslipidemia, and 75% remission in hypertension.[13–15,18] The number of cardiovascular disease risk factors is greatly reduced following surgery, with weight loss and female sex being primary drivers.[19] Additionally, bariatric surgery improves functional mobility and reduces musculoskeletal pain,[20] favorably alters levels of adipokines and cytokines,[21] improves insulin sensitivity and β-cell function,[22] improves kidney function and albuminuria,[23] reduces disorder eating symptoms,[24] and improves weight-related quality of life.[25,26] NAFLD and NASH are highly prevalent among adolescents undergoing MBS (60%–80% prevalence),[27,28] and these can be greatly reduced following bariatric surgery.[29,30] However, at this time, bariatric surgery requires further investigation before it can be provided as a stand-alone treatment for the NAFLD spectrum.[31] Perhaps one of the most important factors observed among bariatric adolescents is the high proportion of youths, who are able to sustain weight loss long term. This is seldomly observed in other pediatric obesity treatments and should be an expectation given the risks and invasive nature of the procedure.[14,16] It is unknown how durable these improvements in comorbid conditions will be following surgery and therefore the necessity for long-term studies. Moreover, whether surgery results in delay of events (e.g., myocardial infarction, stroke) and improvements in outcomes (e.g., mortality) is unknown and will need to be evaluated.

Although weight loss and long-term weight loss maintenance are remarkably similar between youths and adults, comorbidity resolution and risk factor reduction rates are starkly different. For instance, the remission rate of T2D in Teen-LABS at 3 years was 95% versus adult studies showing 50%–70% remission.[32–34] This is remarkable, considering the aggressive nature of adolescent T2D—even best-practice medical management of T2D in youth is notorious for poor outcomes with >40% glycemic failure rates (requiring insulin) within 3 years.[35] Because of the poor results of intensive medical management and the promising outcomes of MBS, adolescents who develop T2D may have surgery be considered as the first line of treatment in the near future. Similarly, reductions in the prevalence of dyslipidemia, hypertriglyceridemia, and hypertension in adult bariatric patients at 3 years range from 30% to 50%,[36] although adolescents experience nearly a twofold (55%–75%) higher chance of remission. The mechanism(s) underlying these discrepancies is currently unknown but cannot be solely attributed to disease duration, weight loss, or other clinical characteristics.[34,37,38] Understanding these mechanisms will be vital for the field of pediatric obesity medicine and surgery to progress as substantial heterogeneity in response occurs, even with MBS.

Despite these many important improvements, MBS is not without risk and not a scalable solution for adolescent severe obesity. It is a life-altering procedure that requires patients to have decisional capacity, which many adolescents have not yet fully developed. Further, the risks of surgery are not inconsequential and may include micronutrient deficiencies, some of which may not be fully prevented by supplementation, future abdominal procedures, higher rates of fracture, excess skin due to weight loss that may require additional surgery for removal, a tendency for increased alcohol abuse, and increased postsurgical loss of controlled eating.[13,14,25,39–42] However, the switch from RYGB to VSG as the primary procedure may reduce the overall risk burden, because preliminary data indicate that VSG results in lower micronutrient deficiencies and a reduced need for surgical revisions than RYGB. Ongoing studies will continue to evaluate the perioperative and long-term risks and benefits of MBS in adolescents. The culmination of these factors likely explains the low uptake of bariatric surgery, which is on the order of 1000–4000 procedures per year in the United States despite the fact that 3–4 million adolescents meet the BMI indications for bariatric surgery. But for now, MBS remains the only treatment option with a high rate of success for weight loss and chronic disease risk reduction for adolescents with severe obesity.

CONCLUSION

Adolescents with severe obesity and the accompanying comorbid conditions may be eligible for MBS. Increasing evidence suggests that although surgery has a higher risk profile than minimally effective lifestyle interventions, the outcomes in terms of weight loss and comorbidity resolution are pronounced. MBS offers sustainable and clinically meaningful weight loss with durable disease remission, which should be the goal of any treatment for adolescent severe obesity. However, the risks of surgery and the potential for long-term complications should be weighed when making decisions about undergoing this expensive, invasive, and life-altering procedure.

OUTLOOK

Cited as being among the biggest barriers to widespread adoption of MBS, among qualifying adolescents, is initial insurance coverage for the procedure and postoperative care. However, studies in adolescents have shown persistence, on the part of providers, in continuing to apply for coverage in spite of rejection results in high success rates

of eventual coverage. Perhaps the biggest barrier to surgery as a scalable solution for treating pediatric severe obesity is the adolescents themselves. Few who medically qualify are ready for such an invasive and life-altering procedure. Moreover, most primary care providers are still hesitant to refer adolescents for surgery, whereas other treatment options are available. This is despite the mounting evidence favoring surgery as a treatment approach for severe obesity. Therefore, until surgery is able to minimize risks and become a treatment option, thus gaining acceptance among primary care practitioners, the uptake of MBS among adolescents with severe obesity will remain low.

REFERENCES

1. Sinha R, Fisch G, Teague B, et al. Prevalence of impaired glucose tolerance among children and adolescents with marked obesity. *N Engl J Med.* 2002;346(11):802–810.
2. Pettitt DJ, Talton J, Dabelea D, et al. Prevalence of diabetes in U.S. Youth in 2009: the SEARCH for diabetes in youth study. *Diabetes Care.* 2014;37(2):402–408.
3. Kelly AS, Barlow SE, Rao G, et al. Severe obesity in children and adolescents: identification, associated health risks, and treatment approaches: a scientific statement from the American Heart Association. *Circulation.* 2013;128(15):1689–1712.
4. Urbina EMKT, McCoy CE, Khoury P, Daniels S, Dolan L. Youth with obesity and obesity-related type 2 diabetes mellitus demonstrate abnormalities in carotid structure and function. *Circulation.* 2009;119:2913–2919.
5. Ryder JR, Kaizer AM, Rudser KD, Daniels SR, Kelly AS. Utility of body mass index in identifying excess adiposity in youth across the obesity spectrum. *J Pediatr.* 2016;177:255–261. e252.
6. Skinner AC, Perrin EM, Moss LA, Skelton JA. Cardiometabolic risks and severity of obesity in children and young adults. *N Engl J Med.* 2015;373(14):1307–1317.
7. Styne DM, Arslanian SA, Connor EL, et al. Pediatric obesity-assessment, treatment, and prevention: an endocrine society clinical practice guideline. *J Clin Endocrinol Metab.* 2017;102(3):709–757.
8. Michalsky M, Reichard K, Inge T, Pratt J, Lenders C. ASMBS pediatric committee best practice guidelines. *Surg Obes Relat Dis.* 2012;8(1):1–7.
9. Pratt JSA, Browne A, Browne NT, et al. ASMBS pediatric metabolic and bariatric surgery guidelines, 2018. *Surg Obes Relat Dis.* 2018;14(7):882–901.
10. Inge TH, Zeller MH, Jenkins TM, et al. Perioperative outcomes of adolescents undergoing bariatric surgery: the Teen-Longitudinal Assessment of Bariatric Surgery (Teen-LABS) study. *JAMA Pediatr.* 2014;168(1):47–53.
11. Danielsson P, Kowalski J, Ekblom O, Marcus C. Response of severely obese children and adolescents to behavioral treatment. *Arch Pediatr Adolesc Med.* 2012;166(12):1103–1108.
12. Kelly AS, Fox CK, Rudser KD, Gross AC, Ryder JR. Pediatric obesity pharmacotherapy: current state of the field, review of the literature, and clinical trial considerations. *Int J Obes.* 2016;40(7):1043–1050.

13. Inge TH, Courcoulas AP, Jenkins TM, et al. Weight loss and health status 3 years after bariatric surgery in adolescents. *N Engl J Med*. 2016;374(2):113–123.

14. Inge TH, Jenkins TM, Xanthakos SA, et al. Long-term outcomes of bariatric surgery in adolescents with severe obesity (FABS-5+): a prospective follow-up analysis. *Lancet Diabetes Endocrinol*. 2017;5(3):165–173.

15. Olbers T, Beamish AJ, Gronowitz E, et al. Laparoscopic Roux-en-Y gastric bypass in adolescents with severe obesity (AMOS): a prospective, 5-year, Swedish nationwide study. *Lancet Diabetes Endocrinol*. 2017;5(3):174–183.

16. Ryder JR, Gross AC, Fox CK, et al. Factors associated with long-term weight loss maintenance following bariatric surgery in adolescents with severe obesity. *Int J Obes*. 2018;42(1):102–107.

17. Ryder JR, Gross AC, Fox CK, et al. Factors associated with long-term weight-loss maintenance following bariatric surgery in adolescents with severe obesity. *Int J Obes*. 2018;42(1):102–107.

18. Beamish AJ, Olbers T, Kelly AS, Inge TH. Cardiovascular effects of bariatric surgery. *Nat Rev Cardiol*. 2016;13(12):730–743.

19. Michalsky MP, Inge TH, Jenkins TM, et al. Cardiovascular risk factors after adolescent bariatric surgery. *Pediatrics*. 2018;141(2):pii: e20172485.

20. Ryder JR, Edwards NM, Gupta R, et al. Changes in functional mobility and musculoskeletal pain after bariatric surgery in Teens with severe obesity: Teen-Longitudinal Assessment of Bariatric Surgery (LABS) study. *JAMA Pediatr*. 2016;170(9):871–877.

21. Kelly AS, Ryder JR, Marlatt KL, Rudser KD, Jenkins T, Inge TH. Changes in inflammation, oxidative stress, and adipokines following bariatric surgery among adolescents with severe obesity. *Int J Obes*. 2015.

22. Inge TH, Prigeon RL, Elder DA, et al. Insulin sensitivity and beta-cell function improve after gastric bypass in severely obese adolescents. *J Pediatr*. 2015;167(5):1042–1048.e1041.

23. Nehus EJ, Khoury JC, Inge TH, et al. Kidney outcomes three years after bariatric surgery in severely obese adolescents. *Kidney International*. 2017;91(2):451–458.

24. Sarwer DB, Dilks RJ, Spitzer JC, et al. Changes in dietary intake and eating behavior in adolescents after bariatric surgery: an ancillary study to the Teen-LABS consortium. *Obes Surg*. 2017;27(12):3082–3091.

25. Zeller MH, Pendery EC, Reiter-Purtill J, et al. From adolescence to young adulthood: trajectories of psychosocial health following Roux-en-Y gastric bypass. *Surg Obes Relat Dis*. 2017;13(7):1196–1203.

26. Zeller MH, Pendery EC, Reiter-Purtill J, et al. From adolescence to young adulthood: trajectories of psychosocial health following Roux-en-Y gastric bypass. *Surg Obes Relat Dis*. 2017;13(7):1196–1203.

27. Xanthakos S, Miles L, Bucuvalas J, Daniels S, Garcia V, Inge T. Histologic spectrum of nonalcoholic fatty liver disease in morbidly obese adolescents. *Clin Gastroenterol Hepatol*. 2006;4(2):226–232.

28. Xanthakos SA, Jenkins TM, Kleiner DE, et al. High prevalence of nonalcoholic fatty liver disease in adolescents undergoing bariatric surgery. *Gastroenterology*. 2015;149(3):623–634. e628.

29. Manco M, Mosca A, De Peppo F, et al. The benefit of sleeve gastrectomy in obese adolescents on nonalcoholic steatohepatitis and hepatic fibrosis. *J Pediatr*. 2017;180:31–37.e32.

30. Nobili V, Carpino G, De Peppo F, et al. Laparoscopic sleeve gastrectomy improves nonalcoholic fatty liver disease-related liver damage in adolescents by reshaping cellular interactions and hepatic adipocytokine production. *J Pediatr*. 2018;194(3):100–108.

31. Xanthakos SA, Schwimmer JB. On a knife-edge—weight-loss surgery for NAFLD in adolescents. *Nat Rev Gastroenterol Hepatol*. 2015;12(6):316–318.

32. Purnell JQ, Selzer F, Wahed AS, et al. Type 2 diabetes remission rates after laparoscopic gastric bypass and gastric banding: results of the longitudinal assessment of bariatric surgery study. *Diabetes Care*. 2016;39(7):1101–1107.

33. Kadera BE, Lum K, Grant J, Pryor AD, Portenier DD, DeMaria EJ. Remission of type 2 diabetes after Roux-en-Y gastric bypass is associated with greater weight loss. *Surg Obes Relat Dis*. 2009;5(3):305–309.

34. Wang G-F, Yan Y-X, Xu N, et al. Predictive factors of type 2 diabetes mellitus remission following bariatric surgery: a meta-analysis. *Obes Surg*. 2015;25(2):199–208.

35. Zeitler P, Hirst K, Pyle L, et al. A clinical trial to maintain glycemic control in youth with type 2 diabetes. *N Engl J Med*. 2012;366(24):2247–2256.

36. Courcoulas AP, King WC, Belle SH, et al. Seven-year weight trajectories and health outcomes in the longitudinal assessment of bariatric surgery (labs) study. *JAMA Surg*. 2018;153(5):427–434.

37. Hatoum IJ, Blackstone R, Hunter TD, et al. Clinical factors associated with remission of obesity-related comorbidities after bariatric surgery. *JAMA Surg*. 2016;151(2):130–137.

38. Benaiges D, Sague M, Flores-Le Roux JA, et al. Predictors of hypertension remission and recurrence after bariatric surgery. *Am J Hypertens*. 2016;29(5):653–659.

39. Staalesen T, Olbers T, Dahlgren J, et al. Development of excess skin and request for body-contouring surgery in postbariatric adolescents. *Plast Reconstr Surg*. 2014;134(4):627–636.

40. Zeller MH, Inge TH, Modi AC, et al. Severe obesity and comorbid condition impact on the weight-related quality of life of the adolescent patient. *J Pediatr*. 2015;166(3):651–659.e654.

41. Zeller MH, Washington GA, Mitchell JE, et al. Alcohol use risk in adolescents 2 years after bariatric surgery. *Surg Obes Relat*. 2017;13(1):85–94.

42. Goldschmidt AB, Khoury J, Jenkins TM, et al. Adolescent loss-of-control eating and weight loss maintenance after bariatric surgery. *Pediatrics*. 2018;141(1).

CHAPTER 25

Staging Model of Eating Disorders

JANET TREASURE, PHD, FRCP, FRCPSYCH • CAROL KAN, BA (CANTAB), MA, MBBS, MRCPSYCH, PHD • KATIE ROWLANDS, BSC

GLOSSARY

Prodrome/prodromal The early signs/symptoms of the disorder.
Staging of illness The progression of an illness following a path of deterioration, increasing in severity and resistance to treatment over time.
Neuroadaptation The rewiring of the brain in which symptomatic behaviors become habitual [e.g., food fears in anorexia nervosa and food wanting (addiction) in binge eating disorder and bulimia nervosa].
Neuroprogression The secondary consequences of poor nutrition on brain structure and function (e.g., reduced neuroplasticity, functional impairment of complex integrative cognitive function).
Precision psychiatry The use of additional information (-omics) to stratify or stage eating disorders to account for variability in prognosis or treatment response, etc.
Stratification This is similar to staging and includes a more precise description and categorization of possible subtypes of illness within the diagnostic categories.

INTRODUCTION

When asked for their views about treatment, patients with eating disorders (EDs) request a more personalized approach.[1] For this to happen, we need to be able to predict the course of the illness and response to treatment of the individual. The premise of staging models is that psychopathology moves along a predictable path from prodromal signs, through to the acute presentation and eventual end-stage manifestations. The implication is that, without early remediation, progressive changes from the active illness may adversely impact the course of the illness. Clinical staging involves determining where the individual presents on this temporal spectrum. The utility of a staging model in psychiatry can be judged by its ability to link to clinical course, treatment outcome, and neurobiology. As such, the aims of this chapter are to consider:

- the level of evidence for a staging model of eating disorders
- the mechanisms contributing to the longitudinal trajectory
- the clinical implications

Before addressing these aims, it is important to define our use of the term "staging," as the term has been used to reflect different meanings within the ED literature. For example, the term "stages of recovery" is often used into compare and contrast people in the acute state of the illness with those following symptom changes in the short or long term.[2,3] By contrast, the term staging has also been used to delineate the progression of the condition as it follows a linear path of deterioration over time, toward a severe and enduring form that is resistant to existing treatments.[4] The latter is considered here.

What Is the Evidence to Support a Staging Model for Eating Disorders?

The staging model builds on evidence from a clinical trial comparing different forms of relapse prevention for anorexia nervosa (AN), in which duration of illness was used to stratify randomization. Treatment outcome differed between those in the early stage (less than 3 years of illness) and those in the late stage (greater than 3 years of illness) at 1 and 5 years.[5,6] Many studies have subsequently found that illness duration predicts prognosis.[7–9]

Eating Disorders and Obesity in Children and Adolescents. https://doi.org/10.1016/B978-0-323-54852-6.00025-2

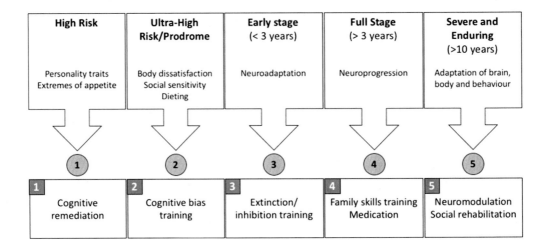

FIG. 25.1 This figure represents the stages of progression of ED over time and suggests some possible stage-matched treatment enhancers. People with high ED risk have impulsive/compulsive and anxious personality disorder traits and extremes of appetite. Environmental triggers such as teasing about weight or shape or social ranking concerns can lead to prodromal symptoms such as food restriction, anxiety disorders, mood disorders, and body dissatisfaction. The cumulative effect of protracted starvation and eating disorder habits leads to progression of the illness. Once the illness persists for over 3 years, it becomes more resistant to treatment. Habits become more strongly engrained, leading to disabilities in the medical, psychological, and social spheres.

The full remission rate for AN at the end of treatment in adolescents (typically with a short duration of illness) is between 33% and 42%.[10,11] In contrast, in adults (many in later stages of illness), only 31% have recovered at 9 years and 68% after 22 years from illness onset.[12]

The staging model in Fig. 25.1 depicts the progression from the pre/clinical phases among those at high risk for developing an eating disorder toward those with a severe and enduring illness.

High eating disorder risk

A number of childhood emotional and behavioral traits, which possibly represent genetic vulnerabilities, increase the risk of developing an ED. Shyness, social difficulties, perfectionism, obsessive-compulsive traits, and autistic-like features are common precursors of all eating disorders.[13] Eating behaviors (appetite/satiety

sensitivity) lie on a continuum[14,15] and picky eating may precede AN, whereas a robust antecedent appetite is seen in BED.[16,17]

Ultrahigh risk/prodrome

The prodromal phase of AN is marked by dieting or "uneasiness and fullness" following food consumption, body dissatisfaction, depression, anxiety,[18,19] social avoidance,[13] and impaired interpersonal functioning.[20]

Early stage of illness

People with AN usually present clinically within a short time window in adolescence (often brought by concerned others).[21] Therefore, child and adolescent services mainly encounter patients with AN in the early stage of their illness. However, in the early stages, many features of eating disorders can be considered transdiagnostic. Thus, a short phase of weight loss can also be followed by a transition to cycles of restrictive and compensatory behaviors that characterize bulimia nervosa (BN).[22]

Full-stage illness

When weight has fallen as a result of persistent restrictive behaviors, the secondary cumulative effects of starvation manifest in the brain, body, and social spheres. The severity of weight loss and chronicity of AN are leading risk factors for developing medical complications in all body systems such as bone loss (osteoporosis).[23] Neuroprogressive changes in the brain accentuate vulnerability traits[4] including social isolation, which also allows ED habits to become more firmly established.

Severe and enduring illness

The final "chronic" phase of AN is characterized by severe emaciation, extreme overexercising, a general debility, and comorbid psychiatric disorders.

The staging model predicts that stage-specific treatment targeting the underlying pathology will optimize outcome. In the early stage of illness, involving the family to focus on weight restoration has been found to be an effective strategy[5,24] and is recommended in the National Institute for Health and Care Excellence (NICE) guidelines; however, there is less certainty about what works best for those who have not accessed treatment in this early phase or who have failed to respond (NICE, 2017).

What Could Be the Underpinning Mechanisms That Contribute to the Longitudinal Trajectory of the Psychopathology?

The staging model predicts that disease progression follows a temporal trajectory. We hypothesize that three processes may be involved: neuroadaptation, neuroprogression, and social alienation. First, ED behaviors become fixed habits (neuroadaptation). Second, poor nutrition and stress reduce neuroplasticity, leading to neuroprogression and a decrease in brain function. Third, social functioning may be profoundly disrupted by these two processes.

Learning and habit formation (neuroadaptation)

Learning is shaped by reward or punishment. Translational science has established that behavioral choices are initially driven by hedonics and goals but, with repetition over time, become fixed into automatic

compulsive habits. This shift to automaticity is associated with reduced activation in prefrontal areas and the ventral striatum to activation in the putamen (dorsal striatum).[25,26] The process of developing learned habits is thought to be an important mechanism explaining how patterns of eating disorder behaviors persist.[27] Thus, one hypothesis to explain the illness trajectory is that sensitivity to punishment accentuates fear learning in AN, which, by over training at a critical period, leads to automated avoidance habits.[28–31,32]

The brain consequences of starvation and poor nutrition (neuroprogression)

Evidence of neuroprogression, from prolonged malnutrition, is seen in both structural and functional changes in the brain. Adolescents in the early stage of AN had increased gray matter volume in areas associated with decision making.[33] However, patients with chronic AN had reduced gray matter, which correlated with duration of illness.[34] Also, in a well-established neuropsychological task, adults with AN demonstrated significantly poorer decision-making abilities in almost all domains measured compared with healthy adults, whereas no significant differences were found between adolescents (AN vs. healthy).[35] The mechanisms underpinning the neuropathological deterioration might include decreased neurotrophins and neurogenesis, epigenetic changes, and inflammation. Indeed, changes in brain-derived neurotrophic factor (BDNF), implicit learning, and event-related potential (ERP) activation have been found in adolescents (early stage) in the acute state of AN.[36–38]

Social functioning

Social difficulties have been identified as both risk and maintaining factors of ED.[13] The underlying assumption of the clinical staging model is that the level of social impairment experienced by patients worsens over time with illness progression. Neuroprogressive changes may be responsible for the reduction in social cognition seen in the acute phase of AN.[39] Some examples include muted emotional receptivity and signalling[40] and impaired mirroring of emotional expressions.[41] Also people with ED attend more to social threats, such as angry[42] and rejecting[43] faces, with an effect size of 0.4 found in a recent metaanalysis.[44] All of these changes in social function can lead to isolation and loneliness, which then leads to further stress as well as hormonal and inflammatory changes[45] driving a vicious cycle of ill health.[46] Additionally, anomalies in emotional and social functioning may alienate others and possibly contribute to the high expressed emotion seen in families.[47] For example, close others can react strongly to the overt changes in physical health, general well-being, and social functioning. Their reactions to this danger (over protection or critical comments) may have the unfortunate effect of reinforcing the illness behaviors.[48] Few studies have directly examined aspects of social functioning across different stages of the illness.

Clinical Implications

The staging model has many clinical implications such as the need to reduce the length of untreated illness. Although there is a tendency to have therapeutic nihilism about people in the late stage of illness, there are glimmers of optimism. For example, the proportion of patients who manage to recover slowly increases even after 10 years of illness.[12] The treatment targets implied by the model are to (1) remediate the continued process of habit learning, (2) prevent a prolonged period of starvation, (3) foster continued social engagement, and (4) manage comorbidities. Some possible types of stage-matched additions to treatment are suggested in Fig. 25.1.

CONCLUSION

The staging model heuristic and exploratory framework offers opportunities to apply a more personalized, targeted approach to treatment for ED. It follows from this model that addressing barriers to early intervention is an important priority for reducing the duration of untreated illness. In the later stages of the illness, it will be helpful to develop a precise formulation to determine the focus for personalized adjuncts to treatment (e.g., cognitive training techniques, improving social connection, and managing comorbidities). This will require a flexible, formulation-based approach augmenting treatment with some of the novel interventions that are now available. In terms of research and development, it would be helpful for individuals to be stratified according to stage (i.e., duration) of illness for research recruitment. It would also be helpful to have a standardized assessment of the typical comorbid traits.[49]

REFERENCES

1. van Furth EF, van der Meer A, Cowan K. Top 10 research priorities for eating disorders. *Lancet Psychiatry.* 2016;3(8):706–707.
2. Fitzsimmons EE, Bardone-Cone AM. Differences in coping across stages of recovery from an eating disorder. *Int J Eat Disord.* 2010;43(8):689–693.
3. Bardone-Cone AM, Sturm K, Lawson MA, Robinson DP, Smith R. Perfectionism across stages of recovery from eating disorders. *Int J Eat Disord.* 2010;43(2):139–148.
4. Treasure J, Stein D, Maguire S. Has the time come for a staging model to map the course of eating disorders from high risk to severe enduring illness? An examination of the evidence. *Early Interv Psychiatry.* 2015;9(3):173–184.
5. Russell GF, Szmukler GI, Dare C, Eisler I. An evaluation of family therapy in anorexia nervosa and bulimia nervosa. *Arch Gen Psychiatry.* 1987;44(12):1047–1056.
6. Eisler I, Dare C, Russell GF, Szmukler G, le Grange D, Dodge E. Family and individual therapy in anorexia nervosa. A 5-year follow-up. *Arch Gen Psychiatry.* 1997;54(11):1025–1030.
7. Zipfel S, Lowe B, Reas DL, Deter HC, Herzog W. Long-term prognosis in anorexia nervosa: lessons from a 21-year follow-up study. *Lancet.* 2000;355(9205):721–722.
8. Vall E, Wade TD. Predictors of treatment outcome in individuals with eating disorders: a systematic review and meta-analysis. *Int J Eat Disord.* 2016;49(4):432–433.
9. Le Grange D, Lock J, Agras WS, Bryson SW, Jo B. Randomized clinical trial of family-based treatment and cognitive-behavioral therapy for adolescent bulimia nervosa. *J Am Acad Child Adolesc Psychiatry.* 2015;54(11):886–894.e882.
10. Agras WS, Lock J, Brandt H, et al. Comparison of 2 family therapies for adolescent anorexia nervosa: a randomized parallel trial. *JAMA Psychiatry.* 2014;71(11):1279–1286.
11. Lock J, Le Grange D, Agras WS, Moye A, Bryson SW, Jo B. Randomized clinical trial comparing family-based treatment with adolescent-focused individual therapy for adolescents with anorexia nervosa. *Arch Gen Psychiatry.* 2010;67(10):1025–1032.
12. Eddy KT, Tabri N, Thomas JJ, et al. Recovery from anorexia nervosa and bulimia nervosa at 22-year follow-up. *J Clin Psychiatry.* 2017;78(2):184–189.
13. Treasure J, Schmidt U. The cognitive-interpersonal maintenance model of anorexia nervosa revisited: a summary of the evidence for cognitive, socio-emotional and interpersonal predisposing and perpetuating factors. *J Eat Disord.* 2013;1:13.
14. Llewellyn CH, Fildes A. Behavioural susceptibility theory: Professor Jane Wardle and the role of appetite in genetic risk of obesity. *Curr Obes Rep.* 2017;6(1):38–45.
15. Llewellyn C, Wardle J. Behavioral susceptibility to obesity: gene-environment interplay in the development of weight. *Physiol Behav.* 2015;152(Pt B):494–501.
16. Jacobi C, Hayward C, de Zwaan M, Kraemer HC, Agras WS. Coming to terms with risk factors for eating disorders: application of risk terminology and suggestions for a general taxonomy. *Psychol Bull.* 2004;130(1):19–65.
17. Nunez-Navarro A, Jimenez-Murcia S, Alvarez-Moya E, et al. Differentiating purging and nonpurging bulimia nervosa and binge eating disorder. *Int J Eat Disord.* 2011;44(6):488–496.
18. Stice E, Ng J, Shaw H. Risk factors and prodromal eating pathology. *J Child Psychol Psychiatry.* 2010;51(4):518–525.
19. Allen KL, Byrne SM, Forbes D, Oddy WH. Risk factors for full- and partial-syndrome early adolescent eating disorders: a population-based pregnancy cohort study. *J Am Acad Child Adolesc Psychiatry.* 2009;48(8):800–809.

20. Stice E, Gau JM, Rohde P, Shaw H. Risk factors that predict future onset of each DSM-5 eating disorder: predictive specificity in high-risk adolescent females. *J Abnorm Psychol*. 2017;126(1):38–51.

21. Micali N, Hagberg KW, Petersen I, Treasure JL. The incidence of eating disorders in the UK in 2000-2009: findings from the General Practice Research Database. *BMJ Open*. 2013;3(5).

22. Anderluh M, Tchanturia K, Rabe-Hesketh S, Collier D, Treasure J. Lifetime course of eating disorders: design and validity testing of a new strategy to define the eating disorders phenotype. *Psychol Med*. 2009;39(1):105–114.

23. Mehler PS, Brown C. Anorexia nervosa - medical complications. *J Eat Disord*. 2015;3:11.

24. Treasure J, Cardi V, Leppanen J, Turton R. New treatment approaches for severe and enduring eating disorders. *Physiol Behav*. 2015;152(Pt B):456–465.

25. Everitt BJ, Robbins TW. From the ventral to the dorsal striatum: devolving views of their roles in drug addiction. *Neurosci Biobehav Rev*. 2013;37(9 Pt A):1946–1954.

26. Voon V, Reiter A, Sebold M, Groman S. Model-based control in dimensional psychiatry. *Biol Psychiatry*. 2017; 82(6):391–400.

27. Walsh BT. The enigmatic persistence of anorexia nervosa. *Am J Psychiatry*. 2013;170(5):477–484.

28. Steinglass J, Walsh BT. Habit learning and anorexia nervosa: a cognitive neuroscience hypothesis. *Int J Eat Disord*. 2006;39(4):267–275.

29. Steinglass JE, Sysko R, Glasofer D, Albano AM, Simpson HB, Walsh BT. Rationale for the application of exposure and response prevention to the treatment of anorexia nervosa. *Int J Eat Disord*. 2011;44(2):134–141.

30. Strober M. Pathologic fear conditioning and anorexia nervosa: on the search for novel paradigms. *Int J Eat Disord*. 2004;35(4):504–508.

31. Guarda AS, Schreyer CC, Boersma GJ, Tamashiro KL, Moran TH. Anorexia nervosa as a motivated behavior: relevance of anxiety, stress, fear and learning. *Physiol Behav*. 2015:466–472.

32. Foerde K, Steinglass JE. Decreased feedback learning in anorexia nervosa persists after weight restoration. *Int J Eat Disord*. 2017;50(4):415–423.

33. Montigny C, Castellanos-Ryan N, Whelan R, et al. A phenotypic structure and neural correlates of compulsive behaviors in adolescents. *PLoS One*. 2013;8(11):e80151.

34. Fonville L, Giampietro V, Williams SC, Simmons A, Tchanturia K. Alterations in brain structure in adults with anorexia nervosa and the impact of illness duration. *Psychol Med*. 2014;44(9):1965–1975.

35. Giannunzio V, Degortes D, Tenconi E, et al. Decision-making impairment in anorexia nervosa: new insights into the role of age and decision-making style. *Eur Eat Disord Rev*. 2018:302–314.

36. Firk C, Mainz V, Schulte-Ruether M, Fink G, Herpertz-Dahlmann B, Konrad K. Implicit sequence learning in juvenile anorexia nervosa: neural mechanisms and the impact of starvation. *J Child Psychol Psychiatry*. 2015;56(11):1168–1176.

37. Zwipp J, Hass J, Schober I, et al. Serum brain-derived neurotrophic factor and cognitive functioning in underweight, weight-recovered and partially weight-recovered females with anorexia nervosa. *Prog Neuro-Psychopharmacol Biol Psychiatry*. 2014;54:163–169.

38. Sfarlea A, Greimel E, Platt B, Bartling J, Schulte-Korne G, Dieler AC. Alterations in neural processing of emotional faces in adolescent anorexia nervosa patients - an event-related potential study. *Biol Psychol*. 2016;119:141–155.

39. Caglar-Nazali HP, Corfield F, Cardi V, et al. A systematic review and meta-analysis of 'Systems for Social Processes' in eating disorders. *Neurosci Biobehav Rev*. 2014;42:55–92.

40. Leppanen J, Cardi V, Paloyelis Y, Simmons A, Tchanturia K, Treasure J. Blunted neural response to implicit negative facial affect in anorexia nervosa. *Biol Psychol*. 2017; 128:105–111.

41. Dapelo MM, Bodas S, Morris R, Tchanturia K. Deliberately generated and imitated facial expressions of emotions in people with eating disorders. *J Affect Disord*. 2016;191:1–7.

42. Harrison A, Tchanturia K, Treasure J. Attentional bias, emotion recognition, and emotion regulation in anorexia: state or trait? *Biol Psychiatry*. 2010;68(8):755–761.

43. Cardi V, Di Matteo R, Corfield F, Treasure J. Social reward and rejection sensitivity in eating disorders: an investigation of attentional bias and early experiences. *World J Biol Psychiatry*. 2013;14(8):622–633.

44. Monteleone AM, Treasure J, Kan C, Cardi V. Reactivity to interpersonal stress in patients with eating disorders: a systematic review and meta-analysis of studies using an experimental paradigm. *Neurosci Biobehav Rev*. 2018;87:133–150.

45. Eisenberger NI, Moieni M, Inagaki TK, Muscatell KA, Irwin MR. Sickness and in health: the Co-regulation of inflammation and social behavior. *Neuropsychopharmacology*. 2017;42(1):242–253.

46. Cacioppo JT, Cacioppo S. Social relationships and health: the toxic effects of perceived social isolation. *Soc Personal Psychol Compass*. 2014;8(2):58–72.

47. Hibbs R, Rhind C, Leppanen J, Treasure J. Interventions for caregivers of someone with an eating disorder: a meta-analysis. *Int J Eat Disord*. 2015;48(4):349–361.

48. Treasure J, Nazar BP. Interventions for the careers of patients with eating disorders. *Curr Psychiatry Rep*. 2016;18(2):16.

49. Carrot B, Radon L, Hubert T, et al. Are lifetime affective disorders predictive of long-term outcome in severe adolescent anorexia nervosa? *Eur Child Adolesc Psychiatry*. 2017;26(8):969–978.

WEB REFERENCE

NICE. *National Institute for Health and Care Excellence. (2017). Eat Disord: Recognition and treatment. National Institute for Health and Clinical Excellence Guideline (NG69)*; 2017:2–41. Website: http://www.nice.org.uk.

CHAPTER 26

Outcomes of Anorexic and Bulimic Eating Disorders

MANFRED M. FICHTER, MD, DIPL-PSYCH • NORBERT QUADFLIEG, PHD

INTRODUCTION

Information about the predictors of unfavorable outcomes following treatment for an anorexic or bulimic eating disorder (ED) can help improve the treatment efficacy over time and promote the development of novel interventions focusing on identified risk factors. Several reviews and many articles have been published, unfortunately with conflicting results due to methodological differences and shortcomings across studies. Many samples were much too small. In other studies, the follow-up time was not sufficient. Outcome measures differed across studies.[1,2] Various samples have been used, such as twin cohort registers[3] or clinical samples, and various definitions of "recovery," "remission," and ED diagnoses have been applied. Therefore, not surprisingly, the published results of studies on ED outcomes are quite contradictory. Recently, a few long-term longitudinal studies of the outcomes of EDs in larger populations have been published, and we will focus this review on recent studies. The length of follow-up [roughly categorized in this chapter as short- (up to 2 years), intermediate- (3–10 years), and long-term (more than 10 years)] plays an important role in increasing recovery rates in long-term follow-up studies.[4]

Outcomes of Anorexia Nervosa

The course of anorexia nervosa (AN) was studied in a number of twin studies. The results of a 10-year follow-up to the FinTwin16 twin cohort study have recently been reported[5]; the twins were then approximately 34 years old. The sample consisted of 2188 women, 40 of whom had a lifetime DSM-IV diagnosis of AN. The authors compared these 40 women with AN with unaffected women from the same cohort. None of these 40 twins with AN died during the follow-up interval. Compared with twins of the same age who were unaffected by AN, twins with AN had a significantly lower body weight at follow-up (22.0 vs. 24.0 kg/m², P = .008).

Among the twins with the disorder, more women were still visiting a university than unaffected twins (15% vs. 4%, P = .003). Consistent with the results of the study by Fichter et al.,[6] fewer women with AN had children (50% compared with 66% of unaffected women, P = .05). However, epidemiologic twin samples usually include persons who have not been treated or whose eating disturbances were not sufficiently severe to seek medical attention. Thus, twin samples may have a different selection mechanism and may therefore not be directly comparable with participants in studies of persons treated on an in- or outpatient basis. Accordingly, patients with AN who are treated on an outpatient basis or, moreover, treated on a self-help basis are more likely to have a more favorable course than persons treated as inpatients.

Generally, patients with AN who are treated at a younger age have a better long-term prognosis than patients with AN who are treated as adults. Similarly, patients who are treated in an institution for children and adolescents show better outcome data and lower mortality rates than patients treated in institutions for adults. Once the course of illness has become chronic and the treatment attempts have become increasingly unsuccessful, the prognosis of further treatment is worse. This finding clearly points to the necessity of quick actions to implement an appropriate treatment.

A study by Lock et al.[7] employed a rather short follow-up period (6–24 months). This study is nevertheless reported here briefly as an example of a follow-up study of randomized controlled trials (RCTs), which usually comprise more selected (homogeneous) samples. The authors used the databases of five different RCTs with adolescents or adults suffering from AN, bulimia nervosa (BN), or binge eating disorder (BED). They concluded that for adolescents with AN, an intervention that achieved a body weight of 95.2% of the expected body weight at the end of treatment appeared to be the best predictor of subsequent recovery. The

Eating Disorders and Obesity in Children and Adolescents. https://doi.org/10.1016/B978-0-323-54852-6.00026-4

most efficient predictor of weight recovery (BMI > 19 kg/m²) for adults with AN at follow-up was a weight gain until the end of treatment period of greater than 85.8% of the ideal body weight. Additionally, the most efficient predictor of psychologic recovery among adults with AN was the achievement of a low weight concern score in the eating disorder examination (EDE) (<1.8).

In a recent study by Fichter et al.,[6] recovery rates were rather low (29.6%) for the total sample after 10 years; the recovery rate was 39.3% for a subsample with a particularly long follow-up period of at least 20 years. Other long-term clinical follow-up studies with large samples reported somewhat more favorable recovery rates. However, the severity of EDs and the definition of recovery differed between the published studies. The use of the same operationalized definition of recovery described by Bardone-Cone et al.[8] in future outcome studies would be very helpful.

An older metaanalysis by Steinhausen[9] that combined 119 patients series with all lengths of follow-up estimated mean percentages of 47% recovery, 33% improvement, and 20% chronicity. A more recent North American study[4] followed 121 adolescent and adult women diagnosed with AN and reported recovery rates of 31.4% at the 9-year follow-up and 62.8% at the 22-year follow-up. A predictor of poor outcomes from the same study at the 22-year follow-up was comorbid depression.[10]

A Swedish study published in 2009 reported the outcomes of *adolescent-onset AN.*[11] Eighteen years after the initial assessment, 12% of patients had a persistent ED. Twenty-five percent of the 51 former patients were unemployed because of their ED or another psychiatric disorder. Premorbid obsessive-compulsive personality disorder, a younger age at onset of AN and autistic traits predicted poor outcomes. In a recent study, Herpertz-Dahlmann et al.[12] reported the outcomes of *childhood AN* (onset < 14 years). Only 1 of 52 patients (1.5%) had died at the 7.5-year follow-up. Patients who were alive at follow-up exhibited 41% good, 35% intermediate, and 24% poor outcomes. The authors concluded that "childhood AN is a serious disorder with an unfavorable course in many patients and high rates of chronicity and psychiatric comorbidity in young adulthood."

Several studies have now confirmed that crossover from AN to BN occurs at a rate of approximately 10%.[6,13] Additionally, at least two studies have shown that crossover from AN to BED virtually does not occur.[6,14] Patients with AN rarely become overweight or even obese. However, an increase in BMI has been observed over decades in the populations of western industrialized countries. For these reasons, a study aiming to determine which patients with AN appear to be largely "immune" to overweight and obesity would be very interesting.

Outcomes of Bulimia Nervosa

BN was defined as an ED in 1979, much later than AN. Consequently, extensive research on BN has only been performed for approximately the past 40 years, and real long-term outcome studies are rare. Thus, we have the opportunity to provide a short but more comprehensive summary of outcomes in the space available than is possible for AN. Most of the limited number of studies on outcomes of BN are based on clinical samples, and we will focus on these patients.

Recovery

In studies addressing the short-term outcomes measured for 2 years after treatment, recovery rates varied between 24% and 60%.[15-17] This range increased to 24%–80% in studies assessing the period from 3 to 5 years after treatment.[14,17-23] A further increase in recovery rates ranging from 48% to 73% was reported by studies examining outcomes 6–10 years after treatment.[4,14,24,25] Long-term studies performed for more than 10 years are rare, and recovery rates of 42%, 66%, and 74% have been reported by Keel et al.,[26] Fichter and Quadflieg,[24] and Abraham et al.,[27] respectively. Eddy et al.[4] reported a recovery rate of 68% after 22 years.

Chronicity and diagnostic crossover

In the same studies, 6%–51% of patients had persistent BN or were rediagnosed with the disorder 2 years after treatment, and 9%–25% were still diagnosed or rediagnosed with BN 6–10 years after treatment. Twelve years after treatment, 11% of patients retained a BN diagnosis in each of the two studies.[24,26] Crossover to AN was observed in 0%–11% of patients after 2 years, in 3%–9% after 6–10 years, and in 1.9% and 0.6% in the two 12-year follow-up studies, respectively. Crossover to BED was rare, and percentages ranged between 1% and 11%. Crossover to eating disorder not otherwise specified (ED-NOS) ranged from 5% to 24%.

Based on these data collected from diverse samples, we concluded that an increasing number of patients recover from BN over time, with a considerable percentage showing chronicity. A small percentage of patients with BN shift to AN, and a still smaller proportion shift to BED over time.

Multiple follow-ups

Data from different studies are inconclusive because of the large overlap in recovery rates obtained for different follow-up periods. Some studies report multiple fol-low-up data from the same patients and provide a bet-ter picture of the course of BN.

Zeeck et al.[17] reported the complete recovery of 15%, 24%, and 33% of patients, partial recovery of 44%, 24%, and 36% of patients, and BN in 41%, 51%, and 31% of patients at 3, 12, and 36 months after treat-ment, respectively.

Milos et al.[28] reported outcomes at 1 and 2.5 years of follow-up. The recovery rate increased from 24% to 31%, and the rate of a BN diagnosis at follow-up decreased from 51% to 37%. Crossover to AN occurred at a rate of 6% at both time points, and crossover to ED-NOS increased from 19% to 27%.

Castellini et al.[14] reported recovery in 24% of patients and a persistence of BN in 54% of patients at 3 years after treatment; 50% recovered after 6 years. Crossover to AN was observed in 4% and 9% of patients, and crossover to BED was reported for 6% and 11% of patients at 3 and 6 years after treatment, respectively.

Fichter and Quadflieg[24] reported outcomes 2, 6, and 12 years after treatment. Recovery rates were 57%, 70%, and 70%, and BN was detected at follow-up in 34%, 22%, and 11% of patients, respectively. Crossover from BN to BED occurred in 0%, 1%, and 2% of patients, whereas crossover of BN to ED-NOS occurred in 7%, 1%, and 14% of patients, respectively.

Eddy et al.[4] reported a recovery rate of 68% for both 9-year and 22-year follow-ups.

In these studies, an increasing proportion of patients achieved recovery during the short to intermediate term after treatment. In the long term, approximately 30% of patients with BN did not achieve complete recovery, with a small percentage of these patients achieving at least partial recovery.

Keel et al.[29] reported relapse rates after complete recovery from BN over a period of 9 years. Of the 110 participants with BN, 83 (75%) achieved complete recovery at some point in the observation period. Of these 83 participants, 29 (35%) relapsed after recovery. In the same study, of the 136 participants with AN, 42 (31%) achieved complete recovery at some point in the observation period. Fifteen (36%) of these patients relapsed after recovery. Although relapse rates did not differ among patients with AN and BN, a considerably lower proportion of participants with AN achieved complete recovery.

Outcomes of Binge Eating Disorder
Recovery
Research on BED outcomes was initiated with the pro-posal of provisional criteria in *DSM-IV* (APA) at the

beginning of the 1990s. Consequently, only very few studies have reported BED outcomes, mostly for shorter time periods than BN and AN. Recovery rates range from 32% to 51% up to 2 years after treatment.[15,30-34] Three studies with a follow-up period from 3 to 5 years reported recovery rates of 27%–82%,[14,18,30] and three studies with 6–10 years of follow-up reported recov-ery rates of 19%–78%.[14,35,36] Only one study reported long-term outcomes at 12 years, with a recovery rate of 67%.[35]

Chronicity and diagnostic crossover
Very few studies have described the persistence of BED after treatment. Approximately one-quarter of patients with BED still had the disorder or were rediagnosed with BED 1 year after treatment.[15,31,32] In the study by Munsch et al.,[36] 8% of patients displayed persis-tent BED at the 6-year follow-up, and Fichter et al.[35] observed BED in 8% of patients 12 years after treat-ment. Crossover to BN was reported in 6% of patients after 3 years and in 9% of patients after 6 years in one study,[14] and in 9% of the sample 12 years after treat-ment in another study.[35] Other ED-NOS diagnoses were reported in 7%–27% of patients at follow-up.

Similar to BN, these data from diverse samples resulted in increasing recovery rates from BED. These data are tentative, based on only a small number of studies. Chronicity was only slightly less than the value reported for BN, and crossover from BED to BN is greater than that from BN to BED. No cases of crossover to AN were reported.

Risk Factors for Unfavorable Outcomes
In a recent systematic review and metaanalysis, Vall and Wade[37] analyzed predictors of treatment outcome for EDs. The review is transdiagnostic and generally com-bines AN, BN, and BED into one category. One conclu-sion of the study was that for patients with EDs, a lesser degree of changes in symptoms during early treatment indicates unfavorable outcomes at follow-up. Further predictors of unfavorable outcomes were a lower BMI at the end of treatment, a higher degree of binge/purge behaviors, a lower motivation to regain a healthy sta-tus, a higher degree of depression, a higher degree of shape/weight concerns, the presence of additional comorbidities, and a greater number of problems in the family environment and problems in interpersonal functioning. O'Brien et al.[38] recently reported on pre-dictors and long-term health outcomes of patients with self-reported EDs (AN or BN). The authors compared participants enrolled in a large study from the United States and Puerto Rico on breast cancer (Sister Study

Cohort). Respondents with self-reported ED were compared with subjects without ED at any time. Two percent of the Sister Study sample (967 participants) reported a history of an ED. Risk factors for having or having had an ED were being of non-Hispanic white descent, having well educated parents, and having a sister with an ED. Subjects who had had an ED were more likely to be underweight, to smoke, and to have had depression in adulthood. A statistical trend for having used birth control was also observed. In addition, a history of an ED was associated with pregnancy-related adverse outcomes: experience with nausea or bleeding during pregnancy, miscarriage, a first birth at an older age, or induced abortion.

Based on a 4- to 9-year follow-up study of patients with ED, Nakai et al.[25] concluded that "the outcome of EDs in Japan is relatively similar to that in western countries, irrespective of social cultural background and health systems" (p. 206).

Ward et al.[39] compared patients with AN subjected to compulsory admission to a specialized ED unit to patients with AN who were voluntarily admitted to the same ward and obtained outcome data over a 20-year period. Although mortality appeared to be higher in patients who were treated on a compulsory basis at the 5-year follow-up, the overall standardized mortality rate between the two groups at 20-year follow-up was not significantly different.

According to Fichter et al.,[6] motherhood is related to a better outcome of AN in the long-term course of the disease (mean: 10 years). In the same study, the percentage of participants who became mothers before or during the follow-up period (27.4%) was significantly less than in females in the German population of the same age and during the same period.

The following predictors of a negative outcome emerged in the study by Fichter et al.[6] using a very large clinical AN sample: (1) a lower BMI at admission, (2) a higher score on the Eating Disorder Inventory subscale "Maturity Fears" at admission, and (3) a lower number of follow-up years. Patients with AN are still more or less unstable at discharge from inpatient treatment. At the time of the study, the patients were not easily able to obtain immediate subsequent outpatient treatment by an experienced psychotherapist. With a longer follow-up, patients appeared to stabilize more, but mortality increased. Therefore, the survivors experienced worse outcomes in the early years after discharge compared with the results of follow-up visits at later time points. Consistent with these data, Ackard et al.[40] stratified 219 female patients with AN who also completed assessments at 1–11 years after the initial assessment

by age and described outcomes for three groups: youth (<18 years), young adults (18–39 years), and midlife adults (40+ years). The authors found that their oldest group of patients with AN (midlife adults) had the highest rates of poor outcomes or death.

A closer investigation of possible indicators of unfavorable courses that were not identified as risk factors in the large clinical study by Fichter et al.[6] is also interesting. Quite a few studies have described psychiatric comorbidities or a higher degree of general psychopathology, depression, or anxiety as possible predictors of an unfavorable course of AN. General psychopathology, as measured by all subscales of the Brief Symptom Inventory (BSI), and depression, as measured by the Beck Depression Inventory (BDI), were not identified as risk factors for an unfavorable course nor were the presence of binge eating/purging behavior nor the extent of eating disorder symptoms at admission. Because the literature about the effectiveness of these variables as predictors of AN outcomes is contradictory, future studies should clarify these issues. Risk factors identified to date can be used to develop innovative treatments in the future.

Among patients with BN, a higher binge frequency at treatment intake is a predictor of unfavorable outcome.[7,41] Other risk factors include a lifetime psychiatric comorbidity,[24,35] alcohol and drug misuse,[40] and ED in the family of origin.[40] With one exception,[42] a longer duration of ED at baseline was a predictor of poor outcomes.[40] Greater disturbances in body image and lower psychosocial functioning predicted relapse after recovery from BN.[29] Bodell et al.[43] reported the 10- and 20-year courses of ED in 1190 female and 509 male college students. A higher degree of bulimic symptoms at the 20-year follow-up was predicted by a greater weight suppression at baseline. This effect was mediated by an increased drive for thinness at the 10-year follow-up.

In a study by Lock et al.,[7] the absence of compensatory behaviors and a greater than 3.4-point reduction in the restraint score (EDE) after treatment were predictors of better outcomes 6–24 months after treatment in adolescent patients with BN. Recovery rates varied according to the number of criteria met. The highest recovery rate was observed in participants meeting both criteria (72%), and lower rates were observed in participants meeting one of the two criteria (35%). No recovery was observed in participants meeting none of these criteria.

Substantial data confirm symptom severity and psychiatric comorbidity (including alcohol and drug misuse) as risk factors for unfavorable outcomes of BN in adolescents and adults.[24,44] Results for the age at the beginning of treatment (or study intake) and age at onset of ED are contradictory in follow-up studies of patients with BN.

Little is known about risk factors for BED outcomes. One study compared participants from the community with BED with participants without any ED[45]; the authors identified parental depression, adverse childhood experiences, exposure to negative comments on weight, shape, and eating, and obesity as risk factors for negative outcomes. Psychiatric comorbidities and self-reported severe sexual abuse were risk factors for BED outcomes 12 years after inpatient treatment.[35] In a questionnaire study, higher scores on the Eating Disorder Inventory bulimia subscale at 6 months follow-up were predicted by lower scores for drive for thinness and hostility, and higher scores for bulimia, interoceptive awareness, anxiety, insufficiency, and a lack of familiarity with one's own body at the end of treatment.[46]

Currently, conclusive evidence for risk factors specific for BED is lacking.

Mortality

Two recent studies reported the mortality of ED. Based on a sample of 5839 inpatients with ED for whom long-term follow-up data on vital status were available, Fichter and Quadflieg[47] reported standardized mortality ratios (SMRs) of 2.39 for narrowly defined eating disorders not otherwise specified (ED-NOS), 1.70 for widely defined ED-NOS, 1.50 for BED, and 1.49 for BN. The highest SMR was observed for AN: 5.35. In a Swedish register study of 8069 female inpatients with AN conducted between 1973 and 2010, the presence of a psychiatric comorbidity increased mortality.[48] Mortality was also increased by the comorbidity of alcohol use disorder with AN. The mortality of EDs has somewhat decreased during the past decade. However, AN is still among the mental disorders with the highest mortality. Because the outcome of AN is generally worse than other EDs, different EDs should be distinguished and analyzed separately and not combined.

CONCLUSIONS

Because of the high rates of chronicity and mortality of EDs (particularly AN), early intervention is necessary for patients by all individuals who can provide assistance (clinicians, administrators, relatives, and friends). Interventions such as psychotherapy should be initiated in an institution by clinicians who are knowledgeable and experienced in the diagnosis and treatment of eating disorders.

REFERENCES

1. Löwe B, Zipfel S, Buchholz C, Dupont Y, Reas DL, Herzog W. Long-term outcome of anorexia nervosa in a prospective 21-year follow-up study. *Psychol Med.* 2001;31:881–890.
2. Zipfel S, Löwe B, Reas DL, Deter HC, Herzog W. Long-term prognosis in anorexia nervosa: lessons from a 21-year follow-up study. *Lancet.* 2000;355:721–722.
3. Keski-Rahkonen A, Raevuori A, Bulik CM, Hoek HW, Rissanen A, Kaprio J. Factors associated with recovery from anorexia nervosa: a population-based study. *Int J Eat Disord.* 2014;47:117–123.
4. Eddy KT, Tabri N, Thomas JJ, et al. Recovery from anorexia nervosa and bulimia nervosa at 22-year follow-up. *J Clin Psychiat.* 2017;78:184–189.
5. Mustelin L, Raevuori A, Bulik CM, et al. Long-term outcome in anorexia nervosa in the community. *Int J Eat Disord.* 2015;48:851–859.
6. Fichter MM, Quadflieg N, Crosby RD, Koch S. Long-term outcome of anorexia nervosa: results from a large clinical longitudinal study. *Int J Eat Disord.* 2017;50:1018–1030.
7. Lock J, Agras WS, Le Grange D, Couturier J, Safer D, Bryson SW. Do end of treatment assessments predict outcome at follow-up in eating disorders? *Int J Eat Disord.* 2013;46:771–778.
8. Bardone-Cone AM, Harney MB, Maldonado CR, et al. Defining recovery from an eating disorder: conceptualization, validation, and examination of psychosocial functioning and psychiatric comorbidity. *Behav Res Ther.* 2010;48:194–202.
9. Steinhausen HC. The outcome of anorexia nervosa in the 20th century. *Am J Psychiat.* 2002;159:1284–1293.
10. Franko DL, Tabri N, Keshaviah A, et al. Predictors of long-term recovery in anorexia nervosa and bulimia nervosa: data from a 22-year longitudinal study. *J Psychiat Res.* 2018; 96:183–188.
11. Wentz E, Gillberg IC, Anckarsäter H, Gillberg C, Rastam M. Adolescent-onset anorexia nervosa: 18-year outcome. *Br J Psychiat.* 2009;194:168–174.
12. Herpertz-Dahlmann B, Dempfle A, Egberts KM, et al. Outcome of childhood anorexia nervosa – the results of a five- tot en-year follow-up study. *Int J Eat Disord.* 2017;51: 295–304.
13. Amemiya N, Takii M, Hata T, et al. The outcome of Japanese anorexia nervosa patients treated with an inpatient therapy in an internal medicine unit. *Eat Weight Disord.* 2012;17:e1–e8.
14. Castellini G, Lo Sauro C, Mannucci E, et al. Diagnostic crossover and outcome predictors in eating disorders according to DSM-IV and DSM-V proposed criteria: a 6-year follow-up study. *Psychosom Med.* 2011;73:270–279.
15. Ekeroth K, Clinton D, Norring C, Birgegard A. Clinical characteristics and distinctiveness of DSM-5 eating disorder diagnoses: findings from a large naturalistic clinical database. *J Eat Disord.* 2013;1:31.
16. Hudson JI, Pope HG, Keck PE, McElroy SL. Treatment of bulimia nervosa with trazodone: short-term response and long-term follow-up. *Clin Neuropharmacol.* 1989;12:38–46.

17. Zeeck A, Weber S, Sandholz A, Joos A, Hartmann A. Stability of long-term outcome in bulimia nervosa: a 3-year follow-up. *J Clin Psychol.* 2011;67:318–327.

18. Agras WS, Crow S, Mitchell JE, Halmi KA, Bryson SA. 4-year prospective study of eating disorder NOS compared with full eating disorder syndromes. *Int J Eat Disord.* 2009;42:565–570.

19. Brewerton TD, Costin C. Long-term outcome of residential treatment for anorexia nervosa and bulimia nervosa. *Eat Disord.* 2011;19:132–144.

20. Helverskov JL, Clausen L, Mors O, Frydenberg M, Thomsen PH, Rokkedal K. Trans-diagnostic outcome of eating disorders: a 30-month follow-up study of 629 patients. *Eur Eat Disord Rev.* 2010;18:453–463.

21. McIntosh VVW, Carter FA, Bulik CM, Frampton CMA, Joyce PR. Five-year outcome of cognitive behavioral therapy and exposure with response prevention for bulimia nervosa. *Psychol Med.* 2011;41:1061–1071.

22. Rowe S, Jordan J, McIntosh V, et al. Dimensional measures of personality as a predictor of outcome at 5-year follow-up in woman with bulimia nervosa. *Psychiat Res.* 2011;185:414–420.

23. Van Son GE, van Hoeken D, van Furth EF, Donker GA, Hoek HW. Course and outcome of eating disorders in a primary care-based cohort. *Int J Eat Disord.* 2010;43:130–138.

24. Fichter MM, Quadflieg N. Twelve-year course and outcome of bulimia nervosa. *Psychol Med.* 2004;34:1395–1406.

25. Nakai Y, Nin K, Noma S, Hamagaki S, Takagi R, Wonderlich SA. Outcome of eating disorders in a Japanese sample: a 4- to 9-year follow-up study. *Eur Eat Disord Rev.* 2014;22:206–211.

26. Keel PK, Mitchell JE, Miller J, Miller KB, Davis TL, Crow SJ. Long-term outcome of bulimia nervosa. *Arch Gen Psychiat.* 1999;56:63–69.

27. Abraham S. Sexuality and reproduction in bulimia nervosa patients over 10 years. *J Psychosom Res.* 1998;44:491–502.

28. Milos G, Spindler A, Schnyder U, Fairburn CG. Instability of eating disorder diagnoses: prospective study. *Br J Psychiat.* 2005;187:573–578.

29. Keel PK, Dorer DJ, Franko DL, Jackson SC, Herzog DB. Postremission predictors of relapse in women with eating disorders. *Am J Psychiat.* 2005;162:2263–2268.

30. Calugi S, Ruocco A, El Ghoch M, et al. Residential cognitive-behavioral weight-loss intervention for obesity with and without binge-eating disorder: a prospective case–control study with five-year follow-up. *Int J Eat Disord.* 2016;49:723–730.

31. De Zwaan M, Herpertz S, Zipfel S, et al. Effect of internet-based guided self-help vs individual face-to-face treatment on full or subsyndromal binge eating disorder in overweight or obese patients. The INTERBED randomized clinical trial. *JAMA Psychiat.* 2017;74:987–995.

32. Friederich HC, Schild S, Wild B, et al. Treatment outcome in people with subthreshold compared with full-syndrome binge-eating disorder. *Obesity.* 2007;15:283–287.

33. Grilo CM, Pagano ME, Stout RL, et al. Stressful life events predict eating disorder relapse following remission: six-year prospective outcomes. *Int J Eat Disord.* 2012;45:185–192.

34. Welch E, Jangmo A, Thornton LM, et al. Treatment-seeking patients with binge-eating disorder in the Swedish national registers: clinical course and psychiatric comorbidity. *BMC Psychiatr.* 2016;16:163.

35. Fichter MM, Quadflieg N, Hedlund S. Long-term course of binge-eating disorder and bulimia nervosa: relevance for nosology and diagnostic criteria. *Int J Eat Disord.* 2008;41:577–586.

36. Munsch S, Meyer AH, Biedert E. Efficacy and predictors of long-term treatment success for cognitive-behavioural treatment and behavioural weight-loss-treatment in overweight individuals with binge-eating disorder. *Behav Res Ther.* 2012;50:775–785.

37. Vall E, Wade TD. Predictors of treatment outcome in individuals with eating disorders: a systematic review and meta-analysis. *Int J Eat Disord.* 2015;48:946–971.

38. O'Brien KM, Whelan DR, Sandler DP, Hall JE, Weinberg CR. Predictors and long-term health outcomes of eating disorders. *PLoS One.* 2017;12:e0181104.

39. Ward A, Ramsay R, Russell G, Treasure J. Follow-up mortality study of compulsorily treated patients with anorexia nervosa. *Int J Eat Disord.* 2015;48:860–865.

40. Ackard DM, Richter S, Egan A, Cronemeyer C. Poor outcome and death among youth, young adults, and midlife adults with eating disorders: an investigation of risk factors by age at assessment. *Int J Eat Disord.* 2014;47:825–835.

41. Wagner G, Penelo E, Nobis G, et al. Predictors for good therapeutic outcome and drop-out in technology assisted guided self-help in the treatment of bulimia nervosa and bulimia like phenotype. *Eur Eat Disord Rev.* 2015;23:163–169.

42. Turnbull SJ, Schmidt U, Troop NA, Tiller J, Todd G, Treasure JL. Predictors of outcome for two treatments for bulimia nervosa: short and long term. *Int J Eat Disord.* 1997;21:17–22.

43. Bodell LP, Brown TA, Keel PK. Weight suppression predicts bulimic symptoms at 20-year follow-up: the mediating role of drive for thinness. *J Abnorm Psychol.* 2017;126:32.

44. Keski-Rahkonen A, Mustelin L. Epidemiology of eating disorders in Europe: prevalence, incidence, comorbidity, course, consequences, and risk factors. *Curr Opin Psychiatry.* 2016;29:340–345.

45. Fairburn CG, Doll HA, Welch SL, Hay PJ, Davis BA, O'Connor ME. Risk factors for binge eating disorder. *Arch Gen Psychiat.* 1998;55:425–432.

46. Lammers MW, Vroling MS, Ouwens MA, Engels RCME, van Strien T. Predictors of outcome for cognitive behaviour therapy in binge eating disorder. *Eur Eat Disord Rev.* 2015;23:219–228.

47. Fichter MM, Quadflieg N. Mortality in eating disorders-results of a large prospective clinical longitudinal study. *Int J Eat Disord.* 2016;49:391–401.

48. Kask J, Ekselius L, Brandt L, Kollia N, Ekbom A, Papadopoulos FC. Mortality in women with anorexia nervosa: the role of comorbid psychiatric disorders. *Psychosom Med.* 2016;78:910–919.

CHAPTER 27

Outcome of Childhood Obesity

DORTHE C. PEDERSEN, MSC • THORKILD I.A. SØRENSEN, MD • JENNIFER L. BAKER, PHD

INTRODUCTION

Alongside with the increasing prevalence of obesity in childhood, the degree of obesity is also increasing, and health effects that used to be limited to adults in middle age are now appearing in children at progressively younger ages. In recognition of the serious concurrent and future health consequences of obesity in childhood, several international organizations have declared it a disease.[1] The declaration is controversial, but it serves to highlight that obesity in childhood is a serious risk to health and that it requires professional and effective treatment. In this era where 18% of children worldwide have overweight or obesity,[2] the impact on global public health is potentially enormous.

Immediate Consequences of Childhood Obesity

Cardiovascular and metabolic complications

Excess childhood body mass index (BMI; kg/m^2) is linked to numerous cardiovascular disease (CVD) risk factors, such as adverse levels of lipids, lipoproteins, inflammatory cytokines, blood pressure, increased arterial stiffness, and endothelial dysfunction.[3] Although direct comparisons across studies are challenging because of the various classification systems used for defining overweight and obesity in childhood, the totality of the evidence supports that the higher the level of excess adiposity, the more likely a child is to have elevated CVD risk factors. These associations are especially evident at the extremes of BMI, such that comparisons of children with BMI values from the 95th to 99th and greater than the 99th percentiles for age and sex show that their risks of having three elevated CVD risk factors increase from 18% to 33%.[4] Although studies have yet to pinpoint the youngest ages at which elevated CVD risk factors emerge, adverse levels of lipids, lipoproteins, and blood pressure can be detected in children with excess BMI at ages as young as 6 years.[5]

Children with obesity are also at increased risks of developing hyperinsulinemia, insulin resistance, and impaired glucose tolerance. The risks of these keep rising with higher levels of BMI. One study showed that 12% of children with moderate obesity (standard deviation score of 2–2.5) had impaired glucose tolerance, whereas 18% of children with severe obesity (standard deviation score above 2.5) had this condition.[6] There are also indications that the risk of having lower glucose tolerance and higher insulin resistance increases with childhood age. Although there can be progression to type 2 diabetes mellitus (T2D), this only manifests in adolescents with severe obesity. Nonetheless, these complications of the hyperglycemic state do not occur in isolation—they tend to cluster with other components of the metabolic syndrome such as high blood pressure and adverse levels of lipids and lipoproteins.[6]

Hepatic complications

The severity of obesity in children is strongly associated with the risk of nonalcoholic fatty liver disease (NAFLD), which ranges from steatosis to steatohepatitis to fibrosis and results in cirrhosis.[3] NAFLD has been reported in young children but is more prevalent among children above age 10 years.[7] Although the prevalence of NAFLD is up to 80% in children with obesity, compared with 3%–10% in the general pediatric population,[7] the more severe cases of the disease can be difficult to estimate as a liver biopsy is needed to make the diagnosis.

Pulmonary complications

A child with obesity is at increased risk of suffering from obstructive sleep apnea syndrome (OSAS). Both the prevalence and the severity of the disease increase with BMI, but the association between obesity and OSAS occurs mainly in adolescents.[8] Associations with asthma and childhood obesity have been reported as well. A metaanalysis of prospective studies found that the risk of physician-diagnosed asthma increased by 50% in children with obesity.[9]

Eating Disorders and Obesity in Children and Adolescents. https://doi.org/10.1016/B978-0-323-54852-6.00027-6

Musculoskeletal complications

Children with obesity are more likely to suffer from knee pain and increased rates of fractures.[3] Furthermore, Blount disease, a growth disorder where the shin bone bows outward, is more prevalent in children with obesity and the risk increases with the severity of obesity.[3] Additionally, children with obesity also have decreased mobility. In turn, this may be related to musculoskeletal fitness as it has been shown to be reduced in children and adolescents with obesity when compared with normal-weight peers. Reduced musculoskeletal fitness may further affect the level of physical activity negatively and thus exacerbate itself.[10]

Psychologic and psychosocial complications

Stigmatization of children with obesity is one of the most well-documented psychosocial aspects of childhood obesity, covered in Chapter 19, but associations with several other psychosocial comorbidities also exist. Age is an important factor for psychosocial complications, as many of these become especially apparent around pubertal ages.

Several studies demonstrate that children with obesity are more likely to have a lower health-related quality of life than normal-weight children[3] and that the impact is stronger in older than younger children.[11] Children with obesity have a four to eight times greater risk of being teased or bullied than their normal-weight peers.[11] Studies have also shown that children and adolescents with obesity are more likely to be involved in bullying behavior. The issue is complex as children and adolescents with obesity, especially boys, may be both perpetrators and victims of bullying.[12] Childhood obesity is also consistently associated with lower self-esteem, and children with obesity are more likely to have lower perceived self-worth than children with normal weight. Also, older children with obesity have lower self-esteem about their physical appearance than younger children with obesity.[11]

Obesity in childhood may be associated with depression, but findings are conflicting. Some studies show no increased risk of depression among children with obesity, whereas other studies find increased risks.[11] Adolescents with obesity are also more likely to have anxiety than children with normal weight. For both depression and anxiety, there are some indications that girls with obesity are more likely to develop these conditions than boys with obesity.[11]

A higher prevalence of loss-of-control eating and binge eating symptoms may be found among children and adolescents with obesity than in children with normal weight.[3] Nonetheless, it remains unclear which comes first—the binge eating or the obesity. Worryingly, 24% of girls with overweight or obesity use extreme weight-control behaviors, which include the abuse of laxatives and diet pills as well as vomiting.[13] Furthermore, the lifetime prevalence of bulimia is higher in individuals who have an onset of obesity in childhood.[11]

SUMMARY

Risks for concurrent health consequences of obesity in childhood strongly depend on the severity of the obesity, with some indications that risks sharply increase among children with the highest BMI values. Furthermore, there are important effects of age; all health complications are more prevalent in older children. Nonetheless, obesity at young ages is harmful as CVD risk factors and NAFLD are identifiable in young children. In concordance with the physical consequences, age is also important for the risks of psychosocial comorbidities, as older children with obesity were more likely to have lower self-esteem and health-related quality of life and engage in extreme weight loss behaviors than younger children. As many of these complications and eating disorders become apparent at adolescent ages, this may be an especially vulnerable life stage for adolescents with obesity.

Long-term Consequences of Childhood Obesity

Obesity

One of the biggest risks of childhood obesity is the risk that the child will also be obese as an adult and thus suffer from all of its associated comorbidities. Although, as described in Chapter 10, not all obese children become obese adults, the risk increases with increasing childhood BMI. Furthermore, the risk increases with childhood age; an adolescent with obesity is more likely to be an obese adult than a young child with obesity.

All-cause mortality

Excess BMI in children and adolescents is associated with an increased risk of all-cause mortality,[14] and these risks appear at levels of BMI that are below current definitions of overweight and obesity.[15] For example, compared with lean men in the Harvard Growth Study with more than 50 years of follow-up, men with a BMI above the 75th percentile in any 2 years at adolescent ages had a relative risk of all-cause mortality of 1.8. When examining long-term health consequences and searching for the underlying mechanisms, considering whether the associations operate through adult BMI is important.

In this study, the association remained statistically significant in the subgroup of men for whom adjustment for adult BMI was possible.[16] This study did not detect an association in women, but other studies did show similar risk estimates as in men, however, without taking adult body size into account.

Cardiovascular disease

Excess child BMI increases risks of coronary heart disease (CHD), and these risks are not limited only to children with overweight or obesity. Using data from a population-based cohort of Danish schoolchildren, we showed that the higher the child's BMI, the higher the risk of CHD morbidity and mortality. Furthermore, these associations strengthened with childhood age from 7 to 13 years.[17] For ischemic stroke, we found that there was a threshold effect of childhood BMI, as below-average BMI values were not associated with the risk, but above-average BMI values were. Compared with children with a BMI in the 25th to 75th percentiles, those with a BMI above the 95th percentile had a 77% increased risk of ischemic stroke at young ages (25–55 years).[18]

Type 2 diabetes mellitus

Obesity in childhood, even among children younger than 6 years of age, increases risks of T2D. A recent meta-analysis found that one standard deviation increase in BMI was associated with an odds ratio of 1.8 and 1.7 among children ages 7–11 years and 12–18 years, respectively.[19] A study in the population-based cohort of Danish schoolchildren showed that, again, there was a threshold effect for the association between child BMI and T2D in adulthood. Below-average BMI values did not have associations with T2D. However, at BMI values above average the association between BMI and T2D increased linearly. For example, a child BMI at one standard deviation above average is associated with a more than doubling of the risk of type 2 diabetes during the ages 30 through 46 years, slightly more so in women than in men (hazard ratios of 2.3 for women and 2.1 for men compared with a hazard ratio of 1.0 at average BMI).[20]

Cancer

Excess BMI in childhood is also linked to increased risks of several forms of cancer. Cancer is a heterogeneous disease, and the strength and directions of the associations depend on the type of cancer. Higher childhood BMI is associated with a decreased risk of premenopausal breast cancer, and this is in accord with the known adult associations.[21] Few studies in this area

on other cancers than breast cancer exist. In our work based on a cohort of Danish schoolchildren, it has been shown that higher childhood BMI values, yet at levels far below internationally accepted definitions of overweight and obesity, are associated with cancer of the liver,[22] thyroid,[23] pancreas (until the age of 70 years),[24] colon,[25] and esophagus.[26] Associations were also found between BMI and endometrial cancer, but there was a threshold effect; substantially increased risks were only observed at high BMI values (>90th percentile).[27]

SUMMARY

Higher childhood BMI values are associated with both adult morbidity and mortality, and obesity, especially in older children, confers the greatest risk for a wide range of chronic diseases. This series of studies gives insights into how early the origins of many diseases may lie, but they do not demonstrate whether child BMI exerts effects on adult disease independently of adult BMI. Nonetheless, they highlight that obesity in childhood is indicative of risks to adult health.

Weight Patterns from Childhood to Adult Ages and Mortality and Morbidity

Relatively, few studies have investigated the association between weight patterns across the life course and risks of morbidity and mortality. A study in Swedish men showed that increases in age-adjusted BMI from age 8 to 20 years increased risks of all-cause and cardiovascular mortality. Men who had overweight at age 8 years, but not at age 20, had similar risk for cardiovascular mortality as men who had normal weight at both ages.[15]

A study in the cohort of Danish school children examined weight patterns in boys (ages 7–13 years) to early adulthood (around ages 19 years) and the risk of T2D and found that boys who gained in BMI had increased risks of adult T2D. Encouragingly, the study found that boys with overweight at age 7 years but who remitted by age 13 and maintained normal weight as young men reduced their risks of T2D to levels observed among men who were normal weight at all ages.[28]

Taken together, the results from these studies suggest that the consequences of childhood obesity are reversible if a child normalizes his weight before adolescence, whereas the consequences of obesity in adolescence are not fully reversible. Furthermore, the studies highlight that a substantial weight gain confers a great risk in itself independent of attained body weight and of age for different diseases.

SUMMARY

Overweight and obesity in childhood and adolescence increase risks of current and future health and well-being. Furthermore, the risk of obesity-related consequences increases with age; childhood and adolescence are two very different developmental phases in life. Because physicians are not exempt from stigmatizing children and adolescents with obesity and their families, special care should be taken to establish a good relationship with both the child and the parents to prevent the avoidance of the medical system, which is of obvious importance for this young patient group.

Although the risk of negative outcomes increases dramatically at overweight and obese BMI values, for many diseases the risks increase across the entire range of BMI, whereas for other diseases there appears to be a threshold effect with increases in risk only for BMI values exceeding the average levels. Although it is intriguing that the adverse effects of childhood obesity seem to be reversible if the weight normalizes before adolescence, interpretations should be made carefully as there is limited evidence in this area.

To improve our knowledge and to allow us to disentangle the effects of the severity of obesity and age, future research should focus on BMI across the range and the timing of when excess BMI emerges across the life course. Future studies should undertake careful examinations of the temporality of these associations, especially for the psychologic and psychosocial complications but others as well, as it is unclear whether overweight and obesity precede or follow the conditions. Furthermore, additional study designs are needed to elucidate the causality of these associations. These considerations are important because we need insight into whether the consequences of excess BMI in childhood can be reversed and whether there is an age, where this is no longer possible, as this would call for different approaches for treatment and prevention.

REFERENCES

1. Farpour-Lambert NJ, Baker JL, Hassapidou M, et al. Childhood obesity is a chronic disease demanding specific health care–a position statement from the Childhood Obesity Task Force (COTF) of the European Association for the Study of Obesity (EASO). *Obes Facts.* 2015;8(5):342–349.
2. NCD Risk Factor Collaboration (NCD-RisC). Data Visualisations, Child & Adolescent Body-Mass Index. http://www.ncdrisc.org/overweight-prevalence-distribution-ado.html. Accessed January 31, 2018.
3. Kelly AS, Barlow SE, Rao G, et al. Severe obesity in children and adolescents: identification, associated health risks, and treatment approaches: a scientific statement from the American Heart Association. *Circulation.* 2013;128(15):1689–1712.
4. Freedman DS, Mei Z, Srinivasan SR, Berenson GS, Dietz WH. Cardiovascular risk factors and excess adiposity among overweight children and adolescents: the Bogalusa Heart Study. *J Pediatr.* 2007;150(1):12–17.e1.
5. Skinner AC, Perrin EM, Moss LA, Skelton JA. Cardiometabolic risks and severity of obesity in children and young adults. *N Engl J Med.* 2015;373(14):1307–1317.
6. Calcaterra V, Klersy C, Muratori T, et al. Prevalence of metabolic syndrome (MS) in children and adolescents with varying degrees of obesity. *Clin Endocrinol.* 2008;68(6):868–872.
7. Alisi A, Feldstein AE, Villani A, Raponi M, Nobili V. Pediatric nonalcoholic fatty liver disease: a multidisciplinary approach. *Nat Rev Gastroenterol Hepatol.* 2012;9(3):152–161.
8. Kohler MJ, Thormaehlen S, Kennedy JD, et al. Differences in the association between obesity and obstructive sleep apnea among children and adolescents. *J Clin Sleep Med.* 2009;5(6):506–511.
9. Egan KB, Ettinger AS, Bracken MB. Childhood body mass index and subsequent physician-diagnosed asthma: a systematic review and meta-analysis of prospective cohort studies. *BMC Pediatr.* 2013;13:121.
10. Thivel D, Ring-Dimitriou S, Weghuber D, Frelut ML, O'Malley G. Muscle strength and fitness in pediatric obesity: a systematic review from the European Childhood Obesity Group. *Obes Facts.* 2016;9(1):52–63.
11. Rankin J, Matthews L, Cobley S, et al. Psychological consequences of childhood obesity: psychiatric comorbidity and prevention. *Adolesc Health Med Therapeut.* 2016;7:125–146.
12. Bacchini D, Licenziati MR, Garrasi A, et al. Bullying and victimization in overweight and obese outpatient children and adolescents: an Italian multicentric study. *PLoS One.* 2015;10(11):e0142715.
13. Neumark-Sztainer DR, Wall MM, Haines JI, Story MT, Sherwood NE, van den Berg PA. Shared risk and protective factors for overweight and disordered eating in adolescents. *Am J Prev Med.* 2007;33(5):359–369.
14. Mossberg HO. 40-year follow-up of overweight children. *Lancet.* 1989;2(8661):491–493.
15. Ohlsson C, Bygdell M, Sonden A, Rosengren A, Kindblom JM. Association between excessive BMI increase during puberty and risk of cardiovascular mortality in adult men: a population-based cohort study. *Lancet Diabetes Endocrinol.* 2016;4(12):1017–1024.
16. Must A, Jacques PF, Dallal GE, Bajema CJ, Dietz WH. Long-term morbidity and mortality of overweight adolescents. A follow-up of the Harvard Growth Study of 1922 to 1935. *N Engl J Med.* 1992;327(19):1350–1355.
17. Baker JL, Olsen LW, Sørensen TIA. Childhood body-mass index and the risk of coronary heart disease in adulthood. *N Engl J Med.* 2007;357(23):2329–2337.

18. Gjærde LK, Gamborg M, Angquist L, Truelsen TC, Sørensen TIA, Baker JL. Association of childhood body mass index and change in body mass index with first adult ischemic stroke. *JAMA Neurol.* 2017;74(11):1312–1318.

19. Llewellyn A, Simmonds M, Owen CG, Woolacott N. Childhood obesity as a predictor of morbidity in adulthood: a systematic review and meta-analysis. *Obes Rev.* 2016;17(1):56–67.

20. Zimmermann E, Bjerregaard LG, Gamborg M, Vaag AA, Sørensen TIA, Baker JL. Childhood body mass index and development of type 2 diabetes throughout adult life-A large-scale Danish cohort study. *Obesity.* 2017;25(5):965–971.

21. Ahlgren M, Melbye M, Wohlfahrt J, Sørensen TIA. Growth patterns and the risk of breast cancer in women. *N Engl J Med.* 2004;351(16):1619–1626.

22. Berentzen TL, Gamborg M, Holst C, Sørensen TIA, Baker JL. Body mass index in childhood and adult risk of primary liver cancer. *J Hepatol.* 2014;60(2):325–330.

23. Kitahara CM, Gamborg M, Berrington de Gonzalez A, Sørensen TIA, Baker JL. Childhood height and body mass index were associated with risk of adult thyroid cancer in a large cohort study. *Cancer Res.* 2014;74(1):235–242.

24. Nogueira L, Stolzenberg-Solomon R, Gamborg M, Sørensen TIA, Baker JL. Childhood body mass index and risk of adult pancreatic cancer. *Curr Dev Nutr.* 2017;1(10).

25. Jensen BW, Gamborg M, Gogenur I, Renehan AG, Sørensen TIA, Baker JL. Childhood body mass index and height in relation to site-specific risks of colorectal cancers in adult life. *Eur J Epidemiol.* 2017;32(12):1097–1106.

26. Cook MB, Freedman ND, Gamborg M, Sørensen TIA, Baker JL. Childhood body mass index in relation to future risk of oesophageal adenocarcinoma. *Br J Cancer.* 2015;112(3):601–607.

27. Aarestrup J, Gamborg M, Ulrich LG, Sørensen TIA, Baker JL. Childhood body mass index and height and risk of histologic subtypes of endometrial cancer. *Int J Obes.* 2016;40(7):1096–1102.

28. Bjerregaard LG, Jensen BW, Angquist L, Osler M, Sørensen TIA, Baker JL. Change in overweight from childhood to early adulthood and risk of type 2 diabetes. *N Engl J Med.* 2018;378(14):1302–1312.

CHAPTER 28

Eating Disorder Prevention Programs

ERIC STICE, BS, MS, PhD • AVIVA JOHNS, MA •
SAMANTHA WILKINSON, BA

INTRODUCTION

Eating disorders (EDs) affect 13% of females[1,2] and are marked by chronicity, relapse, distress, functional impairment, and increased risk for future obesity, depression, suicide, substance abuse, and mortality.[2–4] Given that 80% of individuals with EDs do not receive treatment,[4] a pressing public health priority is to broadly implement ED prevention programs that have been found to reduce future onset of EDs or initial ED symptoms. This chapter first summarizes risk factors that have been found to predict future onset of EDs, as these findings guide which factors prevention programs should seek to reduce, as well as which high-risk subgroups to target with selective prevention programs. Next, it summarizes the evidence base for prevention programs that reduce future ED onset or symptoms. In this context, implementation efforts with selected ED prevention programs are reviewed. Finally, this chapter concludes by offering suggestions for future research on ED prevention.

Risk Factors for Future Onset of Eating Disorders
Anorexia nervosa

Only two truly prospective studies used risk factors assessed at baseline to predict future onset of anorexia nervosa (AN) or subthreshold AN among individuals confirmed to be free of an ED at baseline. This type of prospective design definitively establishes that the risk factors temporally preceded onset of clinically significant eating pathology. Low body mass index (BMI) and low dieting predicted onset of threshold or subthreshold AN over a 5-year follow-up, but early puberty, perceived pressure for thinness, thin-ideal internalization, body dissatisfaction, negative affect, and social support deficits did not.[5] Similarly, over a 3-year follow-up in a high-risk sample of young women with body dissatisfaction, low BMI and impaired psychosocial functioning predicted onset of threshold or subthreshold AN,

but thin-ideal internalization, positive expectances regarding thinness, denying the costs of pursuing the thin ideal, body dissatisfaction, weight control behaviors, dieting, overeating, fasting, excessive exercise, negative affect, and mental health care did not.[6]

Three retrospective studies assessed risk factors during a developmental period that predates typical AN emergence. Vaginal instrumental delivery, cephalhematoma, premature birth, low birth weight, and cobirth correlated with lifetime AN diagnosis, but maternal age at childbirth, number of overall maternal births, diabetes, preterm membrane rupture, cesarean delivery, neonatal jaundice, and pregnancy complications, hypertension, and bleeding did not.[7] In a longitudinal study, childhood eating conflicts correlated with subthreshold AN onset over an 8- to 17-year follow-up, whereas childhood pica, digestive problems, not eating, disinterest in food, picky eating, and eating too little or too slowly did not.[8] Controlling for childhood ED symptoms, perfectionism and low BMI during childhood correlated with lifetime diagnoses of threshold or subthreshold AN, but negative affect, impulsivity, and family functioning did not.[9]

Bulimia nervosa

Seven prospective studies examined risk factors that predicted future onset of bulimia nervosa (BN) or subthreshold BN. Adolescent dieters versus nondieters showed greater threshold or subthreshold BN onset over a 1-year follow-up.[10] Weight concerns, drive for thinness, body dissatisfaction, ineffectiveness, negative affectivity, dieting, alcohol use, and lower interoceptive awareness predicted BN onset over a 4-year follow-up, but perfectionism, maturity fears, interpersonal distrust, and BMI did not.[11] Dieting and psychiatric problems predicted BN onset over a 3-year follow-up, but peer dieting, daily exercise, and parental separation did not.[12] Elevated BMI, social pressure for thinness, thin-ideal internalization, dieting, fasting, negative affect, social support deficits, and early puberty predicted BN onset over a 5-year follow-up, but body dissatisfaction did not.[5,13] Social pressure to be thin and body dissatisfaction predicted BN onset over a 7-year follow-up, but thin-ideal internalization, dieting, negative affect, and depressive symptoms did not.[14] Thin-ideal internalization, positive expectances from thinness, denying costs of pursuing the thin ideal, body dissatisfaction, dieting, overeating, fasting, negative affect, impaired social functioning, and mental health care predicted BN onset over a 3-year follow-up in a high-risk sample of body-dissatisfied young women, but weight control behaviors, excessive exercise, and BMI did not.[6]

Two studies assessed risk factors during a developmental period that predates the typical emergence of BN, although neither study confirmed that participants were free of an ED at baseline. Eating too little during childhood correlated with BN onset over an 8–17 year follow-up, but childhood pica, digestive problems, eating conflicts, not eating, disinterest in food, picky eating, and eating too slowly did not.[8] Controlling for childhood ED symptoms, negative affect during childhood correlated with lifetime diagnoses of BN, but perfectionism, BMI, impulsivity, and family functioning did not.[9]

Binge eating disorder

Only two studies investigated baseline factors that predicted future onset of threshold or subthreshold binge eating disorder (BED). Social pressure for thinness predicted BED onset over a 7-year follow-up, but thin-ideal internalization, body dissatisfaction, dieting, and negative affect/depressive symptoms did not.[14] Thin-ideal internalization, positive expectances regarding thinness, body dissatisfaction, dieting, overeating, negative affect, impaired social functioning, and mental healthcare predicted BED onset over a 3-year follow-up in a high-risk sample of body-dissatisfied young women, but denying costs of pursuing the thin-ideal, weight control behaviors, fasting, excessive exercise, and BMI did not.[6]

Purging disorder

Only two studies investigated baseline risk factors predicting purging disorder (PD) onset. Thin-ideal internalization, body dissatisfaction, and dieting predicted PD onset over a 7-year follow-up, but social pressure to be thin, negative affect, and depressive symptoms did not.[14] Thin-ideal internalization, positive expectances about thinness, denying costs of pursuing the thin ideal, body dissatisfaction, dieting, fasting, overeating, excessive exercise, negative affect, impaired social

functioning, and mental healthcare predicted PD onset over a 3-year follow-up in a high-risk sample of body-dissatisfied young women, but weight control behaviors and BMI did not.[6]

Pursuit of the thin beauty ideal, body dissatisfaction, overeating, dieting, fasting, and psychosocial impairment predicted onset of BN, BED, and PD. These findings suggest that prevention programs should target individuals with elevated levels of these risk factors in selective prevention programs. However, most risk factors reviewed above have not predicted future AN onset. Curiously, low BMI and low dieting predicted AN onset, suggesting individuals who are constitutionally thin, or thin because of other factors, are at risk for AN. These findings imply that current evidence-based ED prevention programs may be ineffective in preventing AN onset and that it might be necessary to target low-weight adolescent girls with programs that promote healthy weight gain.

Current etiologic theories of eating pathology do not implicate impaired psychosocial functioning. However, only impaired psychosocial functioning predicted onset of all four EDs, implying that a prevention program improving psychosocial functioning among young women might effectively prevent the full spectrum of EDs, rather than only those involving binge eating and compensatory behaviors.

Evidence-Based Eating Disorder Prevention Programs

Although dozens of ED prevention programs have been developed and evaluated, most have not reduced future onset of EDs, the ultimate goal of prevention programs, or initial ED symptoms. Herein, we describe ED prevention programs that have produced effects for one or both of these two key outcomes.

Body project

The *Body Project* produced significantly greater reductions in ED symptoms than the *Healthy Weight* ED prevention program, an expressive writing comparison condition, and assessment-only controls and produced significantly greater reductions in future ED onset over a 3-year follow-up than assessment-only controls in a large efficacy trial.[15,16] In this dissonance-based group intervention, young women critique the thin beauty ideal in verbal, written, and behavioral exercises, prompting them to reduce their pursuit of this unrealistic ideal because people align their attitudes with their publically displayed behaviors.[17] Reduced thin-ideal internalization putatively decreases body dissatisfaction, dieting, negative affect, and ED symptoms.

Evidence that *Body Project* produced greater symptom reductions than alternative credible prevention programs provides evidence that effects are not simply due to demand characteristics and expectances inherent to randomized trials. It also produced significantly greater reductions in ED symptoms in other efficacy trials conducted by our team[18,19] and others.[20-23] In support of the intervention theory, participants randomized to versions of *Body Project* designed to maximize versus minimize dissonance induction showed greater ED symptom reductions,[24,25] and the *Body Project* also reduced responsivity of the brain reward region to thin models compared with educational brochure controls.[26] Evidence that *Body Project* reduced objectively measured neural responses further reduces concerns that effects are due to demand characteristics. It is critical that *Body Project* has produced effects in trials conducted by several independent teams because many findings do not replicate.[27]

Effectiveness trials confirmed that *Body Project* reduces ED symptoms when delivered by high school and college counselors under ecologically valid conditions,[28-31] although in the effectiveness trials, *Body Project* did not significantly reduce future ED onset. Of note, other effectiveness trials indicate that *Body Project* produces reductions in ED symptoms when delivered by undergraduate peer educators.[32-36] In the latest effectiveness trial, participants who completed peer-led *Body Project* groups showed a significant 74% reduction in future ED onset over a 6-month follow-up relative to participants who completed an Internet-based version of the *Body Project*.[32] It is important to note that the Internet-based version of the *Body Project* did produce significant reductions in ED symptoms at posttest and a 6-month follow-up, as this is a rare effect for ED prevention programs.

Healthy weight

The *Healthy Weight* prevention program reduced ED onset and symptoms relative to expressive writing and assessment-only controls over a 3-year follow-up.[15,16] Relative to *Body Project*, expressive-writing controls, and assessment-only controls, *Healthy Weight* reduced BMI gain and obesity onset.[15] In this group-based intervention, young women with body image concerns make healthy changes to dietary intake and exercise that bring caloric intake and expenditure into balance, which should reduce weight gain and risk for eating pathology. The lifestyle change plan is participant-driven to promote internalization of health goals and executive control over lifestyle choices. A version of *Healthy Weight*, including nutritional principles, resulted in

greater ED symptom reductions, a 60% reduction in ED onset over a 2-year follow-up versus educational brochure controls, and less BMI gain through a 6-month follow-up in a second efficacy trial.[37] An expanded six-session version of *Healthy Weight* produced greater reductions in ED symptoms and BMI than the cognitive reappraisal–based *Minding Health* prevention program and greater reductions in body fat and ED symptoms than educational video controls in another efficacy trial.[38]

A 6-h dissonance-based version of *Healthy Weight* and *Project Health* added verbal and written exercises to create dissonance regarding unhealthy lifestyle behaviors and produced significantly smaller increases in BMI through a 2-year follow-up versus participants who completed *Healthy Weight* in an effectiveness trial.[39] *Project Health* participants also showed a 41% and 43% reduction in overweight/obesity onset over a 2-year follow-up versus *Healthy Weight* participants and controls, respectively. In response to Socratic questions, participants discuss costs of obesity and an unhealthy lifestyle, as well as benefits of leanness, healthy diets, and exercise in *Project Health*. Engaging in these activities theoretically increases the likelihood that participants' attitudes will align with the perspectives assumed in the sessions, resulting in healthier dietary and exercise choices. *Healthy Weight* and *Project Health* participants showed significantly greater ED symptom reductions than controls through a 2-year follow-up, as well as marginally lower eating disorder onset over a follow-up than controls.[39]

Student bodies

Although the *Student Bodies* ED prevention program did not produce a significant main effect for future ED onset reduction, it reduced future ED onset in certain subsets of participants included in trials. In a large efficacy trial, *Student Bodies* reduced future ED onset in women with weight and shape concerns versus waitlist controls over a 2-year follow-up at one of the two sites.[40] There was also evidence that *Student Bodies* produced a significant reduction in future ED onset among women with elevated BMI and compensatory behaviors at baseline.[40] *Student Bodies* is a cognitive-behavioral Internet-based program, wherein participants journal and engage in clinician-supervised group discussions. It seeks to reduce weight and shape concerns, informs participants about risks associated with EDs, and how to engage in healthy living practices over 8 weeks.[41] One study recruited high school students at or above the 85th percentile BMI for their age and who reported at least one binge episode per week for the past 3 months to receive either a modified, 16-week version of *Student Bodies* focusing on weight stabilization and healthy living practices or a waitlist control.[42] Intervention participants showed a significant reduction in reported binge episodes and BMI from baseline to posttreatment and from baseline to 4-month follow-up compared with the waitlist control group. Of note, the majority of participants in *Student Bodies* condition completed seven or fewer weeks of the online intervention, suggesting the acceptability of this intervention is low. Furthermore, because *Student Bodies* is moderated, it requires more clinician time than other evidence-based prevention programs. To our knowledge, *Student Bodies* has not been evaluated by independent research teams or in effectiveness trials.

Student Athlete Eating Disorder Prevention Program

This ED prevention program targeted at adolescent female and male elite athletes prevented ED symptoms and onset in females over a 1-year follow-up versus assessment-only controls.[43] Using the social-cognitive framework, adolescent male and female high school athletes work on augmenting self-esteem through self-efficacy and understanding intrinsic versus extrinsic motivation[44] and mastery versus performance goals,[45] to emphasize the importance of deriving strength from oneself rather than performance and significant others. At a 1-year follow-up, the program reduced EDs in female athletes, compared with control athletes, who showed a 5.5% increase in diagnoses of *DSM-IV* EDs. Although 26 participants had an ED before starting the intervention (intervention $n = 13$, control $n = 13$), 16 participants (intervention $n = 12$, control $n = 4$) no longer met ED criteria at the 1-year follow up. Upon program completion, intervention female athletes reported fewer EDs symptoms than female control athletes. However, this effect was weakened at the 1-year follow up. Thus, the program was efficacious in preventing and reducing ED symptoms in female athletes but had limited effects on male athletes. To our knowledge, this program has not been evaluated by independent research teams or in effectiveness trials.

Mindfulness eating disorder prevention

In one randomized control trial, women aged 17–31 years who reported body image concerns but did not have an ED were assigned to either a mindfulness-based intervention (MBI), a dissonance-based intervention (DBI), or an assessment-only control.[46] In the MBI, participants practiced mindfulness, discussed barriers to engaging in mindfulness, and completed exercises

aimed at countering negative body image–related thoughts during group sessions and homework.[47] Both group-based programs shared the same program structure—three 1-h group sessions over a period of 3 weeks led by graduate students, with two to four participants in each group. The MBI produced significant reductions in weight and shape concern (WSC), thin-ideal internalization, dietary restraint, ED symptoms, and psychosocial impairment, relative to assessment-only controls at posttreatment; only dietary restraint remained significantly reduced in the MBI relative to control at a 1-month follow-up, with no outcomes maintaining significance at a 6-month follow-up. At posttreatment, thin-ideal internalization was significantly lower in MBI relative to DBI, but this difference disappeared at 1-month and 6-month follow-ups. Participants in the DBI condition improved in dietary restraint and ED symptoms from baseline to posttreatment but did not show any significant differences relative to the assessment-only control at any time point. The sample size in this study was extremely small ($n = 37$). Moreover, the DBI did not include many of the exercises contained in *Body Project*, the training provided to clinicians in this trial was less intensive than the previously described trials, and no supervision was provided to clinicians. These factors may explain why this trial was not able to replicate the positive effects observed for dissonance-based ED prevention programs by most research teams. To our knowledge, MBI has not been evaluated in any additional trials by this research team or other teams, and it has not been evaluated in effectiveness trials.

IMPLEMENTATION EFFORTS

ED prevention programs have been shown to reduce ED onset and symptoms, prompting several exciting implementation efforts by various entities. Tri Delta, a national college sorority, initiated the first large implementation effort of an ED prevention program. Based on evidence that *Body Project* reduced body dissatisfaction and ED symptoms in female students in sororities,[20] the national chapter of sorority (Tri Delta) set the goal of reaching 20,000 young women with a rebranded version of *Body Project* referred to as *Reflections*. Over a 6-year period, Tri Delta supported the training of peer educators in the delivery of *Reflections* at over 100 universities across the United States.[48]

The Dove Self Esteem program also initiated a global implementation project to promote body acceptance in young women. They partnered with ED prevention experts and the World Association of Girl Guides and Girl Scouts to create a dissonance-based body acceptance ED prevention program referred to as *Free Being Me* designed for youth, ultimately reaching over 3.4 million preadolescent and adolescent girls in 125 countries.[48]

The Eating Recovery Center launched a major donor-funded implementation project. They have been underwriting training of peer educators at universities around the United States in the delivery of *Body Project*, hoping to implement this program in 85 universities over a 5-year period.[48]

The National Eating Disorder Association launched an implementation effort by training nearly 200 undergraduate peer leaders to implement *Body Project* in lower income area high schools throughout New York State. There are additional implementation efforts in several other countries, including Mexico, France, and Japan. The free availability and mounting evidence base for certain prevention programs appear to play a critical role in their adoption and implementation.

CONCLUSIONS AND DIRECTIONS FOR FUTURE RESEARCH

Four ED prevention programs have significantly reduced ED onset and/or symptoms, with another program producing these effects in certain subgroups of the larger samples in efficacy trials. Before the year 2000, no ED prevention program had produce either effect. In addition, the evidence base for ED prevention programs often includes rigorous tests of the intervention theory and effectiveness trials that determine whether the program works under ecologically valid conditions. Furthermore, several implementation projects have been launched, which have the potential to reduce the population prevalence of EDs.

There are a number of important directions for future research. First, it is critical to determine how to improve the efficacy of existing evidence-based ED prevention programs, as it is ideal to increase the magnitude and persistence of the intervention effects (e.g., by refining inclusion and exclusion criteria). Second, it would be useful to investigate procedures that promote broad sustained delivery of evidence-based ED prevention programs at universities and high schools. It will be critical to examine factors that influence adoption and implementation of evidence-based ED prevention programs, as well as factors predicting fidelity, competence, and sustainability of intervention delivery. Relatively, little is known about how best to broadly support clinicians and peer educators in sustainable delivery of these prevention programs. Third, emerging evidence suggests that pursuit of the thin beauty ideal, body dissatisfaction, and reported dieting predict future onset of BN, BED, and PD, but not onset of AN.[6] Given that most evidence-based prevention programs target individuals with body dissatisfaction and attempt to reduce pursuit of the thin beauty ideal, body dissatisfaction, and unhealthy weight control behaviors, these new etiologic findings imply that although existing evidence-based prevention programs are appropriate for the binge/compensatory behavior spectrum EDs, they may be less effective in preventing AN. The fact that low BMI, low dieting, and psychosocial impairment predict future onset of AN[6] implies that to optimally prevent restricting EDs, it might be necessary to target low BMI, early adolescent girls, and for the prevention programs to reduce qualitatively different risk factors. Finally, it is vital to continue conducting prospective risk factor studies to advance knowledge of subgroups at elevated risk for ED onset and additional risk factors, including biologic factors that predict ED onset. A more complete understanding of the risk processes that give rise to these pernicious disorders will eventually allow us to even more effectively prevent EDs.

REFERENCES

1. Allen KL, Byrne SM, Oddy WH, Crosby RD. DSM-IV-TR and DSM-5 eating disorders in adolescents: prevalence, stability, and psychosocial correlates in a population-based sample of male and female adolescents. *J Abnorm Psychol*. 2013;122:720–732.
2. Stice E, Marti C, Rohde P. Prevalence, incidence, impairment, and course of the proposed DSM-5 eating disorder diagnoses in an 8-year prospective community study of young women. *J Abnorm Psychol*. 2013;122:445–457. https://doi.org/10.1037/a0030679.
3. Arcelus J, Mitchell A, Wales J, Nielsen S. Mortality rates in patients with anorexia nervosa and other eating disorders: a meta-analysis of 36 studies. *Arch Gen Psychiatr*. 2011;68(7):724–731.
4. Swanson S, Crow S, Le Grange D, Swendsen J, Merikangas K. Prevalence and correlates of eating disorders in adolescents: results from the national comorbidity survey replication adolescent supplement. *Arch Gen Psychiatr*. July 2011;68(7):714–723.
5. Stice E, Bohon C. Eating disorders. In: Beauchaine TP, Hinshaw SP, eds. *Child and Adolescent Psychopathology*. Hoboken, New Jersey: Wiley and Sons; 2013:715–738.
6. Stice E, Gau J, Rohde P, Shaw H. Risk factors that predict future onset of each DSM-5 eating disorder: predictive specificity in high-risk adolescent females. *J Abnorm Psychol*. 2017;126:38–51.
7. Cnattingius S, Hultman C, Dahl M, Sparén P. Very preterm birth, birth trauma, and the risk of anorexia nervosa among girls. *Archiv General Psychiat*. 1999;56(7):634–638.

8. Kotler L, Cohen P, Davies M, Pine D, Walsh B. Longitudinal relationships between childhood, adolescent, and adult eating disorders. *J Am Acad Child Adolesc Psychiat.* 2001;40(12):1434–1440.

9. Tyrka A, Waldron I, Graber J, Brooks-Gunn J. Prospective predictors of the onset of anorexic and bulimic syndromes. *Int J Eating Disorders.* 2002;32(3):282–290.

10. Patton G, Johnson-Sabine E, Wood K, Mann A, Wakeling A. Abnormal eating attitudes in London schoolgirls: a prospective epidemiological study: outcome at twelve month follow-up. *Psychol Med.* 1990;20(2):383–394.

11. Killen J, Taylor C, Strachowski D, et al. Weight concerns influence the development of eating disorders: a 4-year prospective study. *J Consult Clin Psychol.* October 1996; 64(5):936–940.

12. Patton GC, Selzer R, Coffey C, Carlin JB, Wolfe R. Onset of adolescent eating disorders: population based cohort study over 3 years. *Br Med J.* 1999;318:765–768.

13. Stice E, Davis K, Miller NP, Marti CN. Fasting increases risk for onset of binge eating and bulimic pathology: a 5-year prospective study. *J Abnormal Psychol.* 2008;117(4): 941–946.

14. Stice E, Marti C, Durant S. Risk factors for onset of eating disorders: evidence of multiple risk pathways from an 8-year prospective study. *Behav Res Ther.* 2011; 49(10):622–627.

15. Stice E, Marti C, Spoor S, Presnell K, Shaw H. Dissonance and healthy weight eating disorder prevention programs: long-term effects from a randomized efficacy trial. *J Consult Clin Psychol.* 2008;76(2):329–340.

16. Stice E, Shaw H, Burton E, Wade E. Dissonance and healthy weight eating disorder prevention programs: a randomized efficacy trial. *J Consult Clin Psychol.* 2006; 74(2):263–275.

17. Festinger LA. *Theory of Cognitive Dissonance.* Stanford, Calif.: Stanford University Press; 1957.

18. Stice E, Mazotti L, Weibel D, Agras W. Dissonance prevention program decreases thin-ideal internalization, body dissatisfaction, dieting, negative affect, and bulimic symptoms: a preliminary experiment. *Int J Eat Disord.* 2000;27(2):206–217.

19. Stice E, Trost A, Chase A. Healthy weight control and dissonance-based eating disorder prevention programs: results from a controlled trial. *Int J Eat Disord.* 2003;33(1):10–21.

20. Becker C, Smith L, Ciao A. Reducing eating disorder risk factors in sorority members: a randomized trial. *Behav Ther.* 2005;36(3):245–253.

21. Halliwell E, Diedrichs P. Testing a dissonance body image intervention among young girls. *Health Psychol.* 2014; 33(2):201–204.

22. Mitchell K, Mazzeo S, Rausch S, Cooke K. Innovative interventions for disordered eating: evaluating dissonance-based and yoga interventions. *Int J Eat Disord.* 2007; 40(2):120–128.

23. Serdar K, Kelly N, Mazzeo S, et al. Comparing online and face-to-face dissonance-based eating disorder prevention. *Eat Disord: The J Treatment Prevent.* 2014;22(3):244–260.

24. Green M, Scott N, Diyankova I, Gasser C, Pederson E. Eating disorder prevention: an experimental comparison of high level dissonance, low level dissonance, and No-treatment control. *Eat Disord.* 2005;13(2):157–169.

25. McMillan W, Stice E, Rohde P. High- and low-level dissonance-based eating disorder prevention programs with young women with body image concerns: an experimental trial. *J Consult Clin Psychol.* 2011;79(1):129–134.

26. Stice E, Yokum S, Waters A. Dissonance-based eating disorder prevention program reduces reward region response to thin models; how actions shape valuation. *PLoS One.* 2015;10(12).

27. Ioannidis J, Munafò M, Fusar-Poli P, Nosek B, David S. Publication and other reporting biases in cognitive sciences: detection, prevalence, and prevention. *Trends Cognit Sci.* 2014;18(5):235–241.

28. Stice E, Butryn M, Rohde P, Shaw H, Marti C. An effectiveness trial of a new enhanced dissonance eating disorder prevention program among female college students. *Behav Res Ther.* 2013;51(12):862–871.

29. Stice E, Rohde P, Butryn M, Shaw H, Marti C. Effectiveness trial of a selective dissonance-based eating disorder prevention program with female college students: effects at 2- and 3-year follow-up. *Behav Res Ther.* 2015;71:20–26.

30. Stice E, Rohde P, Gau J, Shaw H. An effectiveness trial of a dissonance-based eating disorder prevention program for high-risk adolescent girls. *J Consult Clin Psychol.* 2009;77(5):825–834.

31. Stice E, Rohde P, Shaw H, Gau J. An effectiveness trial of a selected dissonance-based eating disorder prevention program for female high school students: long-term effects. *J Consult Clin Psychol.* 2011;79(4):500–508.

32. Stice E, Rohde P, Shaw H, Gau J. Clinician-led, peer-led, and Internet-delivered dissonance-based eating disorder prevention programs: acute effectiveness of these delivery modalities. *J Consult Clin Psychol.* 2017;85:883–895.

33. Becker C, McDaniel L, Bull S, Powell M, McIntyre K. Can we reduce eating disorder risk factors in female college athletes? A randomized exploratory investigation of two peer-led interventions. *Body Image.* 2012;9:31–42.

34. Ciao A, Latner J, Brown K, Ebneter D, Becker C. Effectiveness of a peer-delivered dissonance-based program in reducing eating disorder risk factors in high school girls. *Int J Eat Disord.* 2015;48(6):779–784.

35. Halliwell E, Jarman H, McNamara A, Risdon H, Jankowski G. Dissemination of evidence-based body image interventions: a pilot study into the effectiveness of using undergraduate students as interventionists in secondary schools. *Body Image.* 2015;14:1–4.

36. Stice E, Rohde P, Durant S, Shaw H, Wade E. Effectiveness of peer-led dissonance-based eating disorder prevention groups: results from two randomized pilot trials. *Behav Res Ther.* 2013;51(4–5):197–206.

37. Stice E, Rohde P, Shaw H, Marti C. Efficacy trial of a selective prevention program targeting both eating disorders and obesity among female college students: 1- and 2-year follow-up effects. *J Consult Clin Psychol.* 2013;81(1):183–189.

38. Stice E, Yokum S, Burger K, Rohde P, Shaw H, Gau JM. A pilot randomized trial of a cognitive reappraisal obesity prevention program. *Physiol Behav.* 2015;138:124–132.

39. Stice E, Rohde P, Shaw H, Gau J. An experimental therapeutics test of whether adding dissonance-induction activities improves the effectiveness of a selected obesity and eating disorder prevention program. *Int J Obes.* 2018; 42:462–468.

40. Taylor C, Bryson S, Wilfley D, et al. Prevention of eating disorders in at-risk college-age women. *Arch Gen Psychiatr.* 2006;63(8):881–888.

41. Winzelberg A, Eppstein D, Taylor C, et al. Effectiveness of an Internet-based program for reducing risk factors for eating disorders. *J Consult Clin Psychol.* 2000;68(2): 346–350.

42. Jones M, Luce K, Taylor C, et al. Randomized, controlled trial of an Internet-facilitated intervention for reducing binge eating and overweight in adolescents. *Pediatrics.* 2008;121(3):453–462.

43. Martinsen M, Bahr R, Borresen R, Holme I, Pensgaard A, Sundgot-Borden J. Preventing eating disorders among young elite athletes: a randomized controlled trial. *Med Sci Sports Exerc.* 2014;46:435–447.

44. Deci EL, Ryan RM. The "what" and "why" of goal pursuits: human needs and the self-determination of behavior. *Psychol Inq.* 2000;11(4):227–268.

45. Nicholls J. *The Competitive Ethos and Democratic Education [e-book].* Cambridge, MA, US: Harvard University Press; 1989.

46. Atkinson M, Wade T. Does mindfulness have potential in eating disorders prevention? A preliminary controlled trial with young adult women. *Early Intervent Psychiat.* 2016; 10(3):234–245.

47. Segal Z, Williams J, Teasdale J. Review of mindfulness-based cognitive therapy for depression: a new approach to preventing relapse. *Psychother Res.* 2003;13(1):123–125.

48. Becker C, Stice E. From efficacy to effectiveness to broad implementation: evolution of the Body Project. *J Consult Clin Psychol.* 2017;85(8):767–782.

Index

A

Acanthosis nigricans, 50
Acne, 50
Addiction
  addiction-like eating, 100
  definition, 99
  dysfunction, 99
  food addiction, 100
  gambling disorder, 100
  media reports, 99
  overeating, 99
  substance use, 99
  substance use disorder, 99
  sugar, 99
Addiction-like Eating Behaviour Scale, 101t
Adolescent eating disorders
  anorexia nervosa
    definition, 39–40
    symptomatology, 40
    treatment outcomes, 160
  bulimia nervosa
    binge eating disorder, 41
    definition, 40
    loss of control (LOC) eating, 41
    symptomatology, 41
  day patient (DP) treatment, 126
  endocrine changes, 42
  enhanced cognitive-behavioral therapy (CBT-E). See Enhanced cognitive-behavioral therapy (CBT-E)
  family-based therapy. See Family-based therapy (FBT)
  inpatient (IP) treatment. See inpatient (IP) treatment
  physical changes, 41t
  psychiatric comorbidity
    anxiety disorders, 43
    attention-deficit/hyperactivity disorder (ADHD), 44
    autism spectrum disorder (ASD), 44
    depression, 43
    obsessive-compulsive disorder, 43
    substance abuse disorder (SAD), 44
    suicidality and self-injurious behavior, 44
  starvation-induced endocrine alterations, 42
Adolescent-focused therapy (AFT), 124

Adolescent Morbid Obesity Surgery (AMOS), 150
Adolescent obesity
  health risk and comorbidity assessment, 48t
  health status and physical well-being, 47
  prevalence rate, 47
  psychological and psychiatric comorbidities
    depression, 50–51
    discrimination, 51
    social anxiety disorder (SAD), 50–51
    stigmatization, 50
  somatic comorbidities
    dermatological disorders, 50
    diabetes mellitus type 2 (T2DM), 47–48
    gastrointestinal disorders, 49–50
    genetic predisposition, 48–49
    metabolic syndrome, 48–49
    orthopedic disorders, 50
    pubertal development disorders, 49
    respiratory disorders, 50
    visceral adipose tissue (VAT), 48–49
Agouti-related peptide (AgRP), 80
α-melanocyte-stimulating hormone (α-MSH), 89
Amylin, 81–82
Anorexia nervosa (AN)
  antipsychotic medications
    aripiprazole, 136
    olanzapine, 136–137
    quetiapine, 136
    risperidone, 136
  atypical, 40
  binge eating/purging type, 40
  body mass index (BMI), 9
  childhood onset, 32
  Crohn's disease, 89
  diagnostic criteria, 39, 39t
  DSM-5 and ICD-11 7 criteria, 2t, 3
  duration of untreated ED (DUED), 130
  early intervention, 129
  enhanced cognitive-behavioral therapy (CBT-E), 115
  food addiction, 100
  genetic mechanisms, 13
  ghrelin, 74–75

Anorexia nervosa (AN) (Continued)
  gut-brain interaction, 89
  gut microbiome alterations, 89–90
  GWASs, 68
  higher percent body fat, 13
  hypoleptinemia, 80
  incidence, 54
  inpatient (IP) treatment
    medication, 125
    nutritional rehabilitation, 124
    psychotherapy, 124–125
    relapse and rehospitalization, 125–126
  leaky gut, 88–89
  leptin concentration, 74
  Medical and Psychosocial Indications for Hospital Admission, 124t
  microbiome interactions, 87, 88f
  multiple family therapy (MFT), 119
  physical hyperactivity, 40
  premorbid body weight, 13
  prevention programs, 171
  proinflammatory markers, 88–89
  psychiatric comorbidity
    anxiety disorders, 43
    attention-deficit/hyperactivity disorder (ADHD), 44
    autism spectrum disorder (ASD), 44
    obsessive-compulsive disorder, 43
    substance abuse disorder (SAD), 44
    suicidal behavior, 44
  reference weight criterion, 39
  reproductive hormones, 73–74
  restricting type, 40
  selective serotonin reuptake inhibitors (SSRIs)
    citalopram, 135–136
    fluoxetine, 135–136
    placebo-controlled trials, 135–136
    randomized clinical trials, 135
    retrospective study, 135
  staging model
    early stage of illness, 154–155
    full stage illness, 155
    high eating disorder risk, 154
    neuroadaptation, 155
    neuroprogression, 155
    remission rate, 153–154
    severe and enduring illness, 155
    social functioning, 155–156

Note: Page numbers followed by "f" indicate figures and "t" indicate tables.

179

Anorexia nervosa (AN) *(Continued)*
    treatment outcome, 153–154
    ultrahigh risk/prodrome, 154
    standardized mortality ratio (SMR),
        123
    starvation, 41–42
    starvation-induced endocrine
        alterations, 42
    symptomatology, 40
    symptom overlap, 135
    treatment outcomes
        adolescent-onset AN, 160
        childhood AN, 160
        lengths of follow-up, 160
        long-term prognosis, 159
        motherhood, 162
        negative outcome predictors,
            162
        psychiatric comorbidities, 162
        randomized controlled trials
            (RCTs), 159–160
        recovery rates, 160
        twin studies, 159
Antidepressant medication
    anorexia nervosa, 135–136
    binge eating disorder, 139
    bulimia nervosa, 138
Antiepileptics
    bulimia nervosa, 138
    for bulimia nervosa, 138
Antipsychotic medications, 136–137
Anxiety disorders, 43
Appetite control
    episodic influences
        satiety cascade, 18–20, 19f
        satiety peptides, 18
    fat-free mass, 20–21
    food availability, 17
    food liking and wanting, 18
    hedonics, 18
    homeostatic, 18
    human food choice, 17–18
    nutritional environment, 17
    tonic effects
        control mechanisms, 18
        energy expenditure and intake, 20
        evolutionary significance, 20
Appetite hormones
    ghrelin, 75
        eating disorders, 74–75
        obesity, 75
    leptin, 74
Aripiprazole, 136
Attention-deficit/hyperactivity disorder
    (ADHD), 44
Atypical anorexia nervosa (AN), 40
Autism spectrum disorder (ASD), 44
Avoidant restrictive food intake
    disorder (ARFID)
    anorexia nervosa, 30
    epidemiology, 29–30
    fear of aversive consequences of
        eating, 30

Avoidant restrictive food intake
    disorder (ARFID) *(Continued)*
    feeding disorder of infancy or early
        childhood (FDIEC), 29
    lack of appetite and limited intake,
        30
    non–fat phobic (NFP) anorexia
        nervosa (AN), 31
    pharmacotherapy, 139
    restricted eating, 30
    subtype, 30
    transdiagnostic approach, 30
    treatment, 31
    underweight, 13

B
Beck Depression Inventory
    (BDI), 162
Behavioral weight loss interventions,
    144
Bifidobacterium, 87–88
Binge eating disorder (BED)
    antidepressant medications,
        139
    characteristics, 41
    criterion of, 41
    food addiction, 100
    mortality rate, 123
    risk factors for future onset, 172
    stimulants, 139
    topiramate, 139
    treatment outcomes
        chronicity and diagnostic
            crossover, 161
        recovery, 161
        risk factors, 163
        weight categories, 13
Bipolar disorder, 129–130
Blount disease, 166
Body image, 23
Body mass index (BMI)
    adult weight categories, 10
    categories, 64t
    childhood obesity
        cardiovascular disease, 167
        type 2 diabetes mellitus, 167
    children and adolescents, 10
    developmental aspects
        fetus, 13
        gender differences, 13
        obese child, 10–13
        underweight and obesity,
            10–13
        young adults, 10–13
    drawback, 9
    and health risks
        obesity, 9–10
        starvation, 9
    and height, 9
    percentiles for, 11f–12f
    tracking, 63
Body mass index-standard deviation
    scores (BMI-SDSs), 10

Body perception
    definition, 23
    female pubertal characteristics
        acne and breast growth, 24–25
        age at menarch, 25
        gender differences, 25
        misconceptions, 25
        pubertal maturation, 25
    gender- and age-specific body
        measurements, 23–24
Body project, 172–173
Body satisfaction, 23
Brain-derived neurotropic factor
    (BDNF), 89
Brief Symptom Inventory (BSI), 162
Bulimia nervosa (BN)
    antidepressant medication, 138
    antiepileptics and mood stabilizers,
        138
    definition, 40
    diagnostic criteria, 40t
    duration of untreated ED (DUED),
        130
    estradiol concentrations, 73
    family-based therapy (FBT), 118–119
    ghrelin, 75
    incidence, 54
    inpatient (IP) treatment, 126
    leptin concentration, 74
    ondansetron, 138
    opiate antagonists, 138
    overweight patients, 40
    progesterone, 73
    psychiatric comorbidity
        attention-deficit/hyperactivity
            disorder (ADHD), 44
        binge eating disorder, 41
        self-injurious behavior, 44
        substance abuse disorder (SAD),
            44
    risk factors for future onset, 171–172
    social phobia, 43
    standardized mortality ratio (SMR),
        123
    symptomatology, 41
    treatment outcomes
        chronicity and diagnostic
            crossover, 160
        higher binge frequency, 162
        multiple follow-ups, 160–161
        recovery rates, 160, 162
        symptom severity and psychiatric
            comorbidity, 162–163
Bullying, 105

C
Cancer, childhood obesity, 167
Cardiovascular disease (CVD)
    adiposity, 165
    childhood BMI, 167
    risk factors, 165
Center for Epidemiological Studies
    Depression Scale (CES-D), 136

Centre for Research on Eating Disorders at Oxford (CREDO), 111
Child and adolescent ED services (CAEDS), 132
Childhood eating disorder
  anorexia nervosa, 32
  avoidant restrictive food intake disorder (ARFID). See Avoidant restrictive food intake disorder (ARFID)
  body development, 63
  body mass index tracking, 63
  overweight and obesity
    incidence, 64
    persistence, 64–65
    prevalence, 63–64
  pica, 31
  rumination disorder (RD), 31
  underweight, 64
Childhood obesity
  immediate consequences
    cardiovascular and metabolic complications, 165
    hepatic complications, 165
    musculoskeletal complications, 166
    psychologic and psychosocial complications, 166
    pulmonary complications, 165
  long-term consequences
    all-cause mortality, 166–167
    cancer, 167
    cardiovascular disease, 167
    obesity, 166
    type 2 diabetes mellitus, 167
  prevalence, 143, 165
  weight patterns, 167
Childhood onset anorexia nervosa, 32
Children's appetite awareness training (CAAT), 37
Child version of the Eating Attitudes Test (ChEAT), 36–37
Child version of the Eating Disorder Examination (ChEDE)
  ChEDE-Q, 36–37
  objective binge eating (OBE), 36
  objective overeating (OO), 36
  semistructured interview, 36
  subjective binge eating (SBE), 36
Child version of the Eating Disorder Examination Questionnaire (ChEDE-Q), 36
Cholecystokinin (CCK), 82
Citalopram, 135–136
Clinical prevalence, 53–54
Cognitive behavioral approach to assessment and treatment (CBT-AR), 30
Composite phenotype analyses, 68
Conventional weight loss programs
  anthropometric measures, 143
  BMI z score, 144
  metaanalysis, 143–144

Conventional weight loss programs (Continued)
  multicomponent weight loss programs, 144–145
  multileveled treatment approach, 145–146, 146f
  preschool children, 144–145
  problems and limitations, 145
  randomized controlled trials, 144
  WHO recommendation, 143–144
Coronary heart disease (CHD), 167
Crohn's disease, 89
Cross-trait analyses, 68–69
C-Terminal Binding Protein 2 (CTBP2), 69

D
Day patient (DP) treatment, 126
Depression, 43, 166
Dermatological disorders, 50
Descriptive epidemiology
  community-based studies, 59
  DSM-5 diagnostic classification, 53
  incidence
    anorexia nervosa, 54
    bulimia nervosa, 54
    community–based study, 54
    nationwide Danish registries, 54–55
  prevalence
    clinical, 53–54
    current prevalence, 55
    information sources, 54
    life-time prevalence, 53, 55, 56t–59t
    mortality and recovery, 53
    true prevalence, 54
  systematic data collection, 59–60
Difficult temperament, 93–94
Dissonance-based intervention (DBI), 174
Dove Self Esteem program, 174–175
Duration of untreated ED (DUED)
  anorexia nervosa, 130
  beat survey, 130
  bulimia nervosa, 130
  lack of consistency, 130
  service/care pathway–related factors, 130–131
  service-led model, 132
  systemic public health intervention, 131–132
Duration of untreated psychosis (DUP), 129–130
Dysthymia, 43

E
Early intervention
  developmental period, 129
  duration of untreated ED (DUED)
    anorexia nervosa, 130
    beat survey, 130
    bulimia nervosa, 130

Early intervention (Continued)
    lack of consistency, 130
    service/care pathway–related factors, 130–131
    service-led model, 132
    systemic public health intervention, 131–132
  duration of untreated psychosis (DUP), 129–130
  full-syndrome disorder, 129
  government-led, country-wide approach, 132
  Model Early Intervention Service for EDs, 131t
  neuroprogression, 129
  stage of illness model, 130
  vs. preventative interventions, 129
Eating addiction, 100
Eating Addiction Questionnaire, 101t
Eating Behaviors Questionnaire, 101t
Eating Disorder Examination (EDE), 112–113, 159–160
Eating disorder not otherwise specified (ED-NOS), 160
Eating Disturbances in Youth-Questionnaire (EDY-Q), 29
11β-hydroxysteroid dehydrogenase type 1 (11β -HSD-1), 48–49
Emetophobia, 30
Endocrine mechanisms in obesity
  amylin, 81–82
  cholecystokinin (CCK), 82
  energy intake and expenditure, 79
  fibroblast growth factor 21 (FGF21), 82–83
  ghrelin, 80–81
  glucagon, 81
  glucagon-like peptide (GLP-1), 82
  insulin, 81
  leptin, 80
  long-term regulators of food, 79–80
  mechanical and enzymatic digestion, 79–80
  neuroendocrine regulation, 79
  short-term regulators of food, 79–80
Energy density, 19–20
Enhanced cognitive-behavioral therapy (CBT-E)
  anorexia nervosa, 115
  Centre for Research on Eating Disorders at Oxford (CREDO), 111
  characteristics, 111
  "coercive" or "prescriptive" procedures, 112
  cognitive change, 112
  features, 111
  goals, 111
  intensive levels of care, 115
  parental involvement, 115
  self-control, 112
  self-empowerment, 112
  structure and procedures

Enhanced cognitive-behavioral therapy (CBT-E) *(Continued)*
  adolescent patient preparation, 112–113
  "broad" form, 112
  collaborative decision, 114
  "focused" form, 112
  homework assignments, 113
  initial interview, 113
  overvaluation of shape and weight, 113–114
  weight changes, 114
  weight maintenance, 115
  transdiagnostic approach, 112
Estrogen
  gut microbiome and inflammation, 87–88
  microbiome interactions, 87–88

F
Family-based interpersonal psychotherapy (FB-IPT), 37
"Family-based multicomponent lifestyle weight management, 143
Family-based therapy (FBT)
  bulimia nervosa (BN), 118–119
  dose of treatment, 118
  implementation
    format, 119
    inpatient setting, 119–120
    levels of care, 119
  phases, 117
  positive outcomes, 117
  principles and techniques
    clinical studies, 118
    externalization of illness, 118
    flexibility, 118
    parent-focused treatment (PFT), 118
    parents' ability to feed, 118
    in vivo family meal, 118
  randomized controlled trial (RCT), 117
  transition age youth (TAY), 119
Fat-free mass (FFM), 20
Fat mass (FM), 20
Feeding disorder of infancy or early childhood (FDIEC), 29
Fibroblast growth factor 21 (FGF21), 82–83
"First Episode Rapid Early Intervention for Eating Disorders (FREED) service, 132
5-hydroxyindoleacetitic acid (5-HIAA), 89
5-hydroxytryptamine (5-HT), 89
Fluoxetine, 135–136
Food addiction
  adversaries, 101
  anorexia nervosa, 100
  binge eating disorder, 100
  controversies, 101, 102t
  measures, 101t
  obesity, 100

Full-syndrome disorder, 129
Functional dysphagia, 30

G
Gambling disorder, 100
Gastroesophageal reflux disease, 49–50
Gastrointestinal disorders, 49–50
Genetic Investigation of ANthropometric Traits consortium (GIANT), 68
Genetics
  heritability, 67
  monogenic forms of obesity, 67
Genome-wide association studies (GWAS)
  anorexia nervosa, 68
  composite phenotype analyses, 68
  cross-trait analyses, 68–69
  elevated BMI, 67
  FTO gene, 67–68
  genetic correlations, 4
  Genetic Investigation of ANthropometric Traits consortium (GIANT), 68
  Japanese subjects, 68
  look-up studies, 69
  polygenes, 67
  single nucleotide polymorphism (SNP), 67
Ghrelin
  acylation, 81
  anorexia nervosa (AN), 80–81
  discovery, 80
  eating disorders, 74–75
  growth hormone secretagogue receptor 1a (GHS-R1a), 80
  microbiome interactions, 87–88
  obesity, 75
  orexigenic effect, 80
Ghrelin-o-acyltransferase (GOAT), 81
Glucagon
  secretion, 81
  thermogenic and lipolytic effect, 81
Glucagon-like peptide (GLP-1), 82
Group psychotherapy, 125
Growth hormone secretagogue receptor 1a (GHS-R1a), 80
Gut-brain interaction, 89
Gut microbiome and inflammation
  anorexia nervosa, 89–90
  gut-brain axis, 87
  gut-brain interaction, 89
  hormone levels, 87–88
  immunology and autoantibodies, 89
  intestinal permeability, 88–89
  metabolism and body weight, 87
  research and therapy, 90

H
Healthy Weight prevention program, 173
High eating disorder risk, 154
Homeostatic appetite control, 18

Hormones
  appetite hormones
    ghrelin, 74–75
    leptin, 74
  puberty
    eating disorders, 75
    obesity, 75
  reproductive. *See* Reproductive hormones
Hyperestrogenemia, 49
Hypoleptinemia, 5, 9, 80
Hypoventilation syndrome, 50

I
Inpatient enhanced cognitive-behavioral therapy (CBT-E), 115
Inpatient (IP) treatment
  admission policies, 123
  bulimia nervosa, 126
  dropout rates, 123
  duration, 123
  multidisciplinary treatment program
    medication, 125
    nutritional rehabilitation, 124
    psychotherapy, 124–125
    relapse and rehospitalization, 125–126
  multimodal approach, 123
  randomized controlled trial (RCT), 123
Insulin, 81
Internalized weight stigma, 105, 107
Intestinal permeability, 88–89
Islet amyloid polypeptide (IAPP), 81–82

L
Lactobacillus, 87–88
"Leaky gut, 88–89
Leptin
  clinical trials, 5
  deficiency, 5
  discovery, 80
  growth hormone, 5
  hypoleptinemia, 5
  hypoleptinemia-induced alterations, 5
  melanocortinergic system, 80
  physiological function, 5
  pro-opiomelanocortin (POMC) neurons, 80
  recombinant, 5
  resistance, 80
  supplementation, 80
Life-time prevalence, 53, 55, 56t–58t
Linkage Disequilibrium SCore (LDSC), 68–69
Lisdexamfetamine (LDX), 139
Lithium, 138
Loss of control (LOC) eating, 41
  definition, 35
  developmental considerations

Loss of control (LOC) eating
  (Continued)
    dietary restraint, 35
    emotion dysregulation and
      distraction, 35–36
    functions, 35
    future aspects, 37–38
    measurement, 36–37
    phenomenology, 35

M
Major depressive disorder (MDD), 3
Maternal anorexia nervosa
  childhood feeding and eating, 96
  temperament, 93–94
Maternal bulimia nervosa (BN)
  childhood feeding and eating, 96
  temperament, 93–94
Maternal eating disorders (EDs)
  child development, 93
  childhood feeding and eating
    anorexia nervosa, 96
    breastfeeding practices, 96
    bulimia nervosa, 96
    dietary pattern, 96–97
    gender specificity, 96
    parenting styles, 96
  children with eating disorder, 97
  cognitive development/
    neuropsychological profile
    child cognitive difficulties, 94–95
    neuropsychological characteristics,
      94
    population-based study, 94–95
    social cognition, 95
    thinking styles, 94
  offspring phenotype, 93, 94f
  perinatal complications, 93
  psychopathology
    AN *vs.* BN, 95
    Child Behavior Checklist, 95
    emotional and behavioral
      disorders, 95
    genetic correlations, 95–96
    homotypic and heterotypic
      transmissions, 95
  temperament
    difficult temperament, 93–94
    emotional reactivity, 93
    maternal anorexia nervosa, 93–94
    maternal bulimia nervosa (BN),
      93–94
    maternal depression and anxiety,
      93
Mayer's law, 79
Metabolic and bariatric surgery (MBS)
  body mass index (BMI), 149
  comorbidities and risk factors, 149
  contraindications, 149
  guidelines, 149
  insurance coverage, 151
  medical effect, 150
  micronutrient deficiencies, 151

Metabolic and bariatric surgery (MBS)
  (Continued)
  psychologic evaluation, 149
  Roux-en-Y gastric bypass (RYGB),
    149–150
  type 2 diabetes (T2D), 150–151
  vertical sleeve gastrectomy (VSG),
    149–150
  vs. non-surgical interventions, 150
Mindfulness-based intervention (MBI),
  174
Mood stabilizers, 138
Multicomponent weight loss programs,
  144–145
Multiple family therapy (MFT), 119
Multitrait analysis of GWAS (MTAG),
  69
Musculoskeletal fitness, childhood
  obesity, 166

N
National Institute for Health and Care
  Excellence (NICE) guidelines, 155
Neuroadaptation, 155
Neuropeptide Y (NPY), 80
Neuroprogression, 155
Nonalcoholic fatty liver disease
  (NAFLD)
  childhood obesity, 165
  metabolic and bariatric surgery
    (MBS), 149–150
  prevalence, 165
Nonalcoholic hepatic steatohepatitis
  (NASH), 150
Non–fat phobic (NFP) anorexia
  nervosa (AN), 31
Nutritional rehabilitation, inpatient
  (IP) treatment, 124

O
Obesity
  ghrelin, 75
  leptin concentration, 74
  puberty, 75
Objective binge eating (OBE), 36
Objective overeating (OO), 36
Obstructive bronchitis, 50
Obstructive sleep apnea syndrome
  (OSAS), 165
Olanzapine, 136–137
Ondansetron, 138
Orthopedic disorders, 50
Outpatient enhanced cognitive-
  behavioral therapy (CBT-E), 115
Overeating, 17
Overweight
  body mass index (BMI), 10
  perception, 23

P
Parent-focused treatment (PFT), 118–119
Partial hospitalization programming
  (PHP), 119

Pharmacotherapy
  anorexia nervosa
    alprazolam, 137
    antidepressant medications,
      135–136
    antipsychotic medications,
      136–137
    D-cycloserine (DCS), 137
    dronabinol, 137
    osteopenia, 137
    oxytocin, 137
  avoidant-restrictive food intake
    disorder (ARFID), 139
  binge eating disorder, 139
  bulimia nervosa
    antidepressant medication, 138
    antiepileptics and mood
      stabilizers, 138
    ondansetron, 138
    opiate antagonists, 138
  pica, 139
  rumination disorder, 139
Pica, 31, 139
Pica, ARFID, Rumination Disorder
  Interview (PARDI), 29
Polygenes, 67
Pramlintide, 81–82
Premeal anxiety, 137
Prevention programs
  body project, 172–173
  future research, 175
  Healthy Weight prevention program,
    173
  implementation efforts,
    174–175
  risk factors for future onset
    anorexia nervosa, 171
    binge eating disorder (BED),
      172
    bulimia nervosa (BN), 171–172
    purging disorder (PD), 172
    student athlete eating disorder, 174
    Student bodies, 173–174
Proinflammatory markers, 88–89
Project Health, 173
Psychobiotics, 90
Pubertal development disorders, 49
Puberty
  eating disorders, 75
  obesity, 75
Purging disorder (PD), 172

Q
Questionnaire on Eating and Weight
  Patterns (QEWP-A), 36–37
Quetiapine
  anorexia nervosa, 136

R
Recombinant leptin, 5
Relational victimization, 105
"Report of the Commission on Ending
  Childhood Obesity, 143

Reproductive hormones
activational effects, 73
estradiol and progesterone
anorexia nervosa, 73–74
hormone concentrations, 73
obesity, 74
ovariectomized animals, 73
psychological symptoms, 73
organizational effects, 73
Respiratory disorders, 50
Resting metabolic rate (RMR), 20
Restricted eating, 30
Risperidone, 136
Roux-en-Y gastric bypass (RYGB),
149–150
Rozin's behavioral science approach,
17–18
Rumination disorder (RD),
31, 139

S
Satiation, 18–19
Satiety, 18–19
Satiety cascade
energy density, 19–20
food properties, 19
physiological sensory factors, 19
psychological factors, 19
satiation, 18–19
satiety, 18–19
Self-injurious behavior, 44
Semistructured interview, 101t
Single family therapy (FT), 119
Social anxiety disorder (SAD), 50–51
Social communication disorders, 95
Social functioning, 155–156
Social phobia, 43
Staging model of eating disorders
anorexia nervosa (AN)
early stage of illness, 154–155
full stage illness, 155
high eating disorder risk, 154
neuroadaptation, 155
neuroprogression, 155
remission rate, 153–154
severe and enduring illness, 155
social functioning, 155–156
treatment outcome, 153–154
ultrahigh risk/prodrome, 154
clinical implications, 156
progression, 154f
Standardized mortality ratio (SMR),
163
anorexia nervosa (AN), 123
bulimia nervosa (BN), 123
Steatosis hepatis, 49–50
Structured interview, 101t

Student bodies, 173–174
Subjective binge eating (SBE), 36
Substance abuse disorder (SAD), 44
Substance use, 99
Substance use disorder, 99
Suicidality, 44

T
Teen-Longitudinal Assessment of
Bariatric Surgery (Teen-LABS),
149
Temperament
difficult temperament, 93–94
emotional reactivity, 93
maternal anorexia nervosa, 93–94
maternal bulimia nervosa (BN),
93–94
maternal depression and anxiety,
93
Teriparatide, 137
Tilt deformity, 50
Tonic effects, appetite control
control mechanisms, 18
energy expenditure and intake, 20
evolutionary significance, 20
Topiramate
for binge eating disorder, 139
for bulimia nervosa, 138
Transition age youth (TAY), 119
Treatment outcomes
anorexia nervosa (AN), 159–160
binge eating disorder
chronicity and diagnostic
crossover, 161
recovery, 161
risk factors, 163
bulimia nervosa (BN)
chronicity and diagnostic
crossover, 160
higher binge frequency, 162
multiple follow-ups, 160–161
recovery rates, 160
symptom severity and psychiatric
comorbidity, 162–163
mortality, 163
self-reported ED, 161–162
unfavorable outcomes, 161–163
Tri Delta, 174
True prevalence, 54
Type 2 diabetes (T2D)
childhood obesity, 167
metabolic and bariatric surgery
(MBS), 150–151

U
Underweight
body mass index (BMI), 10

V
Vertical sleeve gastrectomy (VSG),
149–150
Visceral adipose tissue (VAT), 48–49
Volcravo, 37

W
Weight and eating disorders
classification, 1, 2t
early intervention. See Early
intervention
major depressive disorder (MDD),
3
obesity, 3
overweight, 3
persistent disturbance, 1
pharmacotherapy. See
Pharmacotherapy
phenomenology, 1
polygenic dissection, 4
prevention programs. See Prevention
programs
restricting and binge eating/purging
types, 3
staging model. See Staging model of
eating disorders
symptomatology, 1
treatment outcomes. See Treatment
outcomes
underweight, 1–3
Weight and shape concern (WSC), 174
Weight stigma
children and adolescents
physical health correlates, 106
psychologic correlates, 106–107
definition, 105
education, 105
healthcare, 106
internalized, 105
interpersonal relationships, 106
media, 106
multicomponent interventions, 107
prevalence, 105
reduction strategies, 107
stereotypes, 105
weight-related discrimination, 105

Y
Yale Brown Obsessive Compulsive
Scale (Y-BOCS), 136–137
Yale Food Addiction Scale (YFAS), 100,
101t
Youth Eating Disorder Examination-
Questionnaire (YEDE-Q), 36–37

Z
z-scores, 10

Printed in the United States
By Bookmasters